Parkinson's disease
and parkinsonism
in the elderly

Edited by

Dr Jolyon Meara

University Department of Geriatric Medicine (North Wales)

and

Professor William C Koller

University of Kansas Medical Center, Kansas City

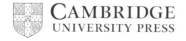
CAMBRIDGE
UNIVERSITY PRESS

PUBLISHED BY THE PRESS SYNDICATE OF THE UNIVERSITY OF CAMBRIDGE
The Pitt Building, Trumpington Street, Cambridge, United Kingdom

CAMBRIDGE UNIVERSITY PRESS
The Edinburgh Building, Cambridge CB2 2RU, UK   http://www.cup.cam.ac.uk
40 West 20th Street, New York, NY 10011–4211, USA   http://www.cup.org
10 Stamford Road, Oakleigh, Melbourne 3166, Australia
Ruiz de Alarcón 13, 28014 Madrid, Spain

First published 2000

Printed in the United Kingdom at the University Press, Cambridge

Typeface Minion 10.5/14pt   *System* QuarkXPress™   [s e]

A catalogue record for this book is available from the British Library

Library of Congress Cataloguing in Publication data

Parkinson's disease and parkinsonism in the elderly / edited by Jolyon Meara and
William C. Koller.
    p. ; cm.
Includes bibliographical references and index.
ISBN 0 521 62884 9 (pb : alk. paper)
1. Parkinson's disease.   2. Aged – Diseases.   I. Meara, Jolyon, 1956–   .   II. Koller, William
C., 1945–   .
[DNLM: 1 Parkinson Disease – Aged. WL 359 P2467 2000]
RC382.P258   2000
618.97′6833–dc21   99–057614

ISBN 0 521 62884 9 paperback

Every effort has been made in preparing this book to provide accurate and up-to-date information which is
in accord with accepted standards and practice at the time of publication. Nevertheless, the authors, editors
and publisher can make no warranties that the information contained herein is totally free from error, not
least because clinical standards are constantly changing through research and regulation. The authors, editors
and publisher therefore disclaim all liability for direct or consequential damages resulting from the use of
material contained in this book. The reader is strongly advised to pay careful attention to information provided by the manufacturer of any drugs or equipment that they plan to use.

Contents

List of contributors   *page* vii
Foreword   ix

1   **A glossary of terms**   1
         Jolyon Meara

2   **Diagnosis of parkinsonism in the elderly**   4
         Robert L. Rodnitzky

3   **Parkinson's disease and parkinsonism in the elderly**   22
         Jolyon Meara and Bimal K. Bhowmick

4   **Drug-induced parkinsonism in the elderly**   64
         Jean P. Hubble

5   **Essential tremor in the elderly**   80
         Rajesh Pahwa and William C. Koller

6   **Gait apraxia and multi-infarct states**   98
         Richard Liston and Raymond C. Tallis

7   **The epidemiology of Parkinson's disease and parkinsonism in elderly
         subjects**   111
         Jolyon Meara and Peter Hobson

8   **Health and social needs of people with Parkinson's disease and the
         worldwide organization of their care**   122
         Peter Hobson

9   **The drug treatment of Parkinson's disease in elderly people**   134
         Theresa A. Zesiewicz and Robert A. Hauser

10 **Rehabilitation in Parkinson's disease and parkinsonism** 165
Christopher D. Ward

11 **Rehabilitation, nursing and elderly patients with Parkinson's disease** 185
Sally Roberts

12 **Rehabilitation, physiotherapy and elderly patients with Parkinson's disease** 198
Hilary Chatterton and Brenda Lövgreen

13 **Rehabilitation, occupational therapy and elderly patients with Parkinson's disease** 217
Jackie Hughes

14 **Rehabilitation, speech and language therapy and elderly patients with Parkinson's disease** 226
Sheena Round

Index 240

Contributors

Bimal K. Bhowmick MD FRCP
Consultant Physician in Geriatric Medicine,
Glan Clwyd District General Hospital, Rhyl,
Denbighshire, North Wales LL18 5UJ, UK.

Hilary Chatterton MSC MCSP
Lecturer, School of Physiotherapy,
Manchester Royal Infirmary, Manchester
M13 9WL, UK.

Robert A. Hauser MD
Associate Professor, College of Medicine,
University of South Florida, Department of
Neurology, Harbour Side, Medical Tower, 4
Columbia Drive, Suite 410, Tampa, Florida
33606, USA.

Peter Hobson BSC
University Department of Geriatric
Medicine, Glan Clwyd District General
Hospital, Rhyl, Denbighshire, North Wales
LL18 5UJ, UK.

Jean P. Hubble MD
Co-Medical Director, The Ohio State
University, University Medical Center, 1581
Dodd Drive, McCampbell Hall, Suite 371,
Columbus, Ohio 43210, USA.

Jackie Hughes Dip COT
Occupational Therapist, Colwyn Bay
Community Hospital, Colwyn Bay, Conwy,
North Wales LL29 8AY, UK.

William C. Koller MD PhD
Professor and Chairman, Department of
Neurology, The University of Kansas
Medical Center, 3901 Rainbow Boulevard,
Kansas City, Kansas 66160, USA.

Richard Liston FRCPI
Consultant Physician in Geriatric Medcine,
Tralee General Hospital, Tralee, County
Kerry, Eire

Brenda Lövgreen MSC MCSP
Lecturer, School of Physiotherapy,
Manchester Royal Infirmary, Manchester
M13 9WL, UK.

Jolyon Meara MD FRCP
Senior Lecturer in Geriatric Medicine,
University of Wales College of Medicine,
Glan Clwyd District General Hospital, Rhyl,
Denbighshire, North Wales LL18 5UJ, UK.

Rajesh Pahwa MD
Assistant Professor, Department of
Neurology, School of Medicine, The
University of Kansas Medical Center,
3901 Rainbow Boulevard, Kansas City,
Kansas 66160, USA.

Sally Roberts RGN
Parkinson's Disease Nurse, Health Care of
the Elderly Department, Glan Clwyd District
Hospital, Rhyl, Denbighshire, North Wales
LL18 5UJ, UK.

Robert L. Rodnitzky M D
Professor of Neurology, The University of
Iowa Hospitals and Clinics, Department of
Neurology, 200 Hawkins Drive, Iowa City,
Iowa 522242–1053, USA.

Sheena Round B S C D i p C C S M C S L T
Speech and Language Therapist, Glan Clwyd
District General Hospital, Rhyl,
Denbighshire, North Wales LL18 5UJ, UK.

Raymond C. Tallis D L i t t F R C P
Professor of Geriatric Medicine, The
University of Manchester, Hope Hospital,
Manchester M6 8HD, UK.

Christopher D. Ward M D F R C P
Professof of Rehabilitation Medicine,
University of Nottingham, Faculty of
Medicine and Health Sciences,
Rehabilitation Research Unit, Derby City
General Hospital, Uttoxeter Road, Derby
DE22 3NE, UK.

Theresa A. Zesiewicz M D
Associate Professor of Neurology, College of
Medicine, University of South Florida,
Department of Neurology, Harbour Side
Medical Tower, 4 Columbia Drive, Suite 410,
Tampa, Florida 33606, USA.

Foreword

No illness can be contained in a vacuum and Parkinson's disease is no exception. Legislation by Governments, awareness and real understanding of this challenging illness by the healthcare professionals, and the change in the demographic profile of our nation will have major implications for the families impacted by this illness.

The population of the world is living longer and with old age there are increasing numbers of chronic neurological illness such as stroke, Alzheimer's and Parkinson's – and yet these people attract scant attention. Parkinson's in the elderly is a common clinical problem. Failure to manage it well results in distress and guilt within a family and expenditure of untargeted resources within the community.

This book examines the diagnosis and the management of Parkinson's in both the UK and USA. The editors are distinguished not only by their expertise in the management of Parkinson's but also well known for their compassion and desire to improve services.

Our elderly population should benefit from the contents of this book and I rejoice that such eminent people have given their time and expertise to contribute to such a worthwhile project.

Mary G Baker MBE
President of the European Parkinson's Disease Association (EPDA)

A glossary of terms

Jolyon Meara

As our knowledge of Parkinson's disease and parkinsonism increases considerable confusion can arise in relation to the terms used to describe these conditions. To maintain consistency in the text the following definitions will be used.

Parkinsonism

A clinical syndrome of akinesia accompanied by rigidity and often tremor. Akinesia includes difficulty with voluntary motor actions, difficulty performing sequential or concurrent motor actions, slowness of voluntary movement, and abnormal fatigability of repetitive motor actions. Rigidity, or 'stiffness', can be defined as the resistance encountered by an examiner when passively stretching relaxed muscles around a joint. Rigidity in parkinsonism can often be detected in the axial skeleton and upper limbs by the examiner performing passive flexion/extension movements of the neck and wrist joint. Tremor is often present at rest when the muscles are fully relaxed and is usually first noted in the upper limb involving the hand and fingers. Leg and jaw tremor may less commonly occur. Parkinson's disease is the most common cause of parkinsonism and arises sporadically and is of unknown cause. Known causes of parkinsonism include drugs, cerebrovascular disease, other sporadic and inherited neurodegenerative disease, infections, head trauma, hydrocephalus, and metabolic diseases, amongst others.

Parkinson's disease (PD)

Levodopa-responsive parkinsonism resulting in a characteristic clinical picture and natural history. When present, a typical 'pill rolling' tremor involving the thumb and index finger is almost pathognomic for PD or drug-induced parkinsonism. The primary neuropathological findings consist of degeneration of cells in the substantia nigra pars compacta resulting in striatal dopamine deficiency and the presence in surviving cells of inclusions called Lewy bodies. Other discrete areas of the brain also demonstrate cell loss and Lewy bodies.

Late stage PD

Late stage PD is associated with significant functional disability and the onset of increasing dependency. The clinical picture in late stage disease is dominated by features that do not respond to dopaminergic drugs, such as poor mobility, falls, confusion, drowsiness, dementia, sialorrhoea, dysarthria, impaired communication, dysphagia, and weight loss.

Late onset PD

Late onset PD can be arbitrarily defined as PD presenting for the first time in subjects who are aged 70 years or older. Even after adjusting for age, late onset PD appears to progress faster and to be associated with the earlier development of cognitive impairment and possibly depression. In late onset disease gait and balance problems appear early in the course of the illness. The pattern of disease at presentation in elderly subjects may reflect the more widespread loss of nigral cells due to aging in addition to the more circumscribed loss due to PD.

Drug-induced parkinsonism (DIP)

Parkinsonism resulting from exposure to antidopaminergic drugs, usually due to blocking of dopamine receptors. The clinical picture can be indistinguishable from PD. Neuroleptic drugs are by far the most common cause of DIP.

Vascular parkinsonism

Parkinsonism resulting from vascular disease of the brain. The clinical picture is dominated by gait disturbance, truncal ataxia with relative sparing of the upper limb and the absence of tremor. There may be associated evidence of upper motor neurone involvement (pseudobulbar palsy, pyramidal deficits) and a history of stroke events. A history of hypertension is often present and brain imaging may demonstrate extensive deep white matter ischaemic changes. Akinesia of the upper limb is absent in most cases. However, basal ganglia infarcts may rarely give rise to a clinical picture indistinguishable from PD.

Parkinsonism in multisystem neurodegenerative disease

Parkinsonism can arise from sporadic disease such as multiple system atrophy, progressive supranuclear palsy, corticobasal degeneration, Alzheimer's disease and dementia with Lewy bodies. Inherited degenerative diseases such as Huntington's disease can cause parkinsonism and familial parkinsonism, although very rare, is now well described. Progressive supranuclear palsy and multiple system atrophy may be mistaken for PD early in the natural history of the disease as both these conditions may initially respond to levodopa treatment.

Dementia with Lewy bodies (DLB)

A progressive fluctuant dementia associated with variable degrees of parkinsonism, visual hallucinations, falls, transient loss of consciousness and neuroleptic sensitivity. Cortical Lewy bodies are prominent at postmortem, particularly in the limbic areas of the mesial temporal lobe. Subcortical changes identical to those found in PD may also be present.

Gait apraxia

Gait apraxia results from a failure of integration of cerebral activity involving high-level sensorimotor systems. The difficulty in walking cannot be explained by motor or sensory abnormalities that can be detected by bedside neurological examination. The term 'high level gait disorder' is often preferred. Lesions of the premotor area, the supplementary motor area, the basal ganglia and their connections appear to be related to the development of gait apraxia.

Essential tremor (ET)

The most common movement disorder in elderly people. A bilateral, persistent postural tremor involving the hands and forearms of longstanding duration is required for a definite diagnosis of ET. A kinetic tremor on movement may also be present. A family history of tremor is elicited, as is a short term improvement of tremor after alcohol. The head, voice and legs may also be involved with decreasing frequency. In elderly subjects ET is commonly misdiagnosed as PD.

Diagnosis of parkinsonism in the elderly

Robert L Rodnitzky

The diagnosis of parkinsonism depends on recognizing its component clinical features. Parkinsonism includes Parkinson's disease (PD) and all the varied conditions with clinical features resembling those of PD. To identify patients with parkinsonism correctly it is important to be able to recognize the cardinal clinical features of PD, namely akinesia, lead-pipe rigidity, rest tremor, and postural instability. The next critically important step is to determine whether they suggest PD or one of the other non-PD causes of parkinsonism (see Table 2.1). This latter distinction will enable effective treatment strategies to be devised and a meaningful discussion of prognosis and genetic implications to be undertaken. The entire process of identifying parkinsonism and assigning a specific clinical diagnosis is particularly challenging in the elderly because many of the motor changes associated with normal ageing resemble parkinsonism. Additionally, several medical conditions that are common in this age group can result in parkinsonism that may incorrectly be considered evidence of PD.

The clinical signs of PD

Of the cardinal motor signs of PD, akinesia is perhaps the most disabling. Slowness, difficulty in initiation, and a reduction in the amount or amplitude of voluntary movement (Rodnitzky and Uc 1997) characterize akinesia (see Table 2.2). A great variety of clinically recognizable signs result from akinesia. A lack of facial expression attended by reduced blink rate is one of the most apparent manifestations of akinesia. Additional findings are diminished arm swing on one or both sides of the body, difficulty arising from a chair, a slow, short stepped gait, en bloc turning, and soft, poorly articulated speech (hypophonia). The clinical signs of akinesia are so striking that their presence alone has been considered by some to be sufficient to establish a diagnosis of PD (Quinn 1995). The more usual view is that additional motor findings are necessary to establish a diagnosis of PD. Rigidity is another common finding in patients with PD (see Table 2.3). Rigidity is felt by an examiner as an increased resistance to passive movement of joints in the fully relaxed limb.

Table 2.1 Stages in the diagnosis of parkinsonism

Stage 1
- Is there clinical evidence of parkinsonism?
- Akinesia must be present for this diagnosis.

Stage 2
- What type of parkinsonism is present?

Table 2.2 Clinical features of PD

Akinesia
- Reduction in spontaneous voluntary motor activity, slow movements, difficulty with sequential and concurrent motor acts, abnormal early fatiguability and reduction in amplitude of movements

Table 2.3 Clinical features of PD

Lead-pipe rigidity
- Abnormal resistance which remains constant throughout the range of movement and is felt when passively stretching muscles around a joint in a relaxed subject

Cog-wheel rigidity
- A ratchet type of fluctuating resistance felt at the wrist in synchrony with tremor bursts

Resistance is unchanged throughout the range of movement of the joint and can be distinguished from spasticity, in which resistance is greatest at the onset of passive movement and then suddenly gives way (clasp knife phenomenon). Often, a ratchet like quality (cog-wheeling) is present as the joint is moved especially when tremor is present. Subtle rigidity can be enhanced by utilizing reinforcement techniques such as instructing the patient to execute repetitive forceful movements in the contralateral limb. True rigidity must be distinguished from gegenhalten in which patients with diffuse encephalopathy or frontal lobe dysfunction exert a force opposite in direction to the examiner's attempted passive movement.

Rest tremor is one of the most easily recognizable signs of PD (see Table 2.4). It usually appears at a frequency of 3–6 Hz when the limb is fully supported and motionless. It also appears in the hands when the arms are suspended at the sides during walking. Typically, the tremor is reduced or totally disappears during action. In PD, tremor is often unilateral at the onset of the illness and remains asymmetrical even though ultimately spreading to the contralateral limbs. The presence or absence of rest tremor is a major consideration when attempting to determine

Table 2.4 Clinical features of PD

Rest tremor
- Classically a 4–5 Hz oscillation involving the distal portion of the upper limb of 'pill rolling' type. Atypical rest tremor can occur and rest tremor is often accompanied by postural and kinetic tremors. The head and trunk are usually spared

---

whether a patient has PD or another form of parkinsonism. Rest tremor is present in the great majority of patients with PD, but in only a smaller percentage of those with other forms of parkinsonism. The distribution of tremor is also important in helping to establish a diagnosis of PD. The tremor of PD commonly begins in the hands and is slightly less common in the lower extremities and mandible. It almost never affects the head or the muscles of articulation. When present, a 'pill rolling' tremor at rest involving the thumb and index finger very strongly suggests a diagnosis of PD or drug-induced parkinsonism. Postural instability has a great number of potential causes other than PD, particularly in the elderly. Patients manifesting this dysfunction are at increased risk of falling since they are unable to generate normal reflex movement to counter even the slightest perturbation to their posture. The clinician can safely demonstrate an absence of postural reflexes by standing behind the patient and applying a brisk backward directed push on the sternum.

Episodes of freezing, also referred to as 'motor blocks', most commonly involve gait. The patient's feet appear 'glued' to the floor when attempting to initiate gait, during turns, or when approaching a real or imagined obstacle such as a narrow passageway or an entrance to a room. Whether this phenomenon represents a severe form of akinesia or is physiologically separate is not known. It is common in late stage PD, but in some other forms of parkinsonism it can be an early, or even a presenting clinical sign (Giladi et al. 1991). Several guidelines have been suggested for utilizing clinical signs to establish a diagnosis of clinically probable PD. Definite diagnosis strictly requires postmortem confirmation of PD. Most guidelines require a certain number of the cardinal motor signs of parkinsonism to be present to make a diagnosis of PD in life. For example, the UK Parkinson's Disease Society Brain Bank criteria (Hughes et al. 1992a) requires the presence of akinesia plus *one* other clinical sign from among rigidity, rest tremor, and postural instability. Koller (1995), on the other hand, suggested that any two of three motor findings from among rigidity, akinesia, and tremor is sufficient to establish a clinical diagnosis of PD. While these criteria increase diagnostic accuracy, they are far from infallible. Several studies have suggested a high level of diagnostic inaccuracy compared to postmortem findings, even when the clinical diagnosis of PD is made by experienced neurologists (Rajput et al. 1991a, Hughes et al. 1992a, de Rijk et al. 1997).

Rajput et al. (1991a) found that only 76% of patients with a final clinical diagnosis of PD during life had evidence of the disease when examined at autopsy. Hughes et al. (1992a) examined 100 brains of patients with a final clinical diagnosis of PD and could confirm such a diagnosis in only 76% of cases. The diagnosis in the remainder included conditions such as progressive supranuclear palsy (PSP), multiple system atrophy (MSA), and Alzheimer's disease (AD). The clinicians in this study had utilized clinical criteria of their choice in arriving at a diagnosis of PD. When systematized diagnostic clinical criteria were retrospectively applied to cases in this study diagnostic accuracy improved to 82%. In clinical practice diagnostic accuracy is likely to be much lower than these figures suggest since these studies only looked at final diagnosis. However, all patients in these studies died at least 10 years ago and in the interim diagnostic awareness may have improved as is suggested by the most recent clinicopathological series (Ansorge et al. 1997). When applying additional computer generated criteria with a high predictive value for diagnostic accuracy (asymmetrical onset, no atypical features and no other possible etiology), the diagnostic accuracy was further increased to 93%, but 32% of pathologically confirmed cases were rejected on this basis. A further study compared eight different sets of diagnostic criteria that might be applied to prevalence studies of PD and found some sets too inclusive and others too restrictive (de Rijk et al. 1997). These authors concluded that the most reasonable inclusion criteria for PD was two of the three cardinal features (tremor, akinesia and rigidity) in the absence of other apparent causes of parkinsonism. It is clear from these studies that PD can be distinguished from other forms of parkinsonism on clinical grounds alone with high, but not total, accuracy. Using the most stringent diagnostic criteria reduces misdiagnosis, but at the expense of misclassifying a significant number of true cases of PD.

Controversy still exists over the condition of 'tremor dominant' PD. In this situation tremor is an isolated finding and this can easily lead to misdiagnosis with the most common cause of isolated tremor, essential tremor. Rest tremor, accompanying the more usual postural and kinetic tremor, can be a late manifestation of essential tremor in elderly subjects (Rajput et al. 1993). Tremor dominant cases of presumed PD could usefully be assessed with an apomorphine challenge test to help distinguish PD from other causes of isolated tremor.

Atypical features suggesting diagnoses other than PD

Despite the caveat that diagnostic criteria can be made so specific as to reduce their clinical utility, the usefulness of incorporating a careful search for atypical features as an exclusionary criterion for PD deserves special mention. Atypical features not only alert the clinician to the possibility that the diagnosis may not be PD, but in a positive sense may suggest another form of parkinsonism and lead the clinician to the correct diagnosis. In this regard it is important to understand which facets of the natural history or clinical examination are to be considered highly atypical for PD as well as which of them singly or in combination strongly suggest another clinical diagnosis within the spectrum of parkinsonism.

There is a reasonably well defined body of clinical signs and symptoms that are distinctly unusual in PD. When one or more of these signs appear in the akinetic–rigid or tremulous patient, they should prompt the clinician to question the diagnosis of PD. The following discussion describes the most important of these atypical signs and indicates which alternative diagnoses each one suggests. Several of these atypical features are much more likely to occur in elderly subjects, making their identification and proper interpretation even more important in this age group.

Early dementia

Dementia is common in PD, having been found in as many as 65% of patients by the age of 85 years (Mayeux et al. 1990). However, the dementia of PD seldom appears at the onset of the illness. Early dementia in the akinetic–rigid patient should prompt consideration of a variety of other syndromes with parkinsonian features, including dementia with Lewy bodies (DLB), PSP, corticobasal ganglionic degeneration (CBGD), normal pressure hydrocephalus, Creutzfeldt–Jacob disease, or AD. The confusion with AD arises from the fact that parkinsonism can appear in some patients with AD (Hughes et al. 1992a, Hulette et al. 1995). These signs are usually thought to occur late in the illness and are most likely to be seen in the elderly patient with severe cognitive impairment (Lopez et al. 1997). However, in the study of Hughes et al. (1992a) AD was a common cause of diagnostic error in PD and it appears from this study that AD, particularly when AD pathology involves the corpus striatum, can present with parkinsonism sufficient to lead to diagnostic confusion with PD. The development of mild parkinsonian features one or more years after the onset of otherwise clinically typical AD, especially in an elderly patient, should be considered to be a case of AD with parkinsonism, rather than PD with dementia. In the elderly patient, the possibility of the concurrent appearance of both PD and AD should also be given consideration, taking into account the high prevalence of both of these conditions in this age group. In this circumstance, the presence of a rest tremor or a significant improvement in parkinsonism after treatment with levodopa lends some support to a diagnosis of PD, rather than parkinsonism due to AD alone.

Certain clinical characteristics of the dementia may also be atypical for PD. Marked fluctuations in cognitive impairment consisting of periods of confusion alternating with lucidity, for example, should suggest DLB (Byrne et al. 1989, Mega et al. 1996). The differentiating characteristics of the dementia associated with AD and those found in PD have been well studied. The dementia of AD is more likely to be associated with abnormalities of memory and language and the presence of anosognosia while that of PD is more commonly characterized by impairment of visuospatial and executive functions (Mohr et al. 1990, Starkstein et al. 1996, Mahieux et al. 1998).

Early hallucinations have implications similar to those of early dementia. Hallucinations occurring in PD typically appear late in the course of the illness and are almost always associated with the chronic use of antiparkinsonian drugs. Hallucinations occurring prior to the initiation of such drugs or with the first administration of these agents strongly suggests another diagnosis, particularly DLB. This phenomenon points out the importance of accurately distinguishing between PD and DLB. Compared to PD, DLB patients are much more likely to suffer behavioural side effects from dopaminergic or anticholinergic agents.

Early falls and postural instability

Falling in PD is typically the result of impaired postural reflexes, postural hypotension or severe large amplitude dyskinesias. Severe freezing with inability to check forward propulsion of the upper trunk is another possible cause. These causes of falling typically appear in late stage PD and seem to occur earlier with late onset PD. However, a variety of other conditions with parkinsonian features may present with early falling.

The condition among those most likely to present with falling is PSP (Jankovic et al. 1990). In these patients, the gait abnormality is quite different from that seen in PD. In PSP patients there is akinesia associated with axial rigidity and nuchal dystonia, often in extension, vertical supranuclear gaze palsy and impaired postural reflexes. This combination results in frequent and early falling. The early appearance of gait freezing in PSP, which sometimes antedates the other motor signs of this condition, is also a major contributing factor to the occurrence of early falling. Postural instability is much more common early in the course of MSA than in PD. These patients may have marked akinesia with a loss of postural reflexes, sometimes associated with truncal dystonia. Wenning et al. (1997) in a review of 203 pathologically proven cases of MSA found that 38% had presented with ataxia. The term 'lower body parkinsonism' has been used to describe a severe isolated gait disorder associated with diffuse cerebral vascular disease (Fitzgerald and Jankovic 1989). This form of vascular parkinsonism is characterized by isolated involvement of the lower extremities and severe freezing of gait, often leading to falls. Normal pressure hydrocephalus can present with an early and predominant gait disorder associated with frequent falls. In this condition the gait is characterized by inability to lift the feet from the floor, short shuffling steps, imbalance while walking, difficulty turning, and gait ignition failure (Marsden and Thompson 1997, Graff-Radford and Godersky 1997, and see Chapter 6).

Severe autonomic dysfunction

Severe autonomic dysfunction early in the course of the illness is not typical of PD. Late in the course of PD patients may develop mild to moderate symptoms of autonomic insufficiency such as constipation, urinary incontinence, orthostatic hypotension, impotence, or impaired lacrimation (Goetz et al. 1986, Beattie et al. 1993). Anticholinergic drugs used to treat PD may contribute to the appearance of constipation or bladder dysfunction, while dopaminergic agents can cause or exacerbate hypotension and, to a lesser extent, constipation. The possibility of MSA should be considered in patients with evidence of early autonomic dysfunction in the absence of other diseases and drug treatments known to effect the autonomic system (Magalhaes 1995). In MSA autonomic dysfunction can predate signs of parkinsonism by several years. In one study of MSA autonomic signs antedated motor symptoms by one to two years in a quarter of cases (Wenning et al. 1994). Two techniques, electromyography of the urethral sphincter (Pramstellar et al. 1995) and formal urodynamic studies (Bonnett et al. 1997) are available to objectively distinguish the autonomic dysfunction of MSA from that of PD. The urethral sphincter is invariably denervated in MSA patients with incontinence, but not in PD patients with similar symptoms. In PD, urodynamic studies reveal an urgency to void without chronic retention, associated with detrussor hyperreflexia and normal urethral sphincter function. In MSA there is often chronic urinary retention, a hypoactive detrusor muscle and lower urethral pressures.

Poor or transient benefit from drug treatment

Dopaminergic drugs, especially levodopa, usually improve the signs of PD. The vast majority of PD patients benefit from levodopa therapy. In one series of pathologically proven cases of PD, 94% had responded to levodopa during life (Rajput et al.1990). The response rate to levodopa in other causes of parkinsonism is much lower. As many as 65% of MSA patients have been reported to respond, at least initially, to levodopa (Hughes et al. 1992b), although in most studies the response is closer to one third (Rajput et al. 1990). Even among those with an initial response, fewer than 5% may continue to benefit in the advanced stages of the illness (Wenning et al. 1997). In PSP, a levodopa response rate of 38% has been reported (Nieforth and Golbe 1993). Patients with multisystem degenerative disease who are initially responsive to levodopa commonly experience a rapid disappearance of benefit within one to two years. In CBGD early benefit from dopaminergic agents is much less common than that seen in PSP or MSA. In other causes of parkinsonism such as vascular parkinsonism and normal pressure hydrocephalus, lack of significant response to levodopa is the rule, but rare exceptions have been reported (Mark et al. 1995). On balance, these observations suggest that total refractoriness to therapeutic doses of levodopa therapy, in the absence of malabsorption, is a strong point against the diagnosis of PD. On the other hand, responsiveness to levodopa at the onset of illness can be considered a mild point in favour of a diagnosis of PD, but does not reliably distinguish between PD and several other forms of parkinsonism.

Striking asymmetry of motor signs

Marked asymmetry is unusual in PD, although mild asymmetry is quite common. When mild to moderate asymmetry does exist in PD, it tends to become less apparent as the illness advances. Profound tremor or rigidity on one side of the body with minimal or no symptoms on the contralateral side suggests a variety of diagnoses other than PD. Marked unilateral limb rigidity is often seen in CBGD (Schneider et al. 1997). A severe and strictly unilateral rest tremor raises the question of structural pathology such as an infarction involving the contralateral cerebellar outflow pathways. This anatomic localization is further suggested when the tremor is worse upon assuming a posture and during action than it is at rest. The syndrome of hemiparkinsonism hemiatrophy results in unilateral levodopa-responsive parkinsonism associated with ipsilateral body atrophy and contralateral brain atrophy, presumably related to brain injury early in life (Giladi et al. 1990). This condition should not be a major source of diagnostic confusion in the elderly since it typically appears before the age of 50 years old. Unilateral parkinsonism of acute onset or parkinsonism associated with pyramidal tract signs should suggest the possibility of an isolated infarction involving the contralateral brain stem or basal ganglia (de la Fuente Fernandez 1995).

Absence of rest tremor

The failure to demonstrate rest tremor does not exclude the diagnosis of PD, but rest tremor is more common in PD than in most other forms of parkinsonism. In two series of pathologically confirmed cases of PD, rest tremor was found to have occurred in 76% (Hughes et al. 1992c) and 100% (Rajput et al. 1991b) of patients during life. However, the incidence of rest tremor in parkinsonism not due to PD in these studies was between 31% and 50%. In autopsy proven cases of MSA only 39% had rest tremor (Wenning et al. 1997), while in 11 autopsy confirmed cases of CBGD only 18 had resting tremor during life (Schneider et al. 1997). It is important to mention that a tremor of the head should not be considered a rest tremor. More commonly, a head tremor is a postural tremor, reflecting the continued activity of axial postural muscles when in the upright position, or a dystonic tremor. In the former instance, a diagnosis of essential tremor should be considered and in the latter instance, cervical dystonia is the likely cause of tremor. In those patients suspected of having PD, but who do not manifest rest tremor, it is useful to engage the patient in mildly stressful activities, such as difficult mental arithmetic, in order to uncover a latent rest tremor.

Other features less common in PD

A variety of other findings cast doubt on a presumptive diagnosis of PD. The presence of more than one similarly affected first degree relative, while not impossible in PD, is unusual. Families with autosomal dominant parkinsonism have been reported but are exceedingly rare (Golbe et al. 1996). Rather, conditions with a known genetic basis for familial occurrence should be considered, such as Wilson's disease, Machado–Joseph disease and adult onset Hallervorden–Spatz disease. In a patient with tremor dominant disease (see above) a positive history of familial tremor may suggest the diagnosis of essential tremor (see Chapter 5). Other than essential tremor, these heritable causes of parkinsonism are unlikely to present in the elderly. Patients with Huntington's disease, an autosomal dominant condition, can manifest signs of parkinsonism at any age, although isolated parkinsonism (the Westphal variant) typically appears as a juvenile form prior to the age of 25 years old. Recent neuroleptic drug therapy precludes a definite diagnosis of PD. Although drug-induced parkinsonism typically remits within a matter of weeks after withdrawal of the offending agent, it can sometimes persist for up to one year (see Chapter 4). A history of oculogyric crisis suggests the possibility of post encephalitic parkinsonism rather than PD.

There are several other clinical signs that may appear in a patient with parkinsonism which are not only atypical for PD, but by themselves strongly suggest another specific diagnosis. These signs, and the conditions they suggest, include supranuclear gaze palsy or eyelid apraxia (PSP), ataxia or other signs of cerebellar dysfunction (MSA), prominent myoclonus (Creutzfeldt–Jakob disease), alien limb phenomenon, or limb apraxia (CBGD) and a marked response to anticholinergic therapy (drug-induced parkinsonism).

Conditions commonly mimicking PD in the elderly

Certain conditions mimic PD so commonly in the elderly that their differentiating features deserve special mention. These conditions have several overlapping clinical features with PD, but for most of them, the relative severity of these signs and their time of appearance in the course of the illness differ from that seen in PD. More importantly the nature of associated neurological signs and symptoms in those conditions usually allow the correct diagnosis to be made.

Vascular parkinsonism

Parkinsonian symptoms can occur as a result of a number of different vascular pathologies. Riley and Lang (1996) identified four categories of cerebral vascular disease that have this potential: multi-infarct disease, etat crible (multiple dilated perivascular spaces), Binswanger's disease (subcortical arteriosclerotic encephalopathy) and single focal infarctions or haemorrhage. These pathologic states become increasingly common with advancing age. It is important to distinguish them from PD so that appropriate therapy can be considered. For vascular parkinsonism, risk factors such as hypertension, hyperlipidemia, and coagulation abnormalities must be identified and reversed, whereas in true PD, specific antiparkinsonian drug therapy will be indicated. A variety of clinical signs and several facets of the clinical course help distinguish vascular parkinsonism from PD. In vascular parkinsonism, a subacute or acute onset of symptoms is sometimes seen, and similarly, the progression of the illness may occur in a stepwise fashion (Hurtig 1993). Rest tremor is rare (Inzelberg et al. 1994) and is almost never the predominant motor sign as can be the case in PD. Pyramidal tract findings such as hyperreflexia and Babinski signs are common in vascular parkinsonism, as are pathological laughing and crying. Rigidity, when present in vascular parkinsonism, is much more likely to be clasp knife in nature secondary to spasticity, rather than the typical lead-pipe variety associated with PD. In patients with widespread bilateral vascular disease, especially that involving the frontal lobes, paratonic rigidity (gegenhalten) may be present and can be distinguished from the rigidity of PD. Many patients with vascular parkinsonism present with a characteristic isolated impairment of ambulation consisting of a hesitant, shuffling gait with a preserved arm swing (Elbe et al. 1996). These patients have extremely poor postural stability and frequent falls are much more common than in PD (Trenkwalder et al. 1995). Parkinsonian symptoms such as hypophonia or facial masking are seldom present (Thompson and Marsden 1987). Patients with vascular parkinsonism demonstrating this predominant involvement of gait and balance with less involvement of the arms and face, have been described as manifesting the syndrome of 'lower body parkinsonism' (Quinn 1995). One of the most important differentiating features between PD and vascular parkinsonism is that there is seldom a significant clinical response to levodopa in patients with the vascular syndrome. Occasional striking, though rare, exceptions to this observation have been reported (Mark et al. 1995). As will be discussed below, brain imaging may help confirm the diagnosis of parkinsonism related to isolated cerebral infarctions or widespread subcortical vascular insults.

Normal pressure hydrocephalus

This condition typically presents with the clinical triad of dementia, urinary incontinence, and a gait disorder (Graff-Radford and Godersky 1997). It can occur at any age, but in adults the majority of cases present after the age of 60 years (Krauss et al. 1997). Although it is usually the gait disorder of normal pressure hydrocephalus (NPH) that results in diagnostic confusion with PD, a variety of other parkinsonian features can also be seen in this condition. In a study of 90 adults with NPH, Krauss et al. 1997 found that 81% had some evidence of akinesia. In the same study, rest tremor and rigidity were relatively rare, each occurring in only 14% of patients. The gait disorder of NPH is commonly referred to as an apraxia of gait, although this label is physiologically incorrect, given the underlying motor abnormality and akinesia seen in this condition. Typically, patients with NPH walk with slow short steps and demonstrate impaired ability to lift their feet off the walking surface (Sudarksy and Simon 1987). Like vascular parkinsonism, the gait in these patients is often impaired out of proportion to upper extremity and facial dysfunction. Aside from this unusual distribution of symptoms, differentiation from PD is aided by a history of antecedent events known to predispose to NPH (meningitis, subarachnoid haemorrhage, serious cranial trauma) and the early appearance of both dementia and bladder dysfunction. Whereas improvement with levodopa therapy is mild and infrequent, removal of 40–50 ml of CSF by lumbar puncture may result in a marked, albeit transient, improvement of symptoms.

The diagnosis of NPH should not be seriously considered unless ventriculomegaly in the absence of cortical atrophy is demonstrated by brain imaging. In properly selected patients, the neurological abnormalities associated with NPH, including the gait disorder, the generalized akinesia and cognitive impairment, can be improved by placement of a cerebrospinal fluid shunt (Black et al. 1985).

Essential tremor

This condition is characterized by a postural tremor that worsens with action (see Chapter 5). It appears predominantly in the arms and to a lesser extent in the lower extremities. The head is commonly involved and there may be an associated voice tremor. Essential tremor (ET) is a common disorder with a prevalence in the general population estimated to be as high as 1.7% (Larsson and Sjogren 1960). More importantly, it is much more common with advancing age. Prevalence rates have been reported to be as high as 13% in individuals between the ages of 70 and 79 years old (Rautakorpi et al. 1982). In individuals experiencing the onset earlier in life, tremor amplitude becomes progressively greater over time. Accordingly, the tremor itself becomes much more apparent in the later years of life.

Because this condition is so common in the elderly, and because it presents with tremor, ET is frequently misdiagnosed as PD. Several clinical features help distinguish it from PD. Perhaps the most important differentiating feature is the nature of the predominant tremor in the two conditions. The tremor of ET appears predominantly when the involved body part is maintained in a fixed posture. It persists or may be accentuated during movement. The classical tremor of PD occurs at rest. In both conditions, however, the opposite form of tremor may appear concurrently, but is almost never the predominant tremor type. Another distinguishing feature is that in ET, tremor commonly affects the head and voice, while in PD this distribution is virtually never seen. Aside from tremor, the associated neurological findings of ET and PD help distinguish the two conditions. ET is a monosymptomatic condition, tremor being the sole manifestation, whereas in fully developed PD, there may be coexistent bradykinesia, postural imbalance, and rigidity. In those cases of tremor dominant PD in which tremor may be the sole presenting sign, the correct diagnosis depends on identifying the tremor's classical circumstance of occurrence (at rest) and distribution (sparing the head and voice). An additional source of diagnostic uncertainty in the elderly patient is the possibility that ET and PD may both be present. Koller et al. (1994), in a study of 678 ET patients, found concurrent PD in 6.1%, an association that is slightly higher than would be predicted by the relatively high prevalence of the two conditions alone. In this regard, it should be noted that the late appearance of rest tremor in an elderly patient previously diagnosed as having ET is not sufficient to diagnose concurrent PD. Rajput et al. (1993) report the finding of resting tremor with no other signs of parkinsonism in three patients with confirmed essential tremor who underwent postmortem study. All three patients had additional postural and/or kinetic tremor of at least 10 years duration before the development of resting tremor. Resting tremor first developed in these three subjects when they were all older than 60 years. Similarly, cogwheel rigidity may appear in ET reflecting the presence of ongoing tremor in muscles that may not be properly relaxed. When other diagnostic criteria have failed to distinguish ET from PD, a trial of therapies that are specific for one or the other of these two conditions may prove useful. Levodopa has the potential to improve PD tremor remarkably, while it has virtually no effect on the tremor of ET. On the other hand, alcohol may dramatically improve the postural tremor of ET (Koller and Biary 1984) but has a less consistent and less impressive effect on the rest tremor of PD.

Senile gait

Significant changes in the mechanics of ambulation appear in the normal elderly individual (Sudarsky 1990, Elble et al. 1992). The resultant pattern of walking has been referred to by a variety of terms, including senile gait, cautious gait, and marche à petit pas. This condition is characterized by a slow short stepped gait carried out on a slightly widespread base. Nutt and Horak (1997) have likened this gait pattern to that of a normal person walking on a slippery surface, and at risk for falling. Elble (1997) reviewed the kinematics of gait in older, healthy adults and found that the major changes were a slower velocity, a shorter stride length, reduced arm swing, a more flexed knee position and reduced toe clearance at initial heel–floor contact. He also observed that these individuals spend a greater proportion of time in a double limb support stance than younger subjects. In this population, arm swing and lower extremity rotations are reduced in proportion to stride length. In addition to these abnormalities, Sudarsky and Tideiksaar (1997) noted that other kinematic investigations of the gait in this population revealed a reduction in velocity and a wider stride. These data clearly indicate that the gait of healthy aged individuals is characterized by a variety of features such as reduced stride length, diminished arm swing and axial flexion that overlaps with several of the typical clinical features of PD. The clinician must therefore not succumb to the temptation to diagnose PD or parkinsonism in an elderly individual solely on the basis of an abnormal gait and impaired mobility. Rather, additional confirmatory signs of a *movement disorder* must be sought, such as a decrease in facial expression, reduced blink rate, significant hypophonia, rest tremor, rigidity and freezing, singly or in combination. The presence of parkinsonism in addition to a gait abnormality is needed to confidently establish a diagnosis of PD or parkinsonism in an elderly individual. A corollary of this is that elderly patients presenting with a primary disorder of gait should not be assigned a diagnosis of senile gait if any of these ancillary clinical findings are present.

Neuroimaging and neurophysiological tests in the diagnosis of parkinsonism

The differentiation of PD from other causes of parkinsonism is largely based on careful clinical observation and examination. However, in some instances neuroimaging or neurophysiologic studies may enhance the certainty of the clinical diagnosis. In conditions for which the causative gene has been identified and can be assayed, the laboratory may provide absolute confirmation of the presumptive clinical diagnosis.

Neurodiagnostic aids are almost never of significant benefit in confirming a diagnosis of PD. Neither magnetic resonance imaging (MRI) of the head nor computed tomography (CT) of the head, reveal any consistent findings. Subtle abnormalities are sometimes found in the region of the substantia nigra in MRI of the brain in late stage PD (Stern et al. 1989) but they are not sufficiently common or definitive to be of great practical benefit in everyday practice. Similarly, neurophysiologic tests such as electroencephalography, evoked potentials, and blink reflex studies, while revealing subtle abnormalities, are seldom useful in establishing a diagnosis of PD. Neuroimaging is occasionally useful in evaluation of patients with other forms of degenerative parkinsonism. This is especially true of advanced cases. Therefore, the primary rationale behind obtaining a neuroimaging study in a patient with parkinsonism is not to confirm a diagnosis of PD, but to determine if a multisystem degenerative or vascular form of parkinsonism is present. In a survey of 49 movement disorder specialists, Anouti and Koller (1996) found that CT or MRI scans were ordered between 76% to 100% of the time to evaluate patients with suspected non-PD akinetic-rigid syndromes. Surprisingly, in the same survey, these studies were ordered 50% to 75% of the time in patients with a clinical diagnosis of PD.

In the late stages of PSP, MRI and CT may reveal atrophy of the dorsal mid brain with associated dilation of the cerebral aqueduct (Schonfeld et al.1987, Yagishita and Oda 1996). A higher instance of multiple cerebral infarcts has also been noted in the scans of patients with PSP, raising the possibility that ischaemia may play an aetiological role in this condition (Dubinsky and Jankovic 1987).

A variety of abnormalities can be uncovered by neuroimaging in multiple system atrophy, again largely in the advanced stages of illness. In the striatonigral form of MSA signal abnormalities in the striatum can be seen, which helps distinguish the syndrome from PD. Most typical is putaminal hypodensity on T2 weighted MRI scans (Olanow 1992). In addition, a narrow band of hyperintensity can be seen in the lateral putamen, a finding not seen in PD (Konagaya et al. 1994). In the olivo-pontocerebellar type of MSA brain CT or MRI may reveal cerebellar atrophy and enlargement of the fourth ventricle (Mark and Sage 1993). In cases of suspected vascular parkinsonism diagnosis can be strongly supported by CT or MRI findings of discrete infarctions, lacunes or diffuse deep white matter signal abnormalities. The latter two abnormalities are much better demonstrated by MRI than CT. The appearance of these imaging abnormalities in elderly patients with clinically typical PD, however, cannot be given too much weight since cerebral vascular disease and PD are both common in this age group and may appear in the same patient independent of one another.

In normal pressure hydrocephalus a definitive diagnosis cannot be made without neuroimaging. Therefore, in patients in whom this diagnosis is being considered, and who are candidates for surgical intervention, CT or MRI must be performed to look for evidence of enlarged ventricles in the absence of significant brain atrophy. The diagnosis of several other less common causes of parkinsonism in elderly subjects is occasionally aided by neuroimaging. In CBGD, CT or MRI can reveal frontoparietal atrophy, which is sometimes asymmetric (Riley et al. 1990). In Hallervorden–Spatz syndrome pallidal hypointensity on T2 weighted MRI scans is greater than that seen in normal individuals (Rodnitzky 1993). In advanced cases the 'eye of the tiger' sign is seen in the globus pallidus, consisting of a central increased signal surrounded by a zone of hypointensity (Sethi et al. 1988).

Positron emission tomography (PET) can provide a powerful research tool to define selective patterns of disruption of regional cerebral metabolism that helps distinguish between PD and other forms of neurodegenerative disease causing parkinsonism (Brooks 1993). PET can also detect early sub-clinical PD in at-risk subjects.

REFERENCES

Anouti A, Koller WC (1996) Diagnostic testing in movement disorders. *Neurological Clinics of North America*, 14, 169–82.

Ansorge O, Lees AJ, Daniel SE (1997) Update on the accuracy of clinical diagnosis of idiopathic Parkinson's disease. *Movement Disorders*, 12, Suppl. 1, S96.

Beattie J, Rodnitzky RL, Dobson JK (1993) Quantitative assessment of lacrimation as a measure of autonomic dysfunction in Parkinson's disease. *Neurology*, 43, A238.

Black PM, Ojeman NRG, Tzouras A (1985) CSF shunts for dementia, incontinence and gait disturbances. *Clinical Neurosurgery*, 32, 632–56.

Bonnett AM, Pichon J, Vidailhet M, Gouider-Khouja N, Robain G, Perrigot M, Agid Y (1997) Urinary disturbances in striatonigral degeneration and Parkinson's disease: Clinical and urodynamic aspects. *Movement Disorders*, 12, 509–13.

Brooks DJ (1993) PET studies on the early and differential diagnosis of Parkinson's disease. *Neurology*, 43, Suppl. 6, S6–S16.

Byrne EJ, Lennox G, Lowe J, Godwin-Austen RB (1989) Diffuse Lewy-body disease: Clinical features in 15 cases. *Journal of Neurology, Neurosurgery, and Psychiatry*, 52, 709–17.

de Rijk MC, Rocca WA, Anderson DW, Melcon MO, Breteler MM, Maraganore DM (1997) A population perspective on diagnostic criteria for Parkinson's disease. *Neurology*, 48, 1277–81.

Dubinsky RM, Jankovic J (1987) Progressive supranuclear palsy and a multi-infarct state. *Neurology*, 37, 570–6.

Elble R (1997) Changes in gait with normal ageing. In: *Gait Disorders of Ageing: Falls and Therapeutic Strategies*, eds. Masdeu JC, Sudarsky L, Wolfson L, pp. 93–105. Philadelphia: Lippincott-Raven.

Elble RJ, Cousins R, Leffler K, Hughes L (1996) Gait initiation by patients with lower-half Parkinsonism. *Brain*, 119, 1705–16.

Elble RJ, Hughes L, Higgins C (1992) The syndrome of senile gait. *Journal of Neurology*, 239, 71–5.

Fitzgerald PM, Jankovic J (1989) Lower body Parkinsonism: Evidence for a vascular etiology. *Movement Disorders*, 4, 249–60.

de la Fuente Fernandez R (1995) Thalamic lacune and contralateral hemiparkinsonism subsequently relieved by spontaneous thalamic–subthalamic hematoma (letters) *Movement Disorders*, 10, 116–7.

Giladi N, Burke RE, Kostic V, Przedborski S, Gordon M, Hunt A, Fahn S (1990) Hemiparkinsonism–hemiatrophy syndrome: Clinical and neuroradiologic features. *Neurology*, 40, 1731–4.

Giladi N, Kao R, Fahn S (1991) Freezing phenomenon in patients with Parkinsonism syndromes. *Movement Disorders*, 12, 302–5.

Goetz CG, Lutge W, Tanner C (1986) Autonomic dysfunction in Parkinson's disease. *Neurology*, 36, 73–5.

Golbe LI, Di Iorio G, Sanges G, Lazzarini AM, La Sala S, Bonavita V, Duvoisin RC (1996) Clinical genetic analysis of Parkinson's disease in the Contursi kindred. *Annals of Neurology*, 40, 767–75.

Graff-Radford NR, Godersky JC (1997) A clinical approach to symptomatic hydrocephalus in the elderly. In: *Gait Disorders of Ageing: Falls and Therapeutic Strategies*, eds. Masdeu JC, Sudarsky L, Wolfson L, pp. 245–59. Philadelphia: Lippincott-Raven.

Hughes AJ, Ben Shlomo Y, Daniel SE, Lees AJ (1992c) What features improve the accuracy of clinical diagnosis in Parkinson's disease: A clinicopathologic study. *Neurology*, 42, 1142–6.

Hughes AJ, Colosimo C, Kleedorfer B, Daniel SE, Lees AJ (1992b) The dopaminergic response in multiple system atrophy. *Journal of Neurology, Neurosurgery, and Psychiatry*, 55, 1009–13.

Hughes AJ, Daniel SE, Kilford L, Lees AJ (1992a) Accuracy of the clinical diagnosis of idiopathic Parkinson's disease: A clinicopathologic study of l00 cases. *Journal of Neurology, Neurosurgery, and Psychiatry*, 55, 181–4.

Hulette C, Mirra S, Wilkinson W, Heyman A, Fillenbaum, Clark C (1995) The consortium to establish a registry for Alzheimer's disease (CERAD) Part IX. A prospective cliniconeuropathologic study of Parkinson's features in Alzheimer's disease. *Neurology*, 45, 1991–5.

Hurtig HI (1993) Vascular parkinsonism. In: *Parkinsonian Syndromes*, eds. Stem MB, Koller WC, pp. 81–93. New York: Marcel-Dekker.

Inzelberg R, Bornstein NM, Reider I, Korczyn AD (1994) Basal ganglia lacunes and parkinsonism. *Neuroepidemiology*, 13, 108–12.

Jankovic J, Friedman DI, Pirozzolo FJ, McCrary JA (1990) Progressive supranuclear palsy: Motor, neurobehaviour and neuro-ophthalmic findings. *Advanced Neurology*, 53, 293–4.

Koller WC (1995) How accurately can Parkinson's disease be diagnosed? *Neurology*, 42, Suppl. 1, 6–16.

Koller WC, Biary N (1984) Effect of alcohol on tremor: Comparison to propranolol. *Neurology*, 34, 221–2.

Koller WD, Busenbark K, Miner K (1994) The relationship of essential tremor to other movement disorders: Report on 678 patients. *Annals of Neurology*, 35, 717–23.

Konagaya M, Konagaya Y, lida M (1994) Clinical and magnetic resonance imaging study of extrapyramidal symptoms in multiple system atrophy. *Journal of Neurology, Neurosurgery, and Psychiatry*, 57, 1528–31.

Krauss JK, Regel JP, Droste DW, Orszagh M, Borremans JJ, Vach W (1997) Movement disorders in adult hydrocephalus. *Movement Disorders*, 12, 53–60.

Larsson T, Sjdogren T (1960) Essential tremor. A clinical and genetic population study. *Acta Psychiatrica et Neurologica Scandinavica*, 36, Suppl. 144, 1–176.

Lopez OL, Wisnieski SR, Becker JT, Boller F, DeKosky ST (1997) Extrapyramidal signs in patients with probable Alzheimer disease. *Archives of Neurology*, 54, 969–75.

Magalhaes M (1995) Autonomic dysfunction in pathologically confirmed multiple system atrophy and idiopathic Parkinson's disease – A retrospective comparison. *Acta Neurologica Scandinavica*, 91, 98–102.

Mahieux F, Fenelon G, Flahault A, Manifacier M-J, Michelet D, Boller F (1998) Neuropsychological prediction of dementia in Parkinson's disease. *Journal of Neurology, Neurosurgery, and Psychiatry*, 64, 178–3

Mark MH, Sage JI (1993) Olivoponto cerebellar atrophy. In: *Parkinsonian Syndromes*, eds. Stern MD, Koller WC, pp. 43–67. New York: Marcel-Dekker.

Mark MH, Sage JI, Walters AS, Duvoisin RC, Miller DC (1995) Binswanger's disease presenting as levodopa-responsive parkinsonism: Clinicopathologic study of three cases. *Movement Disorders*, 10, 450–5.

Marsden CD, Thompson PA (1997) Toward a nosology of gait disorders: descriptive classification. In: *Gait Disorders of Ageing: Falls and Therapeutic Strategies*, eds. Masdeu JD, Sudarsky L, Wolfson L, pp. 135–46. Philadelphia: Lippincott-Raven.

Mayeux R, Chen J, Mirabello E, Marder K, Bell K, Dooneief G, Cote L, Stern Y (1990) An estimate of the incidence of dementia in idiopathic Parkinson's disease. *Neurology*, 40, 1513–16.

Mega MS, Masterman DL, Benson DF. Vinters HV, Tomiyasu U, Craig AH, Foti DJ, Kaufer D, Scharre DW, Fairbanks L, Cummings JL (1996) Dementia with Lewy bodies: Reliability and validity of clinical and pathologic criteria. *Neurology*, 47, 1403–9.

Mohr E, Litvan I, Williams J, Fedio P, Chase TN (1990) Selective deficits in Alzheimer and parkinsonian dementia: Visuospatial function. *Canadian Journal of Neurological Sciences*, 17, 292–7.

Nieforth KA, Golbe LI (1993) Retrospective study of drug response in 87 patients with progressive supranuclear palsy. *Clinical Neuropharmacology*, 16, 338–46.

Nutt JD, Horak FB (1997) Gait and balance disorders. In: *Movement Disorders: Neurologic Principles and Practice*, eds. Watts RL, Keller WC, p. 658. New York: McGraw-Hill.

Olanow CW (1992) Magnetic resonance imaging in Parkinsonism. *Neurologic Clinics*, 10, 405–20.

Pramstellar PP, Wenning GK, Smith SJM, Beck RO, Quinn NP, Fowler CJ (1995) Nerve conduction studies, skeletal muscle EMG, and sphincter EMG in multiple system atrophy. *Journal of Neurology, Neurosurgery, and Psychiatry*, 58, 618–21.

Quinn N (1995) Parkinsonism – Recognition and differential diagnosis. *British Medical Journal*, 310, 447–52.

Rajput AH, Rozdilsky B, Ang L (1991b) Occurrence of resting tremor in Parkinson's disease. *Neurology*, 41, 1298–9.

Rajput AH, Rozdilsky B, Ang L, Rajput A (1993) Significance of Parkinsonian manifestations in essential tremor. *Canadian Journal of Neurological Sciences*, 20, 114–17.

Rajput AH, Rozdilsky B, Rajput A (1991a) Accuracy of clinical diagnosis in parkinsonism – a prospective study. *Canadian Journal of Neurological Sciences*, 18, 275–8.

Rajput AH, Rozdilsky B, Rajput A, Ang L (1990) Levodopa efficacy and pathological basis of Parkinson syndrome. *Clinical Neuropharmacology*, 13, 553–8.

Rautakorpi I, Takala J, Martilla RJ, Sievers K, Rinne UK (1982) Essential tremor in a Finnish population. *Acta Neurologica Scandinavica*, 66, 58–67.

Riley DE, Lang AE (1996) Non-Parkinson akinetic-rigid syndromes. *Current Opinion in Neurology*, 9, 321–6.

Riley DE, Lang AE, Lewis A, Resch L, Ashby P, Hornykiewicz O, Black S (1990) Cortical–basal ganglionic degeneration. *Neurology*, 40, 1203–12.

Rodnitzky RL (1993) Hallervorden–Spatz syndrome. In: *Parkinsonian Syndromes*, eds. Stern MB, Koller WC, pp. 341–58. New York: Marcel-Dekker.

Rodnitzky RL, Uc EY (1997) Approach to the hypokinetic patient. In: *Practical Neurology*, ed. Biller J, pp. 299–311. Philadelphia: Lippincott-Raven.

Schneider JA, Watts RL, Gearing M, Brewer RP, Mirra SS (1997) Corticobasal degeneration: Neuropathologic and clinical heterogeneity. *Neurology*, 48, 959–69.

Schonfeld SM, Golbe LI, Sage JI, Safer JN, Duvoisin RC et al. (1987) Computed tomographic findings in progressive supranuclear palsy: Correlation with clinical grade. *Movement Disorders*, 2, 263–78.

Sethi KD, Adams RJ, Loring DW, El Gammal T (1988) Hallervorden–Spatz syndrome: Clinical and magnetic resonance imaging correlations. *Annals of Neurology*, 24, 692–4.

Starkstein SE, Sabe L, Petracca G, Chemerinski E, Kuzis G, Merello M, Leiguarda R (1996) Neuropsychological and psychiatric differences between Alzheimer's disease and Parkinson's disease with dementia. *Journal of Neurology, Neurosurgery, and Psychiatry*, 61, 381–7.

Stem MB, Braffman BH, Skolnick BE, Hurtig HI, Grossman RI (1989) Magnetic resonance imaging in Parkinson's disease and parkinsonian syndromes. *Neurology*, 39, 1524–6.

Sudarsky L (1990) Gait disorders in the elderly. *New England Journal of Medicine*, 322, 1441–6.

Sudarsky L, Simon S (1987) Gait disorder in late life hydrocephalus. *Archives of Neurology*, 44, 263–7.

Sudarsky L, Tideiksaar R (1997) The cautious gait, fear of falling and psychogenic gait disorders. In: *Gait Disorders of Ageing: Falls and Therapeutic Strategies*, eds. Masdeu JD, Sudarsky L, Wolfson L, pp. 283–95. Philadelphia: Lippincott-Raven.

Thompson PD, Marsden CD (1987) Gait disorder of subcortical arteriosclerotic encephalopathy: Binswanger's disease. *Movement Disorders*, 2, 1–8.

Trenkwalder C, Paulus W, Krafczyk S, Hawken M, Oertel WH, Brandt T (1995) Postural stability differentiates 'lower body' from idiopathic parkinsonism. *Acta Neurologica Scandinavica*, 91, 444–52.

Wenning GK, Ben Shlomo Y, Magalhaes M, Daniel SE, Quinn NP (1994) Clinical features and natural history of multiple system atrophy: An analysis of 100 cases. *Brain*, 117, 835–45.

Wenning GK, Tison F, Ben Shlomo Y, Daniel SE, Quinn NP (1997) Multiple system atrophy: A review of 203 pathologically proven cases. *Movement Disorders*, 12, 133–47.

Yagishita A, Oda M (1996) Progressive supranuclear palsy: MRI and pathological findings. *Neuroradiology*, 38, Suppl. 1, 560–6.

3

Parkinson's disease and parkinsonism in the elderly

Jolyon Meara and Bimal K Bhowmick

Introduction

The syndrome of parkinsonism, defined as akinesia accompanied by rigidity, and often tremor, occurs more frequently as people grow older and may be present in a significant proportion of elderly people (Mayeux et al.1992, Bennett et al. 1996, Meara et al. 1997). Two-thirds of patients with the diagnosis of Parkinson's disease (PD) will be over the age of 70 years, though the proportion of parkinsonism not due to PD increases with age. A further important issue in the care of the elderly with PD is that many patients, particularly women, will be living alone or will be cared for by a spouse who may also suffer from limitations imposed by health problems. The frailty of the diagnosis of parkinsonism and PD is addressed in Chapter 2, the epidemiology of parkinsonism in Chapter 7 and the drug treatment of PD in elderly subjects in Chapter 9.

The neuropathological basis of PD

PD is characterized by cell loss and gliosis in a paired brain stem nucleus called the substantia nigra (Jellinger 1986, Forno 1996). The substantia nigra is a pigmented dopamine rich nucleus that forms part of five closely related deep-seated subcortical brain nuclei, collectively called the basal ganglia (caudate, putamen, globus pallidus, subthalamic nucleus and substantia nigra). The substantia nigra consists of a densely cellular pars compacta, and a less cellular pars reticulata. The neurones in the substantia nigra pars compacta project to the caudate and putamen (together called the striatum) forming the nigrostriatal tract. The substantia nigra pars reticulata forms a major output nucleus of the basal ganglia projecting to specific thalamic nuclei and receiving afferent input from the striatum and subthalamic nucleus.

The cell loss in the substantia nigra occurs in a different distribution to that seen simply as a result of aging changes (Gibb and Lees 1991). Tretiakoff first suggested the causal link between degenerative changes in the substantia nigra and PD in 1919. His hypothesis was not widely accepted until after PD was found to be associated with a dopamine deficiency state in the striatum and the dopamine rich nigrostriatal tract linking the substantia nigra with the the striatum had been located (Bernheimer et al. 1973).

The remaining, but compromised nerve cells in the substantia nigra pars compacta contain typical inclusions in the cytoplasm called Lewy bodies (Jellinger 1986, Forno 1996). Lewy bodies have a dense eosinophilic core and pale halo and demonstrate characteristic staining reactions. Other inclusions have also been described in PD (Gibb et al. 1991). There is still debate about whether the diagnosis of PD can be made in clinically typical cases that fail to show typical neuropathological features. At postmortem, PD that was clinically typical in life may fail to show Lewy body degenerative disease in the substantia nigra (Rajput et al. 1989). In PD, Lewy bodies may be found in other pigmented and nonpigmented nuclei that provide ascending dopaminergic, serotonergic, noradrenergic and cholinergic projections to the cortex and basal ganglia (Agid et al. 1987). Lewy bodies also appear to occur in the cerebral cortex in most cases of PD (Hughes et al. 1992). Pathology outside the nigrostriatal tract presumably accounts for the clinical manifestations in PD of cognitive impairment, dementia, autonomic failure, postural imbalance, freezing, dysphagia and dysarthria.

Large numbers of cortical Lewy bodies in association with senile plaques, a feature of Alzheimer's disease, may suggest the diagnosis of dementia with Lewy bodies or a variant of Alzheimer's disease. Interestingly, cases that fulfil pathological criteria for PD but which have atypical clinical features, often including a poor response to levodopa treatment, tend to have prominent numbers of cortical Lewy bodies or additional vascular disease in the striatum (Hughes et al. 1993). Lewy bodies can also be found in other neurodegenerative conditions such as motor neurone disease and may be present in up to 10% of elderly subjects dying without evidence of PD in life (presumably disease-in-evolution).

Two important clinicopathological brain bank studies have demonstrated that diagnostic accuracy for PD at death is at best only around 76% (Rajput et al. 1991, Hughes et al. 1992). Neuropathological findings in cases misdiagnosed as PD consisted, not unexpectedly, of multisystem degenerative diseases that cause parkinsonism, such as progressive supranuclear palsy and multiple system atrophy, but more surprisingly, a significant number of cases of Alzheimer's disease and Alzheimer type changes. The use of stringent clinical diagnostic criteria can improve the specificity for the diagnosis of PD at the expense of sensitivity. Diagnostic accuracy in more recent cases referred to a brain bank was shown to have improved to around 84% (Ansorge et al. 1997). The second striking finding from these studies is that co-existing neuropathology both within and outside the striatum is extremely common in the brains of elderly subjects with histologically confirmed PD (Hughes et al. 1993).

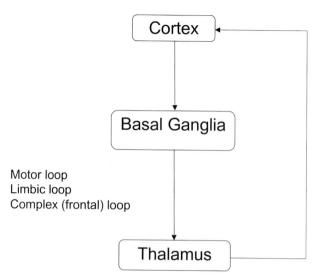

Fig. 3.1   Anatomy of cortical–basal ganglia–cortical loops: motor loop, limbic loop, complex (frontal) loop.

The neurophysiological basis of PD

The loss of dopaminergic modulation in the striatum causes a profound distur-bance of voluntary motor control leading to akinesia, tremor and rigidity. Restoring dopamine levels by the oral administration of the dopamine precursor levodopa can, at least temporarily, improve the motor impairments of PD. Our knowledge of the complex neurochemical, neuroanatomical and neurophysiolog-ical relationships in the basal ganglia in man and animal models has greatly increased in the past decade (Alexander et al. 1986, Alexander and Crutcher 1990, DeLong 1990, Elble 1998, Graybiel 1990, McRae 1998). Widespread cortical areas project to the striatum and pass from there to the globus pallidus/substantia nigra pars reticulata (the output nuclei of the basal ganglia) before passing back to specific cortical areas via the thalamus. Several loops exist linking the cortex, the basal ganglia, the thalamus, and cortex (see Fig. 3.1). The basic output from the thalamus is excitatory to the cortex, though this can be altered by the inputs from the output nuclei of the basal ganglia, which cause tonic inhibition of the thalamus (see Fig. 3.2). The motor signs of PD appear to result from a failure of the motor loop that links the sensorimotor cortex, putamen, globus pallidus/substantia nigra pars reticulata, thalamus, and the supplementary motor area in the cortex.

Normally, tonic thalamic inhibition from the basal ganglia is reduced in prepar-ation for a voluntary movement so that the excitatory thalamic output can increase to the relevant area in the supplementary motor area of the motor cortex. This is

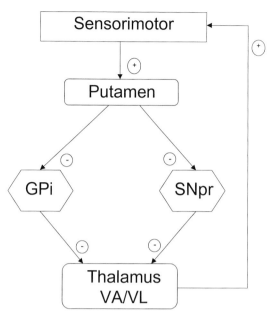

Fig. 3.2   Functional aspects of the motor loop – there is a resting tonic inhibition of VA/VL
(ventroanterior and ventrolateral thalamic nuclei) by GPi (globus pallidus pars interna)
and SNpr (substantia nigra pars reticulata).

achieved by cortical inputs to the putamen that cause inhibition of the output
nuclei (direct pathway). Cortical inputs can also increase the inhibition of the thalamus from the output nuclei by the involvement of a loop between the globus pallidus, subthalamic nucleus and globus pallidus/substantia nigra pars reticulata
(indirect pathway). The flow of activity between the direct and indirect pathways is
modulated by dopaminergic input from the substantia nigra pars compacta via the
ascending nigrostriatal pathway. Normally, dopamine in the striatum excites the
direct pathway and inhibits the indirect pathway. In PD the loss of dopamine
increases activity in the indirect pathway, thereby increasing thalamic inhibition
and reducing cortical excitability (see Fig. 3.3). This provides an explanation, albeit
rather simplistic, for the akinesia of PD and the failure of the proper execution of
automatic learned motor plans (Delwaide and Gonce 1998). Neurophysiological
data broadly support this type of explanation for some aspects of akinesia.
However, the simple model of PD provides no satisfactory explanation for tremor
or rigidity and the neurophysiogical basis for these motor signs is controversial
(Meara and Cody 1992, Hua et al. 1998).

   The subthalamic nucleus appears to play a critical part in the pathophysiology of
PD by providing powerful control over the inhibitory output activity of the basal
ganglia (globus pallidus pars interna/substantia nigra pars reticulata). Surgical

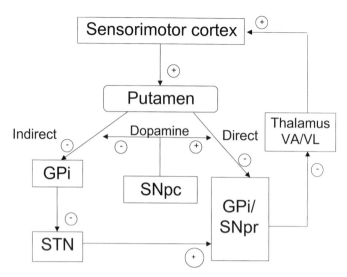

Fig. 3.3   Direct and indirect basal ganglia pathways modulated by dopamine from the nigrostriatal tract. GPi, globus pallidus pars externa; SNpc, substantia nigra pars compacta; SNPr, substantia nigra pars reticulata; STN, subthalamic nucleus; VA/VL, ventroanterior and ventrolateral thalamic nuclei.

lesions of the subthalamic nucleus or subthalamic stimulation can improve and sometimes even abolish all the motor features of PD (Limousin et al. 1995). Vascular damage to this area in elderly subjects without PD has been known for a long time to cause the hyperkinetic movement disorder of hemiballism. In the future, pharmacological manipulation of the excitatory glutamatergic pathway between the subthalamic nucleus and globus pallidus may also offer therapeutic potential.

A case history

The following history gives some account of the difficulties faced by many elderly patients with PD and the stress faced by some caregivers.

Mr R. W. is an 80-year-old retired solicitor and past captain of a golf club, who had continued to work until over 70 years old. His problem first began when he gave up playing golf about eight years ago. He refused to leave the house, saying that he had a bad back and complained to his children that the visits of his young grandchildren made him feel too tired and irritable. One year later he was diagnosed as having 'mild' PD by his general practitioner. He had been made to consult by his wife, who was worried about a tremor of his right hand that she had noticed for about six months and his difficulty with buttoning clothes and drawing cheques. He was commenced on selegiline. Due to lack of benefit, levodopa was added, with improvement of manual dexterity and some improvement of tremor. Still he did not engage in social activities.

Within two years he was requiring increasing doses of levodopa to control stiffness and loss of mobility. A tremor of the left hand developed. His wife noticed that his memory was getting worse. He fell twice, once in the house and once outside in the garden. Since that time he has become reluctant to go outside or venture upstairs.

Dopamine agonist therapy with bromocriptine was started with reduction in akinesia and rigidity. However, this drug had to be stopped due to recurrent complex visual hallucinations at night. The hallucinations consisted of a dog that had been a pet 30 years before.

At present he remains disabled by akinesia, dysarthria, tremor and impairment of postural reflexes. Oxybutynin has been prescribed for nocturia. He self medicates with levodopa and often takes doses in excess of that prescribed though remains dependent on his wife for elements of self-care. He is distressed and agitated at night, calling to his wife, who sleeps in a separate room, several times throughout the night to help him to go to the toilet. At night his wife has found him wandering in the bedroom looking for burglars. His wife notices that he becomes drowsy later in the day, so much so that on occasion he has fallen asleep into his dinner. He has refused to attend at a Day Centre because he believes his wife is having affairs behind his back when he is away.

The effects of aging and comorbidity on PD

Aging directly influences the clinical expression of PD and other diseases that appear with the passage of time. The resulting multiple pathology and polypharmacy of old age act to magnify and modify the disability and handicap of PD (see Table 3.1). In aging, cells from widespread areas of the substantia nigra projecting into the striatum are lost as well as dopamine receptors in the striatum. In PD, cells are primarily lost more specifically from the ventral tier nigral zona compacta cells projecting into the posterior striatum (Gibb and Lees 1991). Aging changes involving muscle, connective tissue, balance, gait, vision and the autonomic nervous system will compound and interact with impairment due to PD.

Clinical heterogeneity with age in PD

As with many diseases, in PD clinical complexity increases with the age of the group of patients studied. Elderly patients with PD will include several groups at very differing stages in the natural history of their disease, posing different problems and challenges (see Table 3.2). In young patients with PD the clinical challenge is that of dealing with a disorder of motor control typified by tremor, akinesia, involuntary movements and drug-induced motor fluctuations. However, in elderly patients akinesia, poor mobility and impaired balance are the most disabling motor features of PD. Additional problems in elderly patients arise from coexisting depression, dementia, autonomic dysfunction and the neuropsychiatric side effects of drug treatment.

Table 3.1 Factors influencing the clinical expression of PD in elderly subjects

• Aging changes in the nervous system	motor pathways
	sensory pathways
	proprioreception
	balance systems
	gait generation
• Aging changes in other organ systems	muscle
	connective tissue
	joints
	vision
• Concurrent disease:	
specific	cerebrovascular disease
	degenerative brain disease
	peripheral neuropathy
	arthritis/myopathy
	depression
nonspecific	immobility/frailty
• Effects of concurrent drug therapy:	
nervous system	cognitive impairment
	confusion
	sedation
	drug-induced
	parkinsonism
cardiovascular	orthostatic hypotension

Late stage PD

Some of the most difficult management challenges are encountered in this group of elderly patients. The clinical picture in late stage disease is dominated by features that do not respond to dopaminergic drugs, such as poor mobility, falls, confusion, drowsiness, dementia, sialorrhoea, dysarthria, impaired communication, dysphagia, and weight loss. With time, palliative care becomes increasingly appropriate for survivors at this stage of the disease.

Subtypes of PD and age at diagnosis

There has been considerable interest in the existence of subtypes of PD (see Table 3.3). Clinical impression suggests that patients with late onset PD (symptoms first starting after the age of 70 years) tend to progress more quickly than patients with early onset disease (symptoms before the age of 40 years). To a large extent clinical

Table 3.2 Clinical heterogeneity of elderly subjects with PD

- Elderly subjects with longstanding PD
- Elderly subjects with symptoms developing after 70 yrs old (late onset PD)
- Elderly subjects with PD of onset before 70 yrs old and of short duration
- Elderly subjects with associated moderate/severe disability/handicap (late stage PD)

Table 3.3 Subtypes of PD

Early onset <50 yrs old	vs.	Late onset >70 yrs old
Tremor dominant	vs.	Postural imbalance and gait disorder
Benign slow progression	vs.	Malignant rapid progression
Unilateral with or without axial disease	vs.	Bilateral disease with or without impaired balance

impressions have been supported by most studies investigating the existence of subtypes in PD (Zetusky et al. 1985, Goetz et al. 1988). The large DATATOP study has analysed the initial clinical findings in a cohort of 800 patients at diagnosis (Jankovic et al. 1990). This study showed that patients with late onset disease progressed at a greater rate and were more cognitively impaired than those with early onset disease. Patients classified as having rapidly progressive PD were older and had more severe bradykinesia and postural imbalance and less tremor when compared to the group with slowly progressive disease. These motor features remained even after adjustment for age. The group of patients with tremor dominant disease had less disability, less cognitive impairment and less depressive symptomatology compared to the group with marked gait and balance impairment. These findings are supported by most (Zetusky et al. 1985, Goetz et al. 1988, Diamond et al. 1989), but not all (Gibb and Lees 1988, Friedman 1994) studies.

Late onset PD

The pattern of disease at presentation in elderly subjects may reflect the more widespread loss of nigral cells due to aging in addition to the more circumscribed loss due to PD. The failure of gait and balance difficulties to respond to levodopa also suggests involvement of other non-dopaminergic neural pathways. The faster progression of PD in late onset disease has been explained by the independent and additive effects of age and disease duration on the natural history of PD. Nigral cell loss due to PD appears to be most rapid in the early stages of disease evolution.

There appears to be a clear association of late onset disease with depression and cognitive impairment. The extent to which this association is attributable to age alone is unclear. The DATATOP analysis suggested that cognitive function and motor deterioration were relatively independent once adjustment for age had taken place (Jankovic et al. 1990). However, patients with late onset disease become demented sooner than patients with early onset disease of similar age (Tanner et al. 1985).

Comprehensive assessment of PD in elderly patients

Optimal management of PD and parkinsonism in elderly patients requires an approach based on the comprehensive assessment of the impact of PD on the physical, mental and social functioning of the individual (Rubenstein et al. 1991, Stuck et al. 1993). Quality of care ultimately depends on timely functional assessment and reassessment from diagnosis, through disease progression and finally to palliative care in advanced PD. The needs and views of the carer should also be addressed in the assessment process.

Specialist clinics with access to a wide range of health and social care expertise can provide this level of assessment, can organize or provide treatment and can monitor outcomes of care. Standardized assessment can be used as the basis for management decisions and for determining treatment outcomes. Assessment in PD should be structured (see Fig. 3.4). The baseline assessment of patients can be undertaken by medical, nursing and therapy staff. In reality, most elderly patients will require referral for specialist assessment by the multidisciplinary team. Swallowing difficulties require assessment by speech therapists, who can also aid communication and language. Dieticians can advise on strategies to improve levodopa absorption, to maintain weight, to maintain safe swallowing and to alleviate constipation. Occupational therapists can assess the physical environment in the home and the patient's functional ability in their normal surroundings. The financial burden and social isolation of PD can be assessed by a social worker who can advise on any financial benefits available and measures to improve social contact. Some patients may require formal psychological and psychiatric assessment.

Elderly patients should initially be assessed by a full clinical history and review of current medication, supported by a general medical and neurological examination. Lying and standing blood pressure and pulse rate are important measures of autonomic function and risk of postural syncope with anti-parkinsonian medication. Selected investigations indicated by the history and examination may be required. Diagnosis should be made based on recommended clinical diagnostic criteria for PD, such as those developed as a result of clinicopathological Brain Bank studies (Hughes et al.1992). The Unified Parkinson's Disease Rating Scale (UPDRS – see Fahn et al. 1987) covers mood, memory, activities of daily living, motor impairment and complications of drug therapy and is used in most large drug research studies in PD. However, the UPDRS takes around 15 minutes to administer in

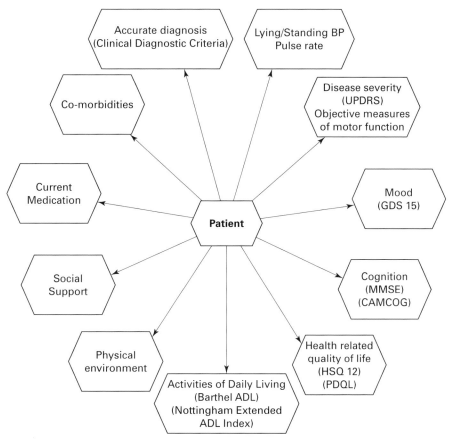

Fig. 3.4   Domains in the assessment of Parkinson's disease.

routine clinical practice. One approach is to select the motor section and complications of therapy from the UPDRS and to use more generic measures for the other domains. Assessment of motor function needs to take place at a defined time in relation to drug treatment, usually when the patient is maximally 'on' in terms of drug response. A simple measure of motor function is a timed ten metre walk with step count and a measure of upper limb akinesia such as the two touch test. The two touch test involves sitting the patient in a straight backed chair with arms. The patient is then asked to touch each arm of the chair in turn with first the right then the left hand. Full excursions over one minute are counted for each hand. Normative values in elderly subjects need to be established.

Activities of daily living, memory and mood are well covered by generic measures, such as the Barthel ADL Scale (Collin et al. 1988), the Nottingham Extended ADL Index (Nouri and Lincoln 1987), the Mini Mental State Examination (MMSE) (Folstein et al. 1975), the CAMCOG assessment of cognitive function (Roth et al.

1986) and the short form of the Geriatric Depression Scale, the GDS-15 (D'Ath et al. 1994).

The GDS-15, has been validated in elderly community dwellers and elderly patients in hospital settings (D'Ath et al. 1994, Lesher and Berryhill 1994). Out of a maximum score of 15 a score of five or more on the GDS-15 has a sensitivity and specificity of around 90% and 70% respectively for depression when compared to formal psychiatric diagnosis (Jackson and Baldwin 1993, D'Ath et al. 1994). The CAMCOG assessment is more sensitive to early cognitive decline than the MMSE (Hobson and Meara 1998) and could be used to assess patients with borderline scores on the MMSE.

Health related quality of life measures are being increasingly used in health care to measure outcome and quality of care. A widely used generic health status measure, the Short-Form 36 (Brazier et al. 1992), contains items inappropriate for elderly subjects and also suffers from missing data when administered by self report in elderly patients with stroke and PD (Hobson and Meara 1997). The Health Status Questionnaire 12 (HSQ-12) is a new measure, derived from the SF-36, which appears to be acceptable to elderly subjects as a brief core measure of health related quality of life (Bowling and Windsor 1997). In addition to generic measures two disease specific tools exist; the PDQL (de Boer et al. 1996) and the PD-39 (Jenkinson et al. 1995).

Frequency of assessment visits

The frequency of clinic visits is determined by the severity and number of functional problems identified and how rapidly patients progress to late stage disease. Patients with stable disease who are managing well may need review only on a yearly basis. Open access to the clinic for patients experiencing difficulties can be an important feature in promoting confidence in the patient and carer. In late stage disease a time will arise when, due to frailty and immobility, clinic visits may no longer be appropriate. In these circumstances home assessment can be performed by the nurse specialist of the team. The need for palliative care can be evaluated and treatment plans agreed with the patient, carer and family doctor. Patients failing to attend at clinic visits are easily lost to follow-up, with resulting fragmentation of care at the terminal stage of their disease.

Specific problems encountered in elderly patients with PD

Motor syndromes

Unlike younger patients with PD, elderly patients are more troubled by gait and balance problems. Dyskinesia and motor fluctuations, apart from 'end of dose' deterioration or 'wearing off', before the next medication is due, are rarely seen in late onset disease. End of dose deterioration is easily overlooked in elderly patients. The two most common motor syndromes seen in elderly patients are, firstly, apparent drug resistant parkinsonian motor signs and secondly, increasing gait and balance problems. Non-drug rehabilitative approaches are an important part of the management of motor disability in elderly patients with PD. Electroconvulsive therapy (ECT) has been found to improve the motor symptoms of PD in elderly patients who are not depressed and ongoing benefit has been reported for nearly three years in some patients (Pridmore and Pollard 1996). Despite evidence of benefit in the majority of the very small number of patients treated with ECT and reported in the literature, it is unlikely that ECT would be widely acceptable to many elderly patients.

Drug resistant motor parkinsonism

Failure of motor signs to respond to levodopa would indicate a diagnosis other than PD. However, motor signs in patients with late onset disease do not appear to respond as well to levodopa as in younger patients. This cannot be explained simply by an inability to tolerate a full therapeutic dose. Patients with long standing PD remain responsive to levodopa, though the duration of response is reduced. Patients with late onset PD should be treated with maximally tolerated doses of levodopa to obtain the best control of symptoms. Patients with long standing PD who have not been under regular medical review may well have been significantly undertreated for several years. In elderly patients standard formulations of levodopa (co-careldopa 25/100 or co-beneldopa 25/100) should be used in a trial of treatment to obtain the best control of disease symptoms. A minimum daily dose of 600 mg levodopa should be reached. A few patients will require higher doses to maximize motor response, though this is unusual. Commonly, a maximally therapeutic levodopa dose may not be tolerated due to side effects of drowsiness, dizziness on standing, and hallucinosis. Patients with late onset disease tend to respond even less well to levodopa and are often poorly tolerant of the nausea and vomiting induced by dopamine and the neuropsychiatric effects of this drug. Poor tolerance of levodopa raises the possibility of parkinsonism not due to PD. The peripheral dopamine antagonist, domperidone, at a dose of 20 mg three times daily taken 30 minutes before levodopa, can be used to control nausea and vomiting. Domperidone may also help postural hypotension, though this requires further study. Depending on the pattern of motor response, dispersible or slow release forms of levodopa can be substituted for standard forms.

Motor fluctuations in elderly patients

With time, levodopa-induced motor complications develop in all patients, though these tend to be less obvious in late onset disease compared to younger patients with PD. How levodopa induces these changes is unknown, but the mechanism probably involves altered dopamine mediated gene regulation in the basal ganglia, coupled with central changes in the pharmacokinetic handling of levodopa.

End of dose fluctuations may respond to the use of tolcapone, a drug that inhibits the peripheral and central metabolism of levodopa, thereby increasing the bioavailability of oral doses, or the use of sustained release levodopa (Sinemet CR, Madopar CR). Elderly patients with a short duration of response to levodopa who remain parkinsonian for long periods of the day may improve with the introduction of oral dopamine agonist drugs (bromocriptine, pergolide, ropinirole, cabergoline) as adjunctive therapy to levodopa (Hindle et al. 1998). The dopamine agonist apomorphine may be useful in selected elderly patients with PD who respond to levodopa, to control severe 'off' period symptoms (Hughes et al. 1993). Apomorphine can also be used perioperatively in elderly patients undergoing surgery, particularly after femur fracture. Those patients with significant cognitive impairment, levodopa-induced hallucinosis, or who are unresponsive to levodopa, will not benefit from the introduction of dopamine agonist therapy.

Severe 'on' period dyskinesia in patients with long standing PD that impairs function may necessitate a reduction in dopaminergic drug treatment. Dopamine agonists and selegiline tend to exacerbate levodopa-induced dyskinesia and should be withdrawn before finally reducing the dose of levodopa itself. Painful 'off' period dystonia, often appearing in the early morning as cramps in the feet and legs, can respond to rapidly absorbed dispersible formulations of levodopa (Madopar dispersible) taken on waking.

Balance and gait problems

In elderly patients mobility deteriorates as a result of impaired gait and balance. Falls inevitably occur, further eroding confidence and increasing immobility. Antiparkinsonian drugs do not help this problem and may make matters worse by impairing cognitive function and increasing postural hypotension.

Good multidisciplinary team working remains the most important aspect in managing this problem. Physiotherapists can work to maintain muscle condition and increase confidence and can instruct patient and carer on the best way to get up after a fall. The team can provide an important source of support, motivation and encouragement to patients facing these difficulties.

Neurosurgery

Neurosurgical approaches to the treatment of PD, involving highly selective lesioning, fetal grafting and deep brain stimulation, are undergoing resurgence at the present time. Unfortunately, it is unlikely that many elderly patients with PD would be suitable candidates for neurosurgical treatment. However, some physiologically fit elderly individuals, particularly if troubled by severe tremor and who respond well to levodopa, may benefit from neurosurgical procedures (Obeso et al. 1997). The major benefit of neurosurgery is to improve 'off' period disability. The quality of the 'on' response to dopaminergic drugs is not improved.

Depression

The most common neuropsychiatric complication of PD is depression, occurring in around 40% of subjects studied (Cummings 1992). However, depression is also the most common psychiatric disorder in older people and community studies of elderly people without PD over 65 years old indicate a prevalence of significant depression of around 15% (Livingstone et al. 1990, Saunders et al. 1993). Furthermore, studies of elderly inpatients suggest a prevalence for depression of around 35% in this group (Jackson and Baldwin 1993).

Diagnostic criteria for depression in PD

The prevalence of depression detected in any study will depend upon the criteria used to diagnose depression. Depression remains, in essence, a clinical judgement based on assessment, observation and clinical experience. Self report 'paper and pencil tests' such as the GDS, structured interviews such as the present state examination and computerized psychiatric assessment schedules have been used in an attempt to standardize and refine this diagnosis. The profile and severity of depressive symptoms has been used in diagnostic systems such as the *Diagnostic and Statistical Manual of Mental Disorders* (American Psychiatric Association 1994) to define 'major depressive disorder' and a persistent but less severe condition called 'dysthymic disorder'. There can be no doubt that self rated questionnaires used to assess mood disorder in PD will inevitably confuse somatic problems due to physical disease with mood disorder and thus will over report mood disturbance. To some extent this has been addressed by the development of self rating scales such as the GDS. The GDS avoids over emphasis on the somatic/vegetative symptoms of depressive illness that could also arise from physical illness and functional disability. Both autonomic failure, which is well recognized in PD, and emotionalism can be mistaken for depression in PD and lead to over diagnosis of this condition (Madeley et al 1992).

Epidemiology of depression in PD

Studies using standardized criteria for both depression and PD in hospital-based (Cummings 1992) and community populations (Tison et al. 1995, Tandberg et al. 1996, Meara et al. 1999) report a prevalence for depression of around 40%, though much lower figures have also been reported (Brown and MacCarthy 1990, Madeley et al. 1993). Depression appears to be more common in elderly patients with PD than would be expected from age alone, though any medical illness is also associated with increased levels of depression. One study comparing a sample of patients with arthritis and PD found that depression scores were similarly high in both disease groups compared with healthy elderly subjects (Gotham et al. 1986). The overall incidence of depression in PD patients over the age of 40 years old has been estimated as around 1.86% per year, with age specific incidence increasing with age of subjects (Doonief et al. 1992). This compares with rates in the general population of 0.17%.

Nature of depression in PD

Although elderly patients with PD express high levels of depressive symptoms the prevalence of major affective disorder, as diagnosed on DSM-III criteria, and other formal psychiatric diagnoses of 'caseness', appears to be low (Madeley et al. 1993, Hantz et al. 1994, Tandberg et al. 1996). The nature of depression in PD may also be characterized qualitatively by pessimism, hopelessness and poor motivation and the absence of guilt, self blame and worthlessness, compared to elderly subjects with primary depressive disease (Gotham et al. 1986). The profile of depressive symptoms may also alter with disease progression (Huber et al. 1990). Psychotic features (hallucinations and delusional ideas) in major depression in PD appear to be rare though have not been specifically studied in depressed patients with PD (Brown and MacCarthy 1990).

Features of PD associated with depression

A complex relationship exists between depression and the disease variables of age at onset, cognitive impairment and the pattern and severity of motor involvement. Patients with early onset disease, starting before the age of 50 years, may have a greater prevalence of depression compared with late onset disease starting after the age of 70 years (Starkstein et al. 1989). The relationship between disease severity and depression is unclear, with some (Gotham et al. 1986, Meara et al. 1999) but not all studies (Huber et al. 1988) supporting a positive association between the two. However, the DATATOP analysis (Jankovic et al. 1990) revealed that patients with unilateral disease were less likely to be depressed than patients with more severe bilateral disease. Depression in PD appears to be associated with disability, particularly at times in the natural history of the disease when disability is rapidly changing (Brown et al. 1988). Stress and social support are also predictors of the risk of depression in PD (Fleminger 1991).

Cognitive impairment appears to be more consistently linked with the expression of depression in PD (Starkstein et al. 1992, Troster et al. 1995, Tandberg et al. 1996) though this may reflect both the impact of depression on cognitive function and the depressing effect of the awareness of impaired cognition. Some evidence suggests that the cognitive function of depressed patients with PD deteriorates more rapidly than in nondepressed patients (Starkstein et al. 1992). The self rated questionnaires used in many studies to diagnose depression may be inappropriate for patients with cognitive impairment and dementia.

The basis of depression in PD

There is no simple unifying mechanism to explain the relationship between depression and PD. It is likely that depression has its origin both in the neurobiology of PD and in the 'reactive' psychological response to living with the unpredictable disability of a progressive neurological disease. However, motor disability is not strongly linked to depression in PD and the treatment of motor disability with antiparkinsonian drugs is not usually associated with resolution of coexisting depressive symptoms.

Evidence exists supporting a link between depression and biological mechanisms that cause PD. Patients may present with depression before the onset of motor symptoms in PD (Mayeux et al. 1981) and mood swings are clearly linked to 'on–off' motor fluctuations in PD (Cantello et al. 1986, Menza et al. 1990). Brain serotonin is reduced in PD and has been implicated in the pathophysiology of depression in PD (D'Amato et al. 1987). An improvement in mood and drive has been reported after the addition of the serotonin precursor L-tryptophan to levodopa (Coppen et al. 1972). Lumbar CSF levels of 5-hydroxyindoleacetic acid have been claimed to be reduced in depressed patients with PD compared with PD patients without depression and normal subjects (Mayeux et al. 1984, Kostic et al. 1987, Mayeux et al. 1988), though values between groups overlap and the reproducibility of these findings is uncertain (Sano et al. 1989). Serotonin precursors have been shown to improve depression in PD patients with concomitant rise in CSF metabolite levels (McCance-Katz et al. 1992). Data from studies of platelet imipramine binding and fenfluramine induced prolactin release, support a greater serotonergic deficit in depressed PD patients compared with nondepressed PD patients and normal age matched subjects without PD (Schneider et al. 1988, Kostic et al. 1993).

A strong case can be made for the involvement of dopamine itself as depression in PD has been shown to be associated with more severe loss of cells in the mesocorticolimbic projection. Furthermore, mood swings are known to complicate rapid changes in striatal dopamine transmission ('on–off' swings) in PD (Menza et al. 1990).

Attempts to define a neuroanatomical basis for depression in PD have produced conflicting results with both right- and left-sided hemiparkinsonism being claimed to be associated with more severe symptoms of depression and anxiety (Starkstein et al. 1990, Fleminger 1991). Studies using positron emission tomography comparing depressed and nondepressed PD patients and depressed and nonde-pressed age matched controls suggest that depression in PD and primary depres-sive illness both reflect abnormal dysfunction in the medial prefrontal cortex (Ring et al. 1994).

Treatment of depression in PD

Depression in PD will respond to the general psychotherapeutic support of a spe-cialist therapy team. More specifically, antidepressant therapy and ECT have been shown to be effective in treating depression in PD (Balldin et al. 1981, Holcomb et al. 1983). Cognitive therapy is also likely to be effective but has not been formally evaluated. ECT can also improve motor symptoms (Fall et al. 1995).

There have been only four double-blind studies of the drug treatment of depres-sion in PD, spanning over 30 years, and involving a total of around 100 PD patients of all ages (Strang 1965, Laitinen 1969, Andersen et al. 1980, Goetz et al. 1984). The primary goal of three of these studies was to confirm the utility of tricyclic anti-depressants (Strang 1965, Laitinen 1969) and bupropion, an indirect dopamine agonist (Goetz et al. 1984), in treating the motor symptoms of PD. The criteria used both for the diagnosis of PD and depression in the two early reports are unclear. The only study using standardized criteria for PD and depression did not report the proportion of patients whose depression clinically responded to drug treatment (Andersen et al. 1980). These studies taken together suggest that drug treatment is effective in the treatment of depression in PD, though side effects to the anti-depressant drugs were reported. The selective serotonin reuptake inhibitors (SSRIs) are better tolerated than tricyclic antidepressant drugs in elderly subjects and are equally effective in treating primary depressive illness. Evidence linking serotonin to depression in PD also indicates that this class of drug should be effective in this group of patients. Some concerns have been raised over evidence indicating that two drugs of this class, fluoxetine and paroxetine, can cause drug-induced parkin-sonism (Steur 1993, Jiminez-Jiminez et al. 1994). The MAO-B inhibitor selegiline, used to treat PD, in combination with SSRI's may cause the toxic serotonin syn-drome. However, the combination of selegiline and fluoxetine, despite these con-cerns, does not appear to be associated with any significant problems in daily clinical use (Waters 1994, Richard et al. 1996). There have been two recent reports of the efficacy and safety of the SSRI sertraline in depressed patients with PD (Meara et al. 1996, Hauser and Zesiewicz 1997). Sertraline has not been reported to cause drug-induced parkinsonism and is in fact a weak dopamine reuptake blocker. We have also studied the long-term use of the drug in a further group of 41 patients with PD reporting high levels of depressive symptoms based on the self report GDS scale. After three months treatment, 39% of this group showed a reduc-tion of 50% or more in the score on the GDS. No deterioration in motor function was observed in any of the patients in the study (unpublished observations). There would appear to be considerable opportunity costs of using the SSRIs to treat depression in PD compared to the older tricyclic antidepressant drugs, although the potential economic advantage remains to be formally evaluated.

Carer distress in PD

The majority of elderly patients with PD living at home receive help from their spouse, or other close family members. An early study found evidence of an association between carer distress and functional impairment in the patient (Calder et al. 1991). However, two recent studies have suggested that distress in carers was best predicted by the level of depression, rather than physical disability, in the recipient of care (Miller et al. 1996, Meara et al. 1999). The former study also demonstrated for the first time that carers of subjects with PD showed significantly elevated levels of distress and strain compared to age matched controls with spouses in good health. The detection and aggressive treatment of depression in patients with PD may be important in treating the distress of their carers. Carer distress could be an important and valid outcome measure for the treatment of depression in the patient.

Detecting and treating depression in PD

Despite the high level of depressive symptomatology in PD and evidence for the efficacy of drug therapy few patients appear to receive specific treatment. In our community-based study of 132 patients over the age of 60 years with PD, only 7% were in receipt of antidepressant medication despite the fact that 64% of this group scored in the depressed range on the GDS-15 (Meara et al. 1999). In this study 79 carer spouses were identified and 35% of this group of carers had significant depressive symptoms. Only around 7% of carers scoring in the depressed range on the GDS were being treated with antidepressant drugs.

Dementia

Dementia is a major factor in the management of PD in elderly subjects, limiting both the drug therapy that can be offered and the quality of life that can be achieved for patient, carer and family. Cognitive impairment in PD, particularly if complicated by hallucinations and delusional ideas, is the most potent risk factor for admission to nursing home care.

Epidemiology of dementia in PD

Dementia is common in patients over the age of 65 years with PD although prevalence figures vary between 10–44% depending on the diagnostic criteria used for dementia, PD, and the nature of the study population (Cummings 1988, Mayeux et al. 1992, Tison et al. 1995, Hobson and Meara 1999). Operational criteria for dementia resulting from AD are usually used to define dementia in PD (American Psychiatric Association 1994), though specific criteria have also been suggested (Cummings and Benson 1983). In simple terms dementia can be defined as global cognitive impairment of sufficient severity to impair social function and employment in the absence of delirium and other general medical disease known to cause cognitive impairment. The risk of developing dementia is at least doubled in patients with PD compared to age matched subjects without the diagnosis of PD. In one study (Biggins *et al.* 1992) there was a cumulative incidence of dementia of 19% in surviving members of a cohort of 87 patients with PD followed up for over four years. The risk of dementia increases exponentially with age such that 65% of surviving members of a cohort of patients with PD over the age of 85 years are likely to be demented (Mayeux et al. 1990).

Risk factors for dementia

Depression, cognitive impairment and age interact in a complex manner and most studies have shown depression to be a risk factor for subsequent dementia (Troster et al. 1995). Risk factors for dementia in PD apart from age and depression have been shown to be: late onset disease, postural imbalance and gait disorder subtype, severe motor deficits, rapid progression of PD, and severe facial akinesia/hypomimia (Ebmeier et al. 1990, Jankovic et al. 1990, Stern et al. 1993, Viitanen et al. 1994, Marder et al. 1995).

Causes of dementia in PD

Elderly patients with dementia predating parkinsonism by at least one year should probably be considered to have a primary dementia, such as AD, or dementia with Lewy bodies complicated by parkinsonism. Parkinsonism predating dementia by at least one year can be considered to be 'PD with dementia'. In this situation dementia can arise from the same causes as for primary dementia as well as from typical brainstem PD pathology alone. Dementia in PD is usually never definitively diagnosed in elderly patients as so few brains are examined in detail after death. There are many causes of dementia in PD. The striking relationship of age to dementia in PD indicates the importance of aging changes and the impact of other concurrent age related dementing disease in the aetiology of dementia in PD. These include the primary changes of PD as well as concurrent pathology due to AD and cerebrovascular disease.

Dementia with Lewy bodies

There remains considerable uncertainty over the nosology of the condition called dementia with Lewy bodies (Okazaki et al. 1961, Kosaka 1978, Gómez-Tortosa et al.

1998, Holmes et al 1999). Some investigators claim that dementia with Lewy bodies is the second commonest cause of dementia and can be detected in life using agreed clinical diagnostic criteria (Byrne et al. 1989, McKeith et al. 1992, McKeith et al. 1995). The primary finding at post mortem in this condition are plentiful Lewy bodies in the limbic areas of the temporal lobe and other cortical areas. Lewy bodies may also be present in subcortical regions. The pathology in older patients with this condition is nearly always complicated by the additional presence of senile plaques and neurofibrillary tangles, similar or identical to those found in AD. This condition is variously felt to be an extension of PD (Gibb et al. 1985, Lieberman 1997), to be a type of AD (Weiner et al. 1996), or to represent a specific type of primary Lewy-body disease (McKeith et al. 1995). As a result the commonest cause of dementia in PD is claimed by some to be AD, and by others to be dementia with Lewy bodies. Cortical Lewy bodies, especially in limbic areas, appear to be present in many if not all PD patients even in the absence of cognitive impairment (Hughes et al. 1992). Furthermore, the density of Lewy bodies in the cortex does not appear to be related to the degree of regional brain atrophy found at post mortem (Mann and Snowden 1995).

Neuropsychological features of dementia and pre-dementia in PD

The characteristics of the neuropsychological deficits in PD patients with dementia or pre-dementia and the relationships of such impairments to the underlying disease processes causing dementia are poorly understood (Brown and Marsden 1990). A classification of dementia into cortical and subcortical dementia has been proposed, based on the results of neuropsychological tests in cortical diseases such as AD and subcortical diseases such as Huntington's chorea. The concept of cortical and subcortical cognitive impairment in PD remains controversial (Starkstein et al. 1996, Lieberman 1997). Many patients with PD demonstrate cognitive deficits that tend to be of subcortical type and may be relatively nonprogressive (Cooper et al. 1991), though a minority of such patients will progress to a full subcortical dementia. Dementia in PD is much more commonly of cortical than subcortical type. Lieberman's (1997) review suggests that two-thirds of dementia in PD is due to AD related changes with or without cortical Lewy bodies, the remaining third being due to Lewy-body pathology. This latter group appears to consist largely of patients with cortical and brainstem Lewy bodies. Patients with presumed dementia with Lewy bodies may show more evidence of impaired attention, executive function and visuospatial difficulty compared to patients with AD. On the whole, most investigators have found little difference between the neuropsychological deficits of AD and PD with dementia. However, impaired visual reasoning (Starkstein et al. 1996, Mahieux et al. 1998) and verbal fluency (Jacobs et al. 1995) have been proposed to be neuropsychological deficits that may serve to distinguish PD with dementia from concurrent AD.

Management of dementia in PD

Elderly patients and their carers need to be told about the risks of cognitive impairment in PD and when cognitive impairment appears to be developing or accelerating, opportunity should be given to address matters such as living wills and advance directives. All drug treatment should be critically reviewed, particularly with regard to any anticholinergic actions of drugs prescribed for other concurrent disease. Most antiparkinsonian drugs further impair cognitive function in dementia, either by impairing alertness or increasing confusion. Patients should be managed on simple regimes of standard levodopa whenever possible. The dose of levodopa should be reduced to the minimum amount that maintains parkinsonian symptoms at levels acceptable to the patient and carer. Reducing antiparkinsonian drug treatment can improve cognitive function by relieving drug-induced delirium and psychosis and increasing alertness. There is no specific drug therapy for dementia in PD. However, the acetylcholinesterase inhibitors tacrine and donepezil may be effective in treating certain types of dementia in PD, though there are no data as yet to support such use.

Psychosis

In both late onset and long standing PD neuropsychiatric complications related to drug therapy are common and result in acute confusional states, sleep abnormalities, hallucinations and paranoid delusions (Celesia and Wanamaker 1972, Nausieda et al. 1984, Factor et al. 1995). Delusions of sexual infidelity are common and may result in elderly patients refusing to attend day centres or be admitted for respite admissions for fear of leaving their partner. A classification of psychosis in PD has recently been suggested (Peyser et al. 1998), which emphasizes the distinction between psychosis associated with and without coexisting delirium and dementia.

Although all antiparkinsonian drugs can provoke these reactions, anticholinergic drugs, dopamine agonists and selegiline appear to cause problems much more commonly than levodopa itself. A strong case can be made for avoiding the use of anticholinergic drugs in PD as these drugs cause cognitive impairment in addition to psychiatric side effects. However, the ability of such drugs to alleviate sialorrhoea in late stage disease, albeit at the expense of a dry mouth, may make patients reluctant to stop such therapy. A balance has to be maintained in late stage disease between mobility and mental clarity. Simple hallucinosis that does not distress the patient or carer may be tolerated without reduction in drug treatment (Haeske-Dewick 1995). Atypical neuroleptic drugs such as clozapine or olanzapine that act on limbic rather than striatal dopamine receptors may be useful in selected patients to specifically control dopaminometic psychosis and allow a larger dose of levodopa to be prescribed to preserve mobility (Kahn et al. 1991, Meltzer et al. 1995,

Wolters et al. 1996). Neither drug is licensed for use in this situation. Demented PD patients with psychosis not clearly related to dopaminergic drug therapy do not tolerate atypical neuroleptic drugs, due to the sedation and delirium such drugs induce.

Autonomic function in elderly patients with PD

Autonomic function involving both the sympathetic and parasympathetic system can be impaired in PD and can lead to a number of prominent and disabling symptoms. These include bladder dysfunction, constipation, dizziness on standing, abnormal sweating, sexual dysfunction and breathlessness. Although tests of autonomic function are normal in early PD, with disease progression increasing evidence of autonomic dysfunction becomes apparent (Gross et al. 1972, Sandyk and Awerbuch 1992, van Dijk et al. 1993, Martin et al. 1993). However, autonomic function also declines with age and is influenced by the presence and drug treatment of concurrent diseases such as diabetes and hypertension. Drugs used to treat PD may also adversely affect the autonomic nervous system. As a result, nearly all elderly patients with PD demonstrate some abnormalities of autonomic function. Symptoms usually attributed to autonomic failure, such as sweating and dizziness on standing, appear to correlate poorly with documented tests of autonomic function (Berrios et al. 1995). The extent of autonomic failure compatible with a diagnosis of PD has not been established, though the development of severe symptoms of autonomic dysfunction in a patient with parkinsonism within two years of the onset of symptoms suggests a diagnosis of multiple system atrophy.

Orthostatic hypotension

Blood pressure and pulse rate need to be carefully monitored in elderly patients with PD and should be assessed lying and standing under controlled conditions with the patient resting supine for ten minutes before standing. The blood pressure and pulse rate should be taken supine and again after two minutes and five minutes standing. A fall in systolic blood pressure of 20 mmHg or more and/or a fall of 10 mmHg or more in the diastolic blood pressure is the most commonly used standard definition for the presence of orthostatic hypotension, whether or not there are any symptoms. Using this definition, orthostatic hypotension was detected in nearly 60% of a group of patients with PD attending a specialist clinic (Senard et al. 1997). Falls in blood pressure occur particularly on rising in the morning and getting up from the meal table. At these times patients are at most risk of syncope and falls. Large drops in systolic and diastolic blood pressure on standing or after exercise do not always cause symptoms, but will do so under any conditions of stress such as the development of any intercurrent infection or prolonged bed rest.

The most common cause of orthostatic hypotension is the drug therapy of patients with PD rather than PD itself, or age related autonomic dysfunction. Levodopa and dopamine agonists cause falls in postural blood pressure by central and peripheral dopaminergic effects. Selegiline may potentiate this effect (Churchyard et al. 1997). Domperidone appears to improve orthostatic hypotension secondary to diabetes and other diseases (Montastruc et al. 1985, Lopes de Faria et al. 1988) though its place in PD remains unclear. As a result of multiple pathology elderly patients with PD are often receiving other hypotensive drugs such as antihypertensive drugs, antianginal drugs, diuretics, sedatives, antidepressants, and anticholinergic drugs. Many of these prescriptions will be unwarranted and can be withdrawn to good effect. It is surprising how many elderly patients with PD and low resting blood pressure are on active treatment with antihypertensive drug therapy. Diuretic drugs are often used inappropriately to treat ankle swelling resulting from immobility rather than cardiac failure.

Elderly patients with PD admitted into hospital with a diagnosis of collapse due to 'transient ischaemic attack' or 'stroke' very often turn out to have syncope due to drug and disease induced orthostatic hypotension. Careful history taking with witness accounts coupled with appropriate assessment of autonomic function, help resolve the diagnostic difficulty in most cases. As prolonged syncope can result in reflex anoxic seizures, a history of 'limb twitching' in the 'funny turn' should not lead to the automatic diagnosis of fits and prescription of inappropriate anticonvulsant therapy. In frail patients with late stage disease orthostatic hypotension can become manifest on transfer from bed to commode or wheelchair even in the seated position. Orthostatic hypotension should initially be treated by simple measures. Raising of the head of the bed at night can help early morning problems, as can drinking strong coffee before rising. Elasticated garments should compress the lower abdomen to be of any value and are rarely practicable. The patient and carer need to be told about the importance of making changes in posture slowly, and the times of greatest risk of postural syncope, such as getting out of bed at night or in the morning and standing up after meals. In reality patients have usually come to such realisations on their own.

Critical review of all prescribed medications can suffice to control symptoms. If this fails to control symptoms a change in antiparkinsonian drug therapy may be necessary, particularly the withdrawal of selegiline and reduction of dopamine agonist drugs. In frail patients on monotherapy with levodopa, reduction of this drug may cause increasing parkinsonism and immobility. In this situation the use of specific drugs to combat orthostatic hypotension such as fludrocortisone (0.1 mg to 1 mg per day) and nonsteroidal anti-inflammatory drugs such as flurbiprofen may be necessary. Most elderly patients with orthostatic hypotension can be managed without resorting to the use of specific drugs.

Bladder symptoms

Symptoms of urge, urge incontinence, frequency and distressing nocturia are common in late stage and longstanding PD. These problems result from bladder detrusor muscle hyperreflexia coupled with abnormalities of the external urethral sphincter. There is still uncertainty about how often urinary dysfunction reflects a specific PD related urinary dysfunction as opposed to the effects of aging on the bladder and external sphincter (Gray et al. 1995). The clinical picture in male patients is often complicated by additional obstructive symptoms suggestive of prostatism. Indeed, many patients may have previously undergone prostatic surgery, which has usually resulted in worsening of urinary symptoms. Urodynamic studies do not support the existence of specific abnormalities in PD and are rarely useful in directing treatment (Khan et al. 1989). An exception to this is in patients referred with prostatism when the demonstration of external sphincter abnormalities should preclude surgery. It is unclear how documented urinary problems respond to antiparkinsonian drug therapy. In most elderly patients bladder dysfunction does not respond predictably to antiparkinsonian drug treatment (Fitzmaurice et al. 1985), though some recent work published only in abstract form suggests that the dopamine agonist pergolide may decrease detrusor instability due to a D1 receptor agonist action. Voiding difficulty in the 'off' state can improve after a subcutaneous apomorphine injection by relaxing the striated urethral sphincter (Christmas et al. 1988, but see Gray et al. 1995).

Urological examination of the patient is necessary before embarking on treatment and this should include a rectal examination, a urinary flow rate and a bladder ultrasound scan to determine residual volume. A bladder specimen of urine by the use of disposable 'lofric' catheter should be obtained for culture. In the absence of a significant residual volume, oxybutynin can help nocturia and urge due to an unstable bladder but at the risk of central and peripheral anticholinergic side effects. In some patients nocturia is so disruptive and tiring that this risk is justified. Desmopressin given intranasally at night may also benefit some patients though blood urea and electrolytes need to be measured. The guidance and support of a specialist nurse continence advisor can be an important part of the long-term management of this problem. Despite the frequency of urinary problems few patients require intermittent self catheterization or suprapubic indwelling urinary catheters.

Bowel symptoms

Constipation, a reduction in normal bowel movements for an individual, is very common in elderly patients with PD (Edwards et al. 1993, Byrne et al. 1994). Immobility, poor diet, drug therapy, poor pelvic floor contractions and autonomic dysfunction with delayed transit time all contribute to the problem of constipation.

Constipation needs to be addressed vigorously to avoid the development of faecal impaction. Loss of the gastrocolic reflex due to constipation may impair levodopa absorption by delaying gastric emptying. Exercise and a good fluid intake are important aspects of bowel maintenance although in most patients aperients will also be required. Osmotic laxatives, such as lactulose, can be effective in some patients, but stimulant laxatives, such as senna, are likely to be needed in most elderly patients. A combination of stool softener and stimulant such as co-danthramer can be particularly useful in elderly patients. Co-danthramer discolours the urine and in the presence of urinary incontinence can cause an irritative dermatitis. Polyethylene glycol, a novel laxative agent that hydrates the stool by osmotic effect, results in a more normal bowel action and has recently become available in the UK. Bulking the stool with fibre in elderly patients can easily provoke faecal incontinence. Cisapride may also be useful in managing constipation in some patients (Jost and Schimrigk 1993). Faecal impaction can occur in frail patients with late stage disease and can present with confusion, nausea and vomiting and overflow diarrhoea. If rectal examination does not demonstrate impacted hard stool then a plain abdominal radiograph will show the level of impaction. A combination of oral laxatives, manual evacuation and phosphate enemas are usually required to resolve the situation. The importance of bowel maintenance in late stage PD needs to be emphasized to the patient, nursing home staff, community nurses and the family.

Speech and swallowing difficulties in PD

With disease progression problems with speech and swallowing soon become apparent in elderly patients (Stroudley and Walsh 1991, Edwards et al. 1993, 1994, Byrne et al. 1994, Bine et al. 1995, and see Chapter 14). Speech problems appear to develop more quickly in late onset PD and communication difficulties are a major source of disadvantage to elderly patients. Response to antiparkinsonian medication is disappointing but evidence exists to support the clinical effectiveness of speech therapy (Ramig et al. 1995). In elderly subjects akinesia and muscle rigidity commonly affect swallowing mechanisms, presenting first as pooling of saliva before progressing in time to cause embarrassing sialorrhoea and choking and coughing at meals. Likewise, response to drug treatment is disappointing, but drug therapy, particularly in previously undiagnosed patients, has been reported to improve swallowing problems (Fonda and Schwarz 1995, Thomas and Haigh 1995). Although causing distress and handicap it is rare for a patient with PD to become anarthric or to require percutaneous gastrostomy feeding. Specialist support is needed from speech and language therapists and from dieticians to minimize disability and handicap and to maintain nutritional status (Davies et al. 1994).

Balance and falls

Impaired balance and an increasing risk of falls is an early feature of late onset PD and of PD in older patients (Klawans and Topel 1974). The pathogenesis of impaired postural reflexes is unknown but may involve neurotransmitter systems other than dopamine as well as age related changes in the brain and peripheral nervous system. Falls are common in elderly patients with PD and such patients are at increased risk of fracture (Johnell et al. 1992). Bone mineral density appears to be lower in PD than that expected from the effects of age alone (Taggart and Crawford 1995). There is also a suggestion that femur fracture in PD is associated with a poorer outcome than in age matched subjects without PD (Gialanella et al. 1990). Falls are life threatening and also further severely restrict mobility due to loss of confidence. This sets in motion a spiral of immobility leading to muscle deconditioning, further immobility and increased risk of falls. Falls are a major cause of institutionalization in PD.

Falls due to akinesia should respond to increasing dopaminergic drug therapy and likewise falls due to drug-induced involuntary movements can be helped by reducing antiparkinsonian drugs. More general gait and balance deterioration is worsened rather than improved by increasing medication because of drug-induced exacerbation of cognitive impairment and drowsiness. Freezing can also result in falls and although noradrenergic drugs have been claimed to reduce freezing episodes in experimental trials no drug therapy has been found to be generally effective.

The best approach is to review drug prescriptions critically and to use a general preventive strategy (Tinetti et al. 1994) coupled with exercise and physiotherapy, (Campbell et al. 1997). Problems with vision and foot care that can be remedied should be urgently addressed.

Sleep disturbances

Most elderly patients with PD complain of disturbed nights though only around a third complain of poor quality of sleep (Lees et al. 1988). In several instances careful questioning can reveal the cause to be motor problems associated with PD (difficulty turning over in bed, painful leg cramps, dystonia, restless legs, leg jerks), more general musculoskeletal problems (back pain), nocturia, vivid dreams, visual hallucinations and mental restlessness or depression. Some of these problems are clearly due to PD and may respond to dopaminergic treatment last thing at night (controlled-release levodopa in the form of Sinemet CR or a dopamine agonist such as pergolide) or antidepressant therapy. Other symptoms such as vivid dreams, dyskinesia and hallucinations will require a reduction in dopaminergic drug treatment later in the day. Hypnotics are best avoided but the use of short acting hypnotics used every few days, or at most in weekly cycles separated by a fortnight, may be justified. In reality at least a third of elderly patients will have already been taking prescribed hypnotic drugs when first assessed and have developed dependency on them to sleep, albeit poorly.

There is increasing evidence to suggest that sleep abnormalities are common in treated PD patients and the term 'sleep fragmentation' has been used to describe this (Nausieda et al. 1984). These abnormalities are in excess of those found simply due to age alone. There is a close association between rapid eye movement sleep (REM sleep) abnormalities in PD, vivid dreams and the presence of dopaminergic drug related hallucinations (Comella et al. 1993). Although polysomnographic sleep measures may be abnormal in untreated PD patients, significant REM abnormalities appear to be related to duration of disease and length of exposure to dopaminergic drug therapy. Comella et al. (1993) found that half of the patients in their study had evidence of REM behaviour disorder. In REM behaviour disorder instead of atonia there is purposeful movement of the limbs and vocalization in REM sleep. This can even amount to sleep violence, as has been reported in a recent study of REM sleep behaviour disorder in which 15% of 61 patients with PD were reported by their caregivers as having kicked and punched the caregiver while asleep (C. Comella, unpublished observations).

Sexual dysfunction

Erectile problems and impotence has been reported by 60% of male patients with PD (Brown et al. 1990). This study took place in a small number of younger patients (mean age 52 years). Sexual dysfunction in older patients has not undergone detailed study. Although motor problems due to PD and autonomic dysfunction may play a small part, it seems likely that the bulk of sexual difficulty expressed by patients and partners is due to psychological factors and stress. Elderly patients are often not approached about sexual problems because of fear of offending a senior citizen, embarrassment on the part of the health care professional or an unjustified assumption that this is not a relevant area for assessment. Enquiries into sexual difficulties in elderly subjects need careful and sensitive handling. Elderly patients are often denied the privacy that such enquiries demand in their encounters with health and social services. An assessment of how important such sexual problems are to the patient and partner is vital to further management. Drug-induced sexual dysfunction should not be overlooked. Commonly prescribed drugs causing this problem are most antidepressant drugs and beta-blockers. After discussion, some patients and their partners will need referral for specialist urological advice.

Palliative care

In late stage disease the time will come when it is evident that a terminal phase of the disease is approaching, as frailty and dependency increase. Often patients will be in nursing homes, particularly if cognitive impairment is advanced. At this time good communication between hospital services, primary health care teams and the general practitioner is essential to optimize management. Treatment plans need to be established in the event of any sudden medical deterioration. These need to be understood and agreed by the patient, family and all the health care professionals involved. Antiparkinsonian drug treatment will need to be reduced if side effects, such as confusion, outweigh any obvious benefit in the patient confined to bed and needing all nursing care. Levodopa can be administered via nasogastric tube in terminal care to control severe rigidity and tremor. Active treatment of bladder, bowel, respiratory and painful symptoms are usually required to relieve distress and suffering.

Parkinsonism not due to PD

The differential diagnosis of parkinsonism has already been discussed (see Chapter 2). The commonest cause of parkinsonism in this group is drug-induced (Gershanik 1994 and see Chapter 4). Excluding long standing prescription of neuroleptic drugs for psychiatric illness, drug-induced parkinsonism (DIP) is most often caused by prochlorperazine prescribed for dizziness and metclopramide for gastrointestinal symptoms. A proportion of elderly patients with presumed DIP will, despite stopping the offending drug, still show signs of parkinsonism and progress to PD.

With the exception of DIP no specific treatment exists for these conditions. Some patients with confirmed multiple system atrophy and progressive nuclear palsy do appear to have responded to levodopa, at least over the initial course of the illness (Hughes et al. 1992). Given this finding and the known difficulties in accurate diagnosis, it would seem reasonable that a trial of levodopa therapy should be undertaken in most cases of parkinsonism even though the presence of PD is thought to be unlikely. In the absence of benefit treatment can be withdrawn. Levodopa is often poorly tolerated by patients with parkinsonism due to multisystem degenerations. Nonpharmacological approaches are the mainstay of treatment and patients in this group need regular assessment, therapy and support.

The specific difficulties faced by elderly patients with parkinsonism are effectively the same as those discussed above, though are usually more severe and progress more rapidly. Parkinsonism due to multisystem degenerations (multiple system atrophy, progressive supranuclear palsy) in elderly subjects is usually a very unpleasant and rapidly progressive disease lasting on average six years from first symptoms. In progressive supranuclear palsy (Litvan et al. 1996) falls and balance problems were the presenting feature in 63% of patients. Falls seemed particularly common in older patients at onset of symptoms. Complaints of disturbed vision are frequently reported due to the characteristic impairment of the voluntary control of eye movements. In this disease there is early involvement of speech and swallowing. Early signs of memory loss and frontal lobe impairment are common. In multiple system atrophy the clinical picture can be very varied, though severe dysarthria, dysphonia, respiratory stridor and autonomic dysfunction is typical of the striato nigral variant (Quinn 1989).

Rehabilitative principles are similar to those used in the management of PD but, in multisystem degenerations, the clinical situation reaches the stage of palliation much more quickly than in PD. Depression needs to be detected and treated, although depression in multisystem degenerations has received little attention (but see Pilo et al. 1996). Patients with parkinsonism due to multisystem degenerative disease are much more likely than patients with PD to be wheelchair bound and to require additional support with gastrostomy feeding, tracheostomy and suprapubic catheterization. Before embarking on life sustaining measures in diseases such as MSA and PSP, careful ethical consideration needs to be given to the implications of such a course of action. Detailed discussion with the patient and carer must take place before a medical decision can be reached and the patient's consent is needed for life sustaining measures to be undertaken or to be withheld. Support for the patient and carer is needed throughout the course of the illness.

Elderly patients with gait disorders due to vascular disease (see Chapter 6) are difficult to treat effectively. Most patients should receive a trial of levodopa, although the drug will not help if the diagnosis is correct. Attempts to retrain gait by treadmill walking are undergoing evaluation. The blood pressure of patients on antihypertensive medication should be carefully monitored to avoid over and under treatment. Antiplatelet drugs are routinely prescribed but are unlikely to be helpful in preventing further gait deterioration, although giving modest protection against vascular events.

Apomorphine treatment in elderly patients with PD

In the UK the dopamine agonist apomorphine has been licensed for the treatment of PD since 1993 and is also widely available in Europe. Neither apomorphine nor domperidone is currently licensed for use in the US, but may be obtained for individual patients.

Apomorphine was first reported to improve the motor symptoms of PD in 1951 (Schwab et al. 1951), but oral administration was associated with uraemia (Cotzias et al. 1970). It was not until the parenteral administration of apomorphine was adopted, coupled with the use of domperidone to reduce the peripheral dopaminergic effects of nausea, vomiting and postural hypotension (Corsini et al. 1979) that apomorphine became a clinically useful drug with which to treat PD (Hardie et al. 1984). Currently apomorphine is administered subcutaneously by intermittent injection (a preloaded adjustable dose pen system for self injection is now available in the UK) or by continuous waking day subcutaneous infusion via a syringe driver system (Stibe et al. 1988). The benefit from apomorphine is maintained over five years' follow-up (Hughes et al. 1993). The major advantage of apomorphine is that, given by intermittent subcutaneous injection, it can rapidly turn a patient back to the 'on' state from an 'off' state that is refractory to oral medication. In addition to open studies, the reduction in 'off' time has been demonstrated in two recent double-blind placebo-controlled studies (van Laar et al. 1993, Ostergaard et al. 1995). Open studies have also reported the ability of continuous infusion of apomorphine to reduce total daily 'off' time (Hughes et al. 1993). The mean age of patients in all these studies has been around 60 years. Like levodopa, apomorphine stimulates both D1 and D2 receptors and the magnitude, though not the duration, of the motor response in PD to these two drugs appears to be very similar (Kempster et al. 1990, Rodriguez et al. 1994). Subcutaneous apomorphine has a rapid onset of action (usually under 20 minutes), which lasts for 20–40 minutes. Patients with 'off' periods lasting longer than this are likely to require continuous infusion therapy. Intermittent injection of apomorphine is usually an adjunctive therapy to levodopa and other oral dopaminergic drugs, though in patients on continuous infusion oral levodopa therapy can be considerably reduced.

Apomorphine is clearly the most potent of all the dopamine agonist drugs and also appears to be less likely than other agonist drugs to cause neuropsychiatric side effects (Ellis et al. 1997) and drug-induced dyskinesia. Continuous apomorphine infusion also appears to cause much less dyskinesia than oral levodopa therapy (Colzi et al. 1997). However, in clinical practice long-term administration of apomorphine is associated with increasing 'on period' dyskinesia (Hughes et al. 1993), which may be attributable to larger coprescribed doses of levodopa in late stage disease.

Despite evidence of clinical effectiveness, apomorphine in the UK still appears to be underused, possibly reflecting the expense of the drug and the need for parenteral administration (Chaudhuri and Clough 1998). This is likely to be particularly true for elderly patients with PD in whom the efficacy and tolerability of apomorphine has not been studied. Criteria for the selection of patients for apomorphine therapy are shown in Table 3.4. Sadly, the majority of patients with late onset PD, and many elderly patients with late stage disease will not meet the suggested criteria for apomorphine use. A combination of factors is usually responsible, including: a variable or poor levodopa response, the absence of identified 'off' periods, significant cognitive impairment/dementia, general physical frailty, concurrent medical disease, and the presence of disabling symptoms such as postural

Table 3.4 Suggested criteria for the selection of elderly patients for apomorphine

- a good response to levodopa that is not maintained by oral therapy throughout the day
- clearly identifiable 'off' motor periods in relation to medication
- 'off' period dystonia and restless legs
- distressing nonmotor 'off' symptoms such as anxiety, panic, breathlessness, abdominal pain, urinary retention
- severe and disabling levodopa-induced dyskinesia
- absence of significant cognitive impairment/dementia
- absence of disabling symptoms such as postural instability and dysarthria that do not respond to dopaminergic drug therapy
- absence of concurrent specific disabling medical disease and general frailty
- ability of the patient, carer or health care support in the community to administer the drug by injection
- availability of resources to fund the drug/administration system

instability and dysarthria that do not respond to dopaminergic drugs. Elderly patients with psychosis clearly related to dopaminergic therapy may benefit from apomorphine as this will allow a reduction to be made in the daily levodopa dose (Ellis et al. 1997).

Suitable elderly patients will need an apomorphine challenge test to establish the effective dose of apomorphine and the tolerability of this treatment. Despite pretreatment with domperidone for three days prior to the test, significant postural hypotension can still occur in frail subjects and preclude the regular use of apomorphine. Elderly patients without a carer may be unable to self administer apomorphine, even with the new pen delivery system, particularly if 'off' periods occur suddenly with little warning. Some elderly patients may have difficulty recognizing when their oral medication is beginning to fail, and again, may rely on a carer to identify this situation. Frail elderly patients may prefer the option of continuous waking day infusion to repeated injections of apomorphine. Clinical impression suggests that apomorphine confers considerable benefit in terms of improved quality of life, though this has not been formally studied. The PD nurse specialist, recently developed in the UK, appears to have an important role in initiating, establishing and monitoring apomorphine therapy.

Apomorphine can also be useful in other situations such as the preoperative management and postoperative rehabilitation in elderly patients with PD. An apomorphine challenge test can also be useful in late stage PD to demonstrate the continuing presence of dopaminergic responsiveness. This can encourage the physician and patient to strive for improved disease control using oral drug therapy and can confirm the diagnosis of PD.

The long-term use of apomorphine results in the development of nodules at the injection site in nearly all patients. These nodules can become painful, and can break down into ulcers with secondary infection. This is usually only seen in patients on continuous infusions, but can occur with intermittent injection regimes. Rotation of injection sites, massage of the skin before and after injection, reduction of apomorphine dose and good injection technique can reduce the incidence of complicated nodules. It is recommended that hepatic and renal function should be monitored periodically. As with levodopa, autoimmune haemolytic anaemia has been reported as a rare occurrence with the long-term use of apomorphine. Apomorphine, although expensive, is effective in maintaining independence in elderly patients with PD and can prevent institutionalization (with considerably greater financial implications) and should not be denied to patients with PD based on age alone. The proportion of elderly patients with late onset and late stage PD that would benefit from and tolerate apomorphine is unknown. In our own specialist clinic based population over the age of 70 years, around 5% are currently prescribed apomorphine.

REFERENCES

Agid Y, Javoy-Agid F, Ruberg M (1987) Biochemistry of neurotransmitters in Parkinson's disease. In: *Movement Disorders 2*, eds. Marsden CD, Fahn S, pp. 166–230. London: Butterworths.

Alexander GE, Crutcher MD (1990) Functional architecture of basal ganglia circuits: neural substrates of parallel processing. *Trends in Neurosciences* 13, 266–71.

Alexander GE, DeLong MR, Strick PL (1986) Parallel organization of functionally segregated circuits linking basal ganglia and cortex. *Annual Review of Neuroscience*, 9, 357–81.

American Psychiatric Association (1994). *Diagnostic and Statistical Manual of Mental Disorders*, 4th ed. Washington DC: American Psychiatric Association.

Andersen J, Aabro E, Gulmann N, Hjelmsted A, Pedersen HE (1980) Anti depressive treatment in Parkinson's disease. A controlled trial of the effect of nortriptyline in patients with Parkinson's disease treated with L-dopa. *Acta Neurologica Scandinavica*, 62, 210–19.

Ansorge O, Lees AJ, Daniel SE (1997) Update on the accuracy of clinical diagnosis of idiopathic Parkinson's disease. *Movement Disorders*, 12, Suppl. 1, S96.

Balldin J, Granerus AK, Lindstedt G, Modigh K, Walinder J (1981) Predictors for improvement after electroconvulsive therapy in parkinsonian patients with on–off symptoms. *Journal of Neural Transmission*, 52, 199–211.

Bennett DA, Beckett LA, Murray AM, Shannon KM, Goetz CG, Pilgrim DM, Evans DA (1996) Prevalence of parkinsonian signs and associated mortality in a community population of older people. *New England Journal of Medicine*, 334, 71–6.

Bernheimer H, Birkmayer W, Hornykiewicz O, Jellinger K, Seitelberger F (1973) Brain dopamine and the syndromes of Parkinson and Huntington – clinical, morphological and neurochemical correlations. *Journal of the Neurological Sciences*, 20, 415–55.

Berrios GE, Campbell C, Politynska (1995) Autonomic failure, depression and anxiety in Parkinson's disease. *British Journal of Psychiatry*, 166, 789–92.

Biggins CA, Boyd JL, Harrop FM, Madeley P, Mindham RHS, Randall JI, Spokes EGS (1992) A controlled, longitudinal study of dementia in Parkinson's disease. *Journal of Neurology, Neurosurgery, and Psychiatry*, 55, 566–71.

Bine JE, Frank EM, McDade HL (1995) Dysphagia and dementia in subjects with Parkinson's disease. *Dysphagia*, 10, 160–4.

Bowling A, Windsor J (1997) Discriminative power of the health status questionnaire 12 in relation to age, sex, and longstanding illness: findings from a survey of households in Great Britain. *Journal of Epidemiology and Community Health*, 51, 564–73

Brazier JE, Jones NMB, O'Cathain A, Thomas KJ, Usherwood T, Westlake L (1992) Validating the SF-36 health survey questionnaire: a new outcome measure for primary care. *British Medical Journal*, 305, 160–4.

Brown RG, Jahanshahi M, Quinn N, Marsden CD (1990) Sexual function in patients with Parkinson's disease and their partners. *Journal of Neurology, Neurosurgery, and Psychiatry*, 53, 480–6.

Brown RG, MacCarthy B (1990) Psychiatric morbidity in patients with Parkinson's disease. *Psychological Medicine*, 20, 77–87.

Brown RG, MacCarthy B, Gothan A-M, Der GJ, Marsden CD (1988) Depression and disability in Parkinson's disease: a follow-up of 132 cases. *Psychological Medicine*, 18, 49–55.

Brown RG, Marsden CD (1990) Cognitive function in Parkinson's disease: from description to theory. *Trends in Neurosciences*, 13, 1, 21–9.

Byrne EJ, Lennox G, Lowe J, Godwin-Austen RB (1989) Diffuse Lewy-body disease: clinical features in 15 cases. *Journal of Neurology, Neurosurgery, and Psychiatry*, 52, 709–17.

Byrne KG, Pfeiffer R, Quigley EMM (1994) Gastrointestinal dysfunction in Parkinson's disease. *Journal of Clinical Gastroenterology*, 19, 1, 11–16.

Calder SA, Ebmeier KP, Stewart L, Crawford JR, Besson JAO (1991) The prediction of stress in carers: The role of behaviour, reported self-care and dementia in patients with idiopathic Parkinson's disease. *International Journal of Geriatric Psychiatry*, 6, 737–42.

Campbell AJ, Robertson MC, Gardner MM, Norton RN, Tilyard MW, Buchner DM (1997) Randomised controlled trial of a general practice programme of home based exercise to prevent falls in elderly women. *British Medical Journal*, 315, 1065–9.

Cantello R, Gilli M, Riccio A, Bergamasco B (1986) Mood changes associated with 'end of dose deterioration' in Parkinson's disease: a controlled study. *Journal of Neurology, Neurosurgery, and Psychiatry*, 49, 1182–90.

Celesia GG, Wanamaker WM (1972) Psychiatric disturbances in Parkinson's disease. *Diseases of the Nervous System*, 33, 577–83.

Chaudhuri KR, Clough C (1998) Subcutaneous apomorphine in Parkinson's disease – effective yet underused. *British Medical Journal*, 316, 641.

Christmas TJ, Chapple CR, Lees AJ, Kempster PA, Frankel JP, Stern GM (1988) Role of subcutaneous apomorphine in parkinsonian voiding dysfunction. *Lancet*, 2, 1451–3.

Churchyard A, Mathias CJ, Boonkongchuen P, Lees AJ (1997) Autonomic effects of selegiline: possible cardiovascular toxicity in Parkinson's disease. *Journal of Neurology, Neurosurgery, and Psychiatry*, 63, 228–34.

Collin C, Wade DT, Davis S, Horne V (1988) The Barthel ADL index: a reliability study. *International Disability Studies*, 10, 61–3.

Colzi A, Turner K, Lees AJ (1997) Continuous waking-day subcutaneous apomorphine therapy in the treatment of levodopa-induced dyskinesias and 'on–off' phenomena in Parkinson's disease. *Movement Disorders*, 12, Suppl. 1, 428.

Comella CL, Tanner CM, Ristanovic RK (1993) Polysomnographic sleep measures in Parkinson's disease patients with treatment-induced hallucinations. *Annals of Neurology*, 34, 710–14.

Cooper JA, Sagar HJ, Jordan N (1991) Cognitive impairment in early untreated Parkinson's disease. *Brain*, 114, 2095–122.

Coppen A, Metcalfe M, Carrol JD, Morris JGL (1972) Levodopa and 1-tryptophan therapy in parkinsonism. Lancet, 1, 654–8.

Corsini GU, Del Zompo M, Gessa GL, Mangoni A (1979) Therapeutic efficacy of apomorphine combined with an extracerebral inhibitor of dopamine receptors in Parkinson's disease. *Lancet*, 1, 954–6.

Cotzias GC, Papavasiliou PS, Fehling C, Kaufman B, Mena I (1970) Similarities between neuro-logic effects of L-dopa and apomorphine. *New England Journal of Medicine*, 282, 31–3.

Cummings JL (1988) Intellectual impairment in Parkinson's disease: Clinical, pathologic, and biochemical correlates. *Journal of Geriatric Psychiatry and Neurology*, 1, 24–36.

Cummings JL (1992) Depression and Parkinson's disease: A review. *American Journal of Psychiatry*, 149, 4, 443–54.

Cummings JL, Benson DF (1983) *Dementia: A Clinical Approach.* Boston: Butterworths.

D'Amato RJ, Zweig RM, Whitehouse PJ, Wenk GL, Singer HS, Mayeux R, Price DL, Snyder SH (1987) Aminergic systems in Alzheimer's disease and Parkinson's disease. *Annals of Neurology*, 22, 229–36.

D'Ath P, Katona P, Mullan E, Evans S, Katona C (1994) Screening, detection and management of depression in elderly primary care attenders. 1: The acceptability and performance of the 15 item Geriatric Depression Scale (GDS-15) and the development of short versions. *Family Practice*, 11, 3, 260–5.

Danielczyk W (1992) Mental disorders in Parkinson's disease. *Journal of Neural Transmission*, Suppl. 38, 115–27.

Davies KN, King D, Davies H (1994) A study of the nutritional status of elderly patients with Parkinson's disease. *Age and Ageing*, 23, 142–5.

de Boer AG, Wijker W, Speelman JD, de Haes JC (1996) Quality of life in patients with Parkinson's disease: development of a questionnaire. *Journal of Neurology, Neurosurgery, and Psychiatry*, 61, 70–4.

DeLong MR (1990) Primate models of movement disorders of basal ganglia origin. *Trends in Neurosciences*, 13, 281–5.

Delwaide PJ, Gonce M (1998) Pathophysiology of Parkinson's signs. In: *Parkinson's Disease and Movement Disorders*, eds. Jankovic J, Tolosa E, pp. 159–76. Baltimore: Williams and Wilkins.

Diamond SG, Markham CH, Hoehn MM, McDowell FH, Muenter MD (1989) Effect of age at onset on progression and mortality in Parkinson's disease. *Neurology*, 39, 1187–90.

Dooneief G, Mirabello E, Bell K, Marder K, Stern Y, Mayeux R (1992) An estimate of the inci-dence of depression in idiopathic Parkinson's disease. *Archives of Neurology*, 49, 305–7.

Ebmeier KP, Calder SA, Crawford JR, Stewart L, Besson JAO, Mutch WJ (1990) Clinical features predicting dementia in idiopathic Parkinson's disease: A follow-up study. *Neurology*, 40, 1222–4.

Edwards LL, Quigley EMM, Harned RK, Hofman R, Pfeiffer RF (1994) Characterization of swallowing and defecation in Parkinson's disease. *American Journal of Gastroenterology*, 89, 1, 15–25.

Edwards LL, Quigley EMM, Hofman R, Pfeiffer RF (1993) Gastrointestinal symptoms in Parkinson disease: 18 month follow-up study. *Movement Disorders*, 8, 1, 83–6.

Elble RJ (1998) Motor control and movement disorders. In: *Parkinson's Disease and Movement Disorders*, eds. Jankovic J, Tolosa E, pp. 15–46. Baltimore: Williams and Wilkins.

Ellis CM, Lemmens G, Parkes JD, Abbott RJ, Pye IF, Leigh PN, Chaudhuri KR (1997) Use of apomorphine in parkinsonian patients with neuropsychiatric complications to oral treatment. *Parkinsonism and Related Disorders*, 3, 103–7.

Factor SA, Molho ES, Podskalny GD, Brown D (1995) Parkinson's disease drug-induced psychiatric states. *Advances in Neurology*, 65, 115–38.

Fahn S, Elton RL, and Members of the UPDRS Development Committee (1987) Unified Parkinson's disease rating scale. In: *Recent Developments in Parkinson's Disease, Vol. 2*, eds. Fahn S, Marsden CD, Calne DB, Goldstein M, Florham Park, NJ, pp. 153–64. Macmillan Health Care Information.

Fall PA, Ekman R, Granerus AK, Thorell LH, Walinder J (1995) ECT in Parkinson's disease. Changes in motor symptoms, monoamine metabolites and neuropeptides. *Journal of Neural Transmission*, 10, 129–40.

Fitzmaurice H, Fowler CJ, Rickards D, Kirby RS, Quinn NP, Marsden CD, Milroy EJ, Turner-Warwick RT (1985) Micturition disturbance in Parkinson's disease. *British Journal of Urology*, 57, 652–6.

Fleminger S (1991) Left-sided Parkinson's disease is associated with greater anxiety and depression. *Psychological Medicine*, 21, 629–38.

Folstein MF, Folstein SE, McHugh PR (1975) Mini mental state: a practical guide for grading the mental state of patients for the clinician. *Journal of Psychiatric Research*, 12, 189–98.

Fonda D, Schwarz J (1995) Parkinsonian medication one hour before meals improves symptomatic swallowing: A case study. *Dysphagia*, 10, 165–6.

Forno LS (1996) Neuropathology of Parkinson's disease. *Journal of Neuropathology and Experimental Neurology*, 55, 3, 259–72.

Friedman A (1994) Old-onset Parkinson's disease compared with young-onset disease: clinical differences and similarities. *Acta Neurologica Scandinavica*, 89, 258–61.

Gershanik OS (1994) Drug-induced parkinsonism in the aged: Recognition and prevention. *Drugs and Aging*, 5, 2, 127–32.

Gialanella B, Mattioli F, D'Alessandro G, Bonomelli, Luisa A (1990) Prognosis of femur fractures in parkinsonian patients. In: *Parkinson's Disease and Extrapyramidal Disorders*, proceedings of the European Conference on Parkinson's Disease and Pyramidal Disorders, Rome, eds. Agnoli A, Fabbrini G, Stocchi F, pp. 591–4. London: J Libbey.

Gibb WRG, Esiri MM, Lees AJ (1985) Clinical and pathological features of diffuse cortical Lewy-body disease (Lewy-body dementia). *Brain*, 110, 1131–53.

Gibb WRG, Lees AJ (1988) A comparison of clinical and pathological features of young and old-onset Parkinson's disease. *Neurology*, 38, 1402–6.

Gibb WRG, Lees AJ (1991) Anatomy, pigmentation, ventral and dorsal subpopulations of the substantia nigra, and differential cell death in Parkinson's disease. *Journal of Neurology, Neurosurgery, and Psychiatry*, 54, 5, 388–96.

Gibb WRG, Scott T, Lees AJ (1991) Neuronal inclusions of Parkinson's disease. *Movement Disorders*, 6, 2–11.

Goetz CG, Tanner CM, Klawans HL (1984) Buproprion in Parkinson's disease. *Neurology*, 34, 1092–4.

Goetz CG, Tanner CM, Stebbins GT, Buchman AS (1988) Risk factors for progression in Parkinson's disease. *Neurology*, 38, 1841–4.

Gómez-Tortosa E, Ingraham AO, Irizarry MC, Hyman BT (1998) Dementia with Lewy bodies. *Journal of the American Geriatrics Society*, 46, 1449–58.

Gotham A-M, Brown RG, Marsden CD (1986) Depression in Parkinson's disease: a quantitative and qualitative analysis. *Journal of Neurology, Neurosurgery, and Psychiatry*, 49, 381–9.

Gray R, Stern G, Malone-Lee J (1995) Lower urinary tract dysfunction in Parkinson's disease: Changes relate to age and not disease. *Age and Ageing*, 24, 499–504.

Graybiel AM (1990) Neurotransmitters and neuromodulators in the basal ganglia. *Trends in Neurosciences*, 13, 244–54.

Gross M, Bannister R, Godwin-Austen R (1972) Orthostatic hypotension in Parkinson's disease. *Lancet*, 1, 4–18.

Haeske-Dewick HC (1995) Hallucinations in Parkinson's disease: Characteristics and associated clinical features. *International Journal of Geriatric Psychiatry*, 10, 487–95.

Hantz P, Caradoc-Davies G, Caradoc-Davies T, Weatherall M, Dixon G (1994) Depression in Parkinson's disease. *American Journal of Psychiatry*, 151, 7, 1010–14.

Hardie RJ, Lees AJ, Stern GM (1984) 'On–off' fluctuations in Parkinson's disease. A clinical and neuropharmacological study. *Brain*, 107, 487–96.

Hauser RA, Zesiewicz TA (1997) Sertraline for the treatment of depression in Parkinson's disease. *Movement Disorders*, 12, 5, 756–9.

Hindle JV, Meara RJ, Sharma JC, Medcalf P, Forsyth DR, Huggett IM, Cassidy TP, Morris J, Dunn A, Hobson JP (The Pergolide Study Group) (1998) Prescribing pergolide in the elderly – an open label study of pergolide in elderly patients with Parkinson's disease. *International Journal of Geriatric Psychopharmacology*, 1, 78–81.

Hobson JP, Meara RJ (1997) Is the SF-36 Health Survey Questionnaire suitable as a self report measure of the health status of older adults with Parkinson's disease. *Quality of Life Research*, 3, 6, 213–16.

Hobson P, Meara J (1998) Screening for 'cognitive impairment, no dementia' in older adults. *Journal of the American Geriatrics Society*, 46, 5, 659–60.

Hobson P, Meara J (1999) The detection of dementia and cognitive impairment in a community population of elderly Parkinson's disease subjects by use of the CAMCOG neuropsychological test. *Age and Ageing*, 28, 39–43.

Holcomb HH, Sternberg DE, Heninger GR (1983) Effects of electroconvulsive therapy on mood, parkinsonism, and tardive dyskinesia in a depressed patient: ECT and dopamine systems. *Biological Psychiatry*, 18, 865–73.

Holmes C, Cairns N, Lantos P, Mann A (1999) Validity of current clinical criteria for Alzheimer's disease, vascular dementia and dementia with Lewy bodies. *British Journal of Psychiatry*, 174, 45–50.

Hua S, Reich SG, Zirh AT, Perry V, Dougherty PM, Lenz FA (1998) The role of the thalamus and basal ganglia in parkinsonian tremor. *Movement Disorders*, 13, Suppl. 3, 40–2.

Huber SJ, Freidenberg DL, Paulson GW, Shuttleworth EC, Christy JA (1990) The pattern of depressive symptoms varies with progression of Parkinson's disease. *Journal of Neurology, Neurosurgery, and Psychiatry*, 53, 275–8.

Huber SJ, Paulson GW, Shuttleworth EC (1988) Relationship of motor symptoms, intellectual impairment, and depression in Parkinson's disease. *Journal of Neurology, Neurosurgery, and Psychiatry*, 51, 855–8.

Hughes AJ, Bishop S, Kleedorfer B, Turjanski, Fernadez A, Lees AJ, Stern GM (1993) Subcutaneous apomorphine in Parkinson's disease: Response to chronic administration for up to five years. *Movement Disorders*, 8, 2, 165–70.

Hughes AJ, Daniel SE, Kilford L, Lees AJ (1992) Accuracy of clinical diagnosis of idiopathic Parkinson's disease: a clinicopathological study of 100 cases. *Journal of Neurology, Neurosurgery, and Psychiatry*, 55, 181–4.

Hughes AJ, Daniel SE, Blankson S, Lees AJ (1993) A clinicopathological study of 100 cases of Parkinson's disease. *Archives of Neurology*, 50, 140–8.

Jackson R, Baldwin B (1993) Detecting depression in elderly medically ill patients: the use of the Geriatric Depression Scale compared with medical and nursing observations. *Age and Ageing*, 22, 349–53.

Jacobs DM, Marder K, Cote LJ, Sano M, Stern Y, Mayeux R (1995) Neuropsychological characteristics of preclinical dementia in Parkinson's disease. *Neurology*, 45, 1691–6.

Jankovic J, McDermott M, Carter J, Gauthier S, Goetz C, Golbe L, Huber S, Koller W, Olanow C, Shoulson I, Stern M, Tanner C, Weiner W and the Parkinson Study Group (1990) Variable expression of Parkinson's disease: A base-line analysis of the DATATOP cohort. *Neurology*, 40, 1529–34.

Jellinger K (1986) Overview of morphological changes in Parkinson's disease. *Advances in Neurology*, 45, 1–18.

Jenkinson C, Peto V, Fitzpatrick R, Greenhall R, Hyman N (1995) Self-reported functioning and well-being in patients with Parkinson's disease: Comparison of the short form health survey (SF-36) and the Parkinson's disease questionnaire (PDQ-39). *Age and Ageing*, 24, 505–9.

Jiminez-Jiminez FJ, Tejeiro J, Martinez-Junquera G, Cabrera-Valdivia F, Alarcon J, Garicia-Albea E (1994) Parkinsonism exacerbated by paroxetine. *Neurology*, 44, 2406.

Johnell O, Melton J, Atkinson EJ, O'Fallon WM, Kurland LT (1992) Fracture risk in patients with parkinsonism: A population-based study in Olmsted County, Minnesota. *Age and Ageing*, 21, 32–8.

Jost WH, Schimrigk K (1993) Cisapride treatment of constipation in Parkinson's disease. *Movement Disorders*, 8, 339–43.

Kahn N, Freeman A, Juncos JL, Manning D, Watts RL (1991) Clozapine is beneficial for psychosis in Parkinson's disease. *Neurology*, 41, 1699–1700.

Kempster PA, Frankel JP, Stern GM, Lees AJ (1990) Comparison of motor response to apomorphine and levodopa in Parkinson's disease. *Journal of Neurology, Neurosurgery, and Psychiatry*, 53, 1004–7.

Khan Z, Starer P, Bhola A (1989) Urinary incontinence in female Parkinson's disease patients: pitfalls of diagnosis. *Urology*, 33, 486–9.

Klawans HL, Topel JL (1974) Parkinsonism as a falling sickness. *Journal of the American Medical Association*, 230, 11, 1555–7.

Kosaka K (1978) Lewy bodies in cerebral cortex. Report of three cases. *Acta Neuropathologica*, 42, 127–34.

Kostic VS, Djuricic BM, Covickovic-Sternic N, Bumbasirevic L, Nikolic M, Mrsulja BB (1987) Depression and Parkinson's disease: possible role of serotonergic mechanisms. *Journal of Neurology*, 234, 94–6.

Kostic VS, Lecic D, Filipovic S, Sternic N (1993) Prolactin and cortisol responses to fenfluramine in depressed parkinsonians: diminished responsivity of central serotonergic function. Abstract. *European Congress on Mental Dysfunction in Parkinson's disease*, IV-8, 42.

Laitinen L (1969) Desipramine in treatment of Parkinson's disease. *Acta Neurologica Scandinavica*, 45, 109–13.

Lees AJ, Blackburn NA, Campbell VL (1988) The nighttime problems of Parkinson's disease. *Clinical Neuropharmacology*, 11, 6, 512–19.

Lesher EL, Berryhill JS (1994) Validation of the Geriatric Depression Scale – short form among inpatients. *Journal of Clinical Psychology*, 50, 2, 256–60.

Lieberman AN (1997) Point of view: Dementia in Parkinson's disease. *Parkinsonism and Related Disorders*, 3, 3, 151–8.

Limousin P, Pollak P, Benazzouz A, Hoffman D, Le Bas J-F, Broussolle E, Perret JE, Benabid A-L (1995) Effect on parkinsonian signs and symptoms of bilateral subthalamic nucleus stimulation. *Lancet*, 345, 91–5.

Litvan I, Mangone CA, Mckee A, Verny M, Parsa A, Jellinger K, D'Olhaberriague L, Chaudhuri KR, Pearce RKB (1996) Natural history of progressive supranuclear palsy (Steele–Richardson–Olszewski syndrome) and clinical predictors of survival: a clinicopathological study. *Journal of Neurology, Neurosurgery, and Psychiatry*, 61, 615–20.

Livingstone G, Hawkins A, Graham N, Blizard B, Mann A (1990) The Gospel Oak Study: prevalence rates of dementia, depression and activity limitation among elderly residents in inner London. *Psychological Medicine*, 20,137–46.

Lopes de Faria SR, Zanella MT, Andriolo A, Ribeiro AB, Chacra AR (1988) Peripheral dopaminergic blockade for the treatment of diabetic orthostatic hypotension. *Clinical Pharmacology and Therapeutics*, 44, 6, 670–4.

Madeley P, Biggins CA, Boyd JL, Mindham RHS, Spokes EGS (1992) Emotionalism in Parkinson's disease. *Irish Journal of Psychological Medicine*, 9, 24–5.

Madeley P, Biggins CA, Mindham RHS (1993) The psychiatry of Parkinson's disease. In: *Recent Advances in Clinical Psychiatry*, ed. Granville-Grossman K, pp. 63–77. London: Churchill Livingstone.

Mahieux F, Fenelon G, Flahault A, Manifacier M, Michelet D, Boller F (1998) Neuropsychological prediction of dementia in Parkinson's disease. *Journal of Neurology, Neurosurgery, and Psychiatry*, 64, 178–83.

Mann DMA, Snowden JS (1995) The topographic distribution of brain atrophy in cortical Lewy-body disease: comparison with Alzheimer's disease. *Acta Neuropathologica*, 89, 178–83.

Marder K, Tang MX, Cote L, Stern Y, Mayeux R (1995) The frequency and associated risk factors for dementia in patients with Parkinson's disease. *Archives of Neurology*, 52, 695–701.

Martin R, Manzanares R, Molto JM, Canet T, Ruiz C, Matías-Guiu J (1993) Cardiovascular reflexes in Parkinson disease. *Italian Journal of Neurological Sciences*, 14, 437–42.

Mayeux R, Chen J, Mirabello E, Marder K, Bell K, Dooneief G, Cote L, Stern Y (1990) An estimate of the incidence of dementia in idiopathic Parkinson's disease. *Neurology*, 40, 1513–17.

Mayeux R, Denaro J, Hemenegildo N, Marder K, Tang M, Cote LJ, Stern Y (1992) A population-based investigation of Parkinson's disease with and without dementia. *Archives of Neurology*, 49, 492–7.

Mayeux R, Stern Y, Cote L, Williams JBW (1984) Altered serotonin metabolism in depressed patients with Parkinson's disease. *Neurology*, 34, 642–6.

Mayeux R, Stern Y, Rosen J, Leventhal J (1981) Depression, intellectual impairment and Parkinson's disease. *Neurology*, 31, 645–50.

Mayeux R, Stern Y, Sano M, Williams JBW, Cote LJ (1988) The relationship of serotonin to depression in Parkinson's disease. *Movement Disorders*, 3, 3, 237–44.

McCance-Katz EF, Marek KL, Price LH (1992) Serotonergic dysfunction in depression associated with Parkinson's disease. *Neurology*, 42, 1813–14.

McKeith IG, Galasko D, Wilcock GK, Byrne EJ (1995) Lewy-body dementia – diagnosis and treatment. *British Journal of Psychiatry*, 167, 709–17.

McKeith IG, Perry RH, Fairbairn AF, Jabeen S, Perry EK (1992) Operational criteria for senile dementia of Lewy-body type (SDLT). *Psychological Medicine*, 22, 911–22.

McRae A (1998) Neurotransmitters and pharmacology of the basal ganglia. In: *Parkinson's Disease and Movement Disorders*, eds. Jankovic J, Tolosa E, pp. 47–66. Baltimore: Williams and Wilkins.

Meara RJ, Cody FWJ (1992) Relationship between electromyographic activity and clinically assessed rigidity studied at the wrist joint in Parkinson's disease. *Brain*, 115, 1167–80.

Meara RJ, Bhowmick BK, Hobson JP (1996) An open uncontrolled study of the use of sertraline in the treatment of depression in Parkinson's disease. *Journal of Serotonin Research*, 4, 243–9.

Meara RJ, Bisarya S, Hobson JP (1997) Screening in primary health care for undiagnosed tremor in an elderly population in Wales. *Journal of Epidemiology and Community Health*, 51, 574–5.

Meara RJ, Mitchelmore E, Hobson JP (1999) Use of the GDS-15 geriatric depression scale as a screening instrument for depressive symptomatology in patients with Parkinson's disease and their carers in the community. *Age and Ageing*, 28, 35–8.

Meltzer HY, Kennedy J, Dai J, Parsa M, Riley D (1995) Plasma clozapine levels and the treatment of L-dopa-induced psychosis in Parkinson's disease: A high potency effect of clozapine. *Neuropsychopharmacology*, 12, 39–45.

Menza MA, Sage J, Marshall E, Cody R, Duvoisin R (1990) Mood changes and 'on–off' phenomena in Parkinson's disease. *Movement Disorders*, 5, 2, 148–51.

Miller E, Berrios GE, Politynska BE (1996) Caring for someone with Parkinson's disease: Factors that contribute to distress. *International Journal of Geriatric Psychiatry*, 11, 263–8.

Montastruc JL, Chamontin B, Senard JM, Rascol A (1985) Domperidone in the management of orthostatic hypotension. *Clinical Neuropharmacology*, 8, 2, 191–2.

Nausieda PA, Glantz R, Weber S, Baum R, Klawans HL (1984) Psychiatric complications of lev-odopa therapy of Parkinson's disease. *Advances in Neurology*, 40, 271–7.

Nouri FM, Lincoln NB (1987) An extended activities of daily living scale for stroke patients. *Clinical Rehabilitation*, 1, 301–5.

Obeso JA, Guridi J, Obeso JA, DeLong M (1997) Surgery for Parkinson's disease. *Journal of Neurology, Neurosurgery, and Psychiatry*, 62, 2–8.

Okazaki H, Lipkin LE, Aronson SM (1961) Diffuse intracytoplasmic ganglionic inclusions (Lewy type) associated with progressive dementia and quadriparesis in flexion. *Journal of Neuropathology and Experimental Neurology*, 20, 237–44.

Ostergaard L, Werdelin L, Odin P, Lindvall O, Dupont E, Christensen PB, Boisen E, Jensen NB, Ingwersen SH, Schmiegelow M (1995) Pen injected apomorphine against off phenomena in late Parkinson's disease: a double-blind, placebo-controlled study. *Journal of Neurology, Neurosurgery, and Psychiatry*, 58, 681–7.

Peyser CE, Naimark D, Zuniga R, Jeste DV (1998) Psychoses in Parkinson's disease. *Seminars in Clinical Neuropsychiatry*, 3, 41–50.

Pilo L, Ring H, Quinn N, Trimble M (1996) Depression in multiple system atrophy and in idio-pathic Parkinson's disease: A pilot comparative study. *Biological Psychiatry*, 39, 803–7.

Pridmore S, Pollard C (1996) Electroconvulsive therapy in Parkinson's disease: 30 month follow-up. *Journal of Neurology, Neurosurgery, and Psychiatry*, 61, 693–700.

Quinn N (1989) Multiple system atrophy – the nature of the beast. *Journal of Neurology, Neurosurgery, and Psychiatry*, Special Supplement, 78–89.

Rajput AH, Rozdilsky B, Rajput A (1991) Accuracy of clinical diagnosis in parkinsonism – a pros-pective study. *Canadian Journal of Neurological Sciences*, 18, 275–8.

Rajput AH, Uitti RJ, Sudhakar S, Rozdilsky B (1989) Parkinsonism and neurofibrillary tangle pathology in pigmented nuclei. *Annals of Neurology*, 25, 602–66.

Ramig LO, Countryman S, Thompson LL, Horii Y (1995) Comparison of two forms of intensive speech treatment for Parkinson's disease. *Journal of Speech and Hearing Research*, 38, 1232–51.

Richard I, Kurlan R, Tanner C (1996) Serotonin syndrome and the combined use of deprenyl and an antidepressant in Parkinson's disease. *Neurology*, 46, A374.

Ring HA, Bench CJ, Trimble MR, Brooks DJ, Frackowiak RSJ, Dolan RJ (1994) Depression in Parkinson's disease – a positron emission study. *British Journal of Psychiatry*, 165, 333–9.

Rodriguez M, Lera G, Vaamonde A, Luquin MR, Obeso JA (1994) Motor response to apomor-phine and levodopa in asymmetric Parkinson's disease. *Journal of Neurology, Neurosurgery, and Psychiatry*, 57, 562–6.

Roth M, Tym E, Mountjoy CQ, Huppert FA, Hendrie H, Verma S, Goddard R (1986) CAMDEX: A standardized instrument for the diagnosis of mental disorder in the elderly with special ref-erence to elderly detection of dementia. *British Journal of Psychiatry*, 149, 698–709.

Rubenstein LZ, Stuck AE, Siu AL, Wieland D (1991) Impacts of geriatric evaluation and man-agement programs on defined outcomes: overview of the evidence. *Journal of the American Geriatrics Society*, 39, Suppl. 8–16.

Sandyk R, Awerbuch GI (1992) Dysautonomia in Parkinson's disease: Relationship to motor dis-ability. *International Journal of Neuroscience*, 64, 23–31.

Sano M, Stern Y, Williams J, Cote L, Rosenstein R, Mayeux R (1989) Coexisting dementia and depression in Parkinson's disease. *Archives of Neurology*, 46, 1284–6.

Saunders PA, Copeland JRM, Dewey ME, Gilmore C, Larkin BA, Phaterpekar H, Scott A (1993) The prevalence of dementia, depression and neurosis in later life: The Liverpool MRC-ALPHA study. *International Journal of Epidemiology*, 22, 5, 838–47.

Schneider LS, Chui HC, Severson JA, Sloane RB (1988) Decreased platelet binding in Parkinson's disease. *Biological Psychiatry*, 24, 348–51.

Schwab RS, Amador LV, Lettvin JY (1951) Apomorphine in Parkinson's disease. *Transcripts of the American Neurological Association*, 76, 251–3.

Senard JM, Rai S, Lapeyre-Mestre M, Brefel C, Rascol O, Rascol A, Montastruc JL (1997) Prevalence of orthostatic hypotension in Parkinson's disease. *Journal of Neurology, Neurosurgery, and Psychiatry*, 63, 584–9.

Starkstein SE, Berthier ML, Bolduc PL, Preziosi TJ, Robinson RG (1989) Depression in patients with early versus late onset of Parkinson's disease. *Neurology*, 39, 1441–5.

Starkstein SE, Bollduc PL, Mayberg HS, Preziosi TJ, Robinson RG (1992) Cognitive impairments and depression in idiopathic Parkinson's disease. *Archives of Neurology*, 49, 305–7.

Starkstein SE, Preziosi TJ, Bollduc PL, Robinson RG (1990) Depression in Parkinson's disease. *Journal of Nervous and Mental Disease*, 178, 27–31.

Starkstein SE, Sabe L, Petracca G, Chemerinski E, Kuzis G, Merello M, Leiguarda R (1996) Neuropsychological and psychiatric differences between Alzheimer's disease and Parkinson's disease with dementia. *Journal of Neurology, Neurosurgery, and Psychiatry*, 61, 381–7.

Stern Y, Marder K, Tang MX, Mayeux R (1993) Antecedent clinical features associated with dementia in Parkinson's disease. *Neurology*, 43, 1690–2.

Steur EN (1993) Increase of parkinson disability after fluoxetine medication. *Neurology*, 43, 211–13.

Stibe CMH, Lees AJ, Kempster PA, Stern GM (1988) Subcutaneous apomorphine in parkinsonian 'on–off' oscillations. *Lancet*, 1, 403–6.

Strang RR (1965) Imipramine in treatment of parkinsonism: a double-blind placebo study. *British Medical Journal*, 2, 33–4.

Stroudley J, Walsh M (1991) Radiological assessment of dysphagia in Parkinson's disease. *British Journal of Radiology*, 64, 890–3.

Stuck AE, Siu AL, Wieland GD, Adams J, Rubenstein LZ (1993) Comprehensive geriatric assessment: a meta-analysis of controlled trials. *Lancet*, 342, 1032–6.

Taggart H, Crawford V (1995) Reduced bone density of the hip in elderly patients with Parkinson's disease. *Age and Ageing*, 24, 326–8.

Tandberg E, Larsen JP, Aarsland D, Cummings JL (1996) The occurrence of depression in Parkinson's disease: a community-based study. *Archives of Neurology*, 53, 175–9.

Tanner CM, Kinoria I, Goetz CG, Carvey PM, Klawans HL (1985) Age at onset and clinical outcome in idiopathic Parkinson's disease. *Journal of Neurology*, 232, Suppl. 25.

Thomas M, Haigh RA (1995) Dysphagia, a reversible cause not to be forgotten. *Postgraduate Medical Journal*, 71, 94–5.

Tinetti ME, Baker DI, McAvay G, Claus EB, Garrett P, Gottschalk M, Koch ML, Trainor K, Horwitz RI (1994) A multifactorial intervention to reduce the risk of falling among elderly people living in the community. *New England Journal of Medicine*, 331, 821–7.

Tison F, Dartigues JF, Auriacombe S, Letenneur L, Boller F, Alperovitch A (1995) Dementia in

Parkinson's disease: A population-based study in ambulatory and institutionalized individuals. *Neurology*, 45, 705–8.

Troster AI, Paolo AM, Lyons KE, Glatt SL, Hubble JP, Koller WC (1995) The influence of depression on cognition in Parkinson's disease: A pattern of impairment distinguishable from Alzheimer's disease. *Neurology*, 45, 672–6.

van Dijk JG, Haan J, Zwinderman K, Kremer B, van Hilten BJ, Roos RAC (1993) Autonomic nervous system dysfunction in Parkinson's disease: relationships with age, medication, duration, and severity. *Journal of Neurology, Neurosurgery, and Psychiatry*, 56, 1090–5.

van Laar T, Steur EN, Essink AWG, Neef C, Oosterloo S, Roos RAC (1993) A double-blind study of the efficacy of apomorphine and its assessment in 'off' periods in Parkinson's disease. *Clinical Neurology and Neurosurgery*, 95, 231–5.

Viitanen M, Mortimer JA, Webster DD (1994) Association between presenting motor symptoms and the risk of cognitive impairment in Parkinson's disease. *Journal of Neurology, Neurosurgery, and Psychiatry*, 57, 1203–7.

Waters CH (1994) Fluoxetine and selegiline. *Canadian Journal of Neurological Sciences*, 21, 259–61.

Weiner MF, Risser RC, Cullum CM, Honig L, White C, Speciale S, Rosenberg RN (1996) Alzheimer's disease and its Lewy-body variant: A clinical analysis of postmortem verified cases. *American Journal of Psychiatry*, 153, 10, 1269–73.

Wolters EC, Steur EN, Tuynman-Qua HG, Bergmans PLM (1996) Olanzapine in the treatment of dopaminomimetic psychosis in patients with Parkinson's disease. *Neurology*, 47, 1085–7.

Zetusky WJ, Jankovic J, Pirozzolo FJ (1985) The heterogeneity of Parkinson's disease: Clinical and prognostic implications. *Neurology*, 35, 522–6.

4

Drug-induced parkinsonism in the elderly

Jean P Hubble

Introduction

Drug-induced parkinsonism (DIP) is probably the most common form of parkinsonism after Parkinson's disease (PD) in terms of overall prevalence (Hubble 1993). Elderly subjects have the greatest risk of developing DIP. The reason for this susceptibility is unknown. In some older individuals DIP may represent pharmacological exposure of latent PD (preexisting nigrostriatal degeneration). Alternatively, less specific pathological changes in the aging brain may simply increase the risk of DIP and other types of drug-induced side effects. While drugs of various classes can produce DIP, the antipsychotic or neuroleptic drugs are most often the agents responsible (Montastruc et al. 1994). DIP is attributed to the primary pharmacological action of this class of drugs, i.e. dopamine receptor blockade. Other medications without overt antidopaminergic action only rarely produce parkinsonism (Hubble 1997). These occurrences are so infrequent that single case reports are often the only documentation of these phenomena. Not surprisingly, DIP due to drugs falling outside the antidopaminergic class of medications is not well understood. This chapter will deal first and most extensively with DIP secondary to antidopaminergic drugs and, subsequently, will review reports of other causative drugs. It is important to emphasize that this chapter cannot serve as a complete or final treatise on DIP because of the ongoing development of new medications and the constantly evolving recognition of drug-induced side effects (Marti-Masso et al. 1996).

Neuroleptic-induced parkinsonism

In the early 1950s, following its introduction for the treatment of psychiatric illness, reports were issued linking the neuroleptic chlorpromazine with various neurological side effects including parkinsonism (Anton-Stephens 1954, Lehmann and Hanrahan 1954). In these early series, the incidence of DIP was in the range of 4–40% (Kinross-Wright 1954, Goldman 1955, Hall et al. 1956). Whilst investigators agreed on the clinical manifestations of the syndrome, they varied in their opinions regarding causative mechanism and identification of at risk individuals. A clear relationship between the occurrence of parkinsonian signs and dose of chlorpromazine administered could not be demonstrated (Hall et al. 1956). It was initially suggested that DIP may be related to chlorpromazine induced liver damage. However, there did not appear to be any relationship between abnormalities of liver function tests and the occurrence of this syndrome (Hall et al. 1956). Similarly, these investigators were unable to corroborate the claim made by others that patients whose psychosis responded well to drug benefit were most prone to develop DIP.

In subsequent years, as additional neuroleptic compounds were developed and as the number of individuals exposed to this class of drugs grew, several distinct adverse reactions involving abnormalities in movement and tone were described. In 1961, Ayd reported extrapyramidal reactions including DIP, dyskinesia and akathisia in 39% of 3775 patients on neuroleptic medication (Ayd 1961). In searching for clues to the cause of DIP, Ayd found that the syndrome developed over a shorter time period in individuals treated with the piperazine and fluorinated phenothiazine compounds.

Specific neuroleptic agents

It is now recognized that parkinsonism can result from the use of numerous drugs among the various types of neuroleptics (see Table 4.1). Certain neuroleptics, such as thioridazine, have fewer reported extrapyramidal side effects and as a result the risk of DIP may be less with their use. However, well controlled comparison studies substantiating this notion are lacking. In one series thioridazine was the third most commonly offending drug following haloperidol and amitriptyline/perphenazine among 125 patients followed for drug-induced movement disorders. The atypical neuroleptic clozapine causes less extrapyramidal side effects, including DIP (Baldessarini and Frankenburg 1991), a characteristic which is attributed to the relative specificity of clozapine's dopamine receptor blockade. The introduction of clozapine offered particular promise for the treatment of psychosis in PD (Scholz and Dichgans 1985, Friedman and Lannon 1989). Confusion, agitation and hallucinations can occur in PD due to dopaminergic drug therapy, the primary disease process, or as a result of unrelated psychiatric disorders. Conventional antipsychotics are poorly tolerated in PD due to their dopamine receptor blocking effects. Clozapine may also reduce tremor and motor fluctuations in PD (Friedman and Lannon 1990, Bennett et al. 1993). However, clozapine at doses of around 75–250 mg daily in elderly PD patients has been associated with sedation, delirium and worsening of motor signs and symptoms (Wolters et al. 1990). The association of this drug with haematological abnormalities including fatal agranulocytosis has

Table 4.1 Common neuroleptic drugs and related agents

	Trade names	Generic names
Phenothiazines	Compazine	prochlorperazine
	Triavil	amitriptyline/perphenazine
	Mellaril	thioridazine
	Phenergan	promethazine
	Prolixin	fluphenazine
	Norzine	thiethylperazine
	Serentil	mesoridazine
	Sparine	promaxine
	Stelazine	trifluoperazine
	Thorazine	chlorpromazine
	Torecan	thiethylperazine
	Trilafon	perphenazine
Butyrophenones	Haldol	haloperidol
	Fentanyl	droperidol
Thioxanthenes	Navane	thiothixene
	Taractran	chlorprothixene
Benzamides	Reglan	metoclopramide
Dihydroindolone	Moban	molindone
Dibenzoxazepine	Loxitane	loxapine
Thienobenzodiazepine	Zyprexa	olanzapine
Benzisoxazole	Risperdal	risperidone
Dibenzodiazepine	Clozaril	clozapine

necessitated weekly blood counts in all treated individuals (Kane et al. 1988). The concern over the potential for neutropenia coupled with the cost and inconvenience of frequent blood tests has limited the use of this agent. Several atypical neuroleptic agents are currently available in the UK (risperidone, sertindole, olanzapine and quetiapine) which, like clozapine, rarely cause acute extrapyramidal side effects, but, unlike clozapine, are less likely to have an adverse influence on the neutrophil count (Kerwin and Taylor 1996). High dose treatment with risperidone has been found to cause DIP. Other atypical neuroleptic drugs (ziprasidone, zotepine and amisulpride) have not yet been licensed for use in the UK, but both ziprasidone and amisulpride can at high dosage result in DIP. While neuroleptics are used primarily as antipsychotic agents, it is important to recognize that these drugs are sometimes prescribed for depression, anxiety, and insomnia. Although typically used to control nausea and vomiting, prochlorperazine and related agents belong to the neuroleptic class of drugs and can produce DIP (Bateman et al. 1986). Metoclopramide, an atypical neuroleptic belonging to the benzamide class, is used to ameliorate gastric stasis and is employed as an antiemetic and various extrapyramidal reactions, including DIP, have been associated with its use (Grimes et al. 1982, Sethi et al. 1989, Miller and Jankovic 1989). In one series, five out of 2557 metoclopramide treated patients developed parkinsonism. All such affected individuals were over 40 years old (Bateman et al. 1989).

Clinical features of neuroleptic-induced parkinsonism

Clinical descriptions of neuroleptic-induced parkinsonism date back to the original reports in the 1960s. In 1961, Ayd reported on DIP's responsiveness to anticholinergic medications, noted its usual abatement with the discontinuation of the offending drug, and distinguished it clinically from PD (Ayd 1961). Ayd also reported it to be more common in women and in the elderly. It was initially suggested that neuroleptic-induced parkinsonism resembled postencephalitic parkinsonism rather than PD (Steck 1954). However, subsequent work suggests that the clinical manifestations of this syndrome can be identical to those seen in PD (Marsden et al. 1975). Akinesia, rigidity, postural abnormalities, and tremor may occur. Akinesia is the earliest, most common, and frequently the only manifestation of DIP, accounting for the expressionless face, loss of associated movements, slow initiation of motor activity, and disturbed speech. Rigidity of the extremities, neck, or trunk, usually without a cogwheel phenomenon, may occur after the onset of bradykinesia. While the characteristic parkinsonian pill rolling tremor may be present, postural tremor resembling essential tremor may also be seen (Indo and Ando 1982, Hershey et al. 1982).

Although DIP may be clinically indistinguishable from PD, some differentiating characteristics may occur (see Table 4.2). The signs and symptoms of PD usually have a unilateral onset before involving, over time, the opposite side. The disease demonstrates mild persistent asymmetry with the first side affected always being more severely impaired (Klawans et al. 1973). Postural instability with episodic freezing and start hesitation frequently occurs in late stage PD but rarely complicates DIP (Giladi et al. 1997). The manifestations of neuroleptic-induced DIP are frequently bilateral and symmetrical and often develop acutely or subacutely. In one series, the signs of DIP emerged within a few days of neuroleptic treatment with a gradual increase in incidence so that 50–70% of cases appeared by one month and 90% of cases within three months (Marsden et al. 1975). It is often stated that with time neuroleptic-induced DIP can spontaneously diminish. However, prospective studies to verify this phenomenon are lacking. The only

Table 4.2 Distinguishing drug-induced parkinsonism from PD

	Drug-induced parkinsonism	Parkinson's disease
Symptom onset	Bilateral and symmetric	Unilateral or asymmetric
Course	Acute or subacute	Insidious, chronic
Tremor type	Bilateral symmetric postural or rest tremor	Unilateral or asymmetric rest tremor
Freezing or start hesitation	Rare	Frequent feature with disease progression
Anticholinergic drug response	May be pronounced	Usually mild–moderate
Withdrawal of suspected offending drug	Remittance within weeks to months	Symptoms and signs slowly progress

evidence for this assumption is the observation that withdrawal of anticholinergic drugs coadministered for several months with neuroleptics is followed by the appearance of relatively few cases of DIP.

After the discontinuation of neuroleptic medication the majority of patients are free of parkinsonian signs within a few weeks. However, the effects may last longer, in some cases up to several years (Klawans et al. 1973). Metoclopramide-induced parkinsonism has been reported to take several months to resolve completely (Weiden et al. 1987, Yamamoto et al. 1987). The potentially long duration of neuroleptic-induced parkinsonism is important to appreciate so that one can avoid diagnostic error. DIP will usually improve slowly over time with reduction or discontinuation of the offending drug whereas the signs and symptoms of PD will progressively worsen.

Neuroleptic-induced movement disorders including DIP frequently go unrecognized. Miller and Jankovic (1989) in their review of metoclopramide-induced movement disorders found that the drug was continued for an average of six months after the onset of extrapyramidal symptoms. Other investigators found that psychiatry physicians in training diagnosed DIP in 11% of neuroleptic treated patients, while researchers determined the prevalence to be 26% in the same population (Hansen et al. 1992). Approximately 32% of 192 individuals newly diagnosed with parkinsonism were found to have DIP using a large neurology outpatient referral registry in Madrid (Perez Gilabert et al. 1994). It has been estimated that 4% of all neurology outpatient clinic patients have DIP (Gershanik 1994). The correct diagnosis of DIP depends on a high index of suspicion, and cases have been described where DIP has resulted from the covert administration of neuroleptic drugs by a spouse to their partner (Albanese et al. 1992).

Pathogenesis of neuroleptic-induced parkinsonism

The primary neurochemical determinant of PD is striatal dopamine depletion (Ehringer and Hornykiewicz 1960). Since neuroleptic drugs function as dopamine receptor blockers, it is not surprising that clinical features of parkinsonism can result from their use. However, DIP cannot simply be a result of dopamine receptor blockade. If this were true, the incidence and severity of DIP should correlate to drug dosage and length of exposure. Attempts to link total drug dosage with the occurrence of parkinsonism have failed to show such a relationship (Hall et al. 1956). Furthermore, plasma neuroleptic drug levels do not appear to correlate with the severity of DIP (Crowley et al. 1978). Parkinsonism appearing within several days of treatment with relatively small drug doses is a common clinical experience, but other patients are successfully maintained on relatively high doses for several years without developing parkinsonism. It has been suggested that DIP is simply idiopathic PD occurring by chance in neuroleptic treated individuals. The reported prevalence of neuroleptic-induced parkinsonism varies, but clinically significant parkinsonism reportedly occurs in 10–15% of treated individuals (Korczyn and Goldberg 1976, Moleman et al. 1986). These rates of DIP are probably underestimates (McClelland 1976). Thus, coincidental PD could not account for all cases of DIP since the occurrence rate of parkinsonism in neuroleptic treated individuals is much greater than estimates of PD in the general populace.

The mechanisms determining individual susceptibility to DIP remain unclear. Some studies suggest that women are at an increased risk for the development of neuroleptic-induced movement disorders, including tardive dyskinesia and DIP (Ayd 1961, Korczyn and Goldberg 1976, Kane and Smith 1982). Oestrogen related dopamine receptor blockade has been offered as the explanation for this female preponderance (Glazer et al. 1983). Others have not found a gender influence (Kennedy et al. 1971, Moleman et al. 1982). Differences in case ascertainment, medication prescription and drug usage based on sex in these studies may explain these findings. In one report low urinary levels of free dopamine were associated with the subsequent development of phenothiazine-induced parkinsonism, suggesting that an inherent metabolic defect may increase the risk of DIP (Crowley et al. 1976). HLA B44 is reported to be common in DIP suggesting a genetic influence (Metzer et al. 1989). In one series, five out of 16 patients with metoclopramide-induced movement disorders had family members with reported parkinsonism, tremor, or chorea (Miller and Jankovic 1989). However, the precise role of genetics in DIP remains uncertain.

The possibility that increased susceptibility to DIP might be related to subclinical PD has also been considered (Delay and Deniker 1968, Duvoisin 1977). In some instances it appears that PD becomes clinically overt during neuroleptic therapy and then subsides when the drug is discontinued, only to reappear years later. At least nine such cases have been documented in the medical literature (Goetz 1983, Stephen and Williamson 1984, Hardie and Lees 1988). In addition, two instances of DIP that completely remitted upon drug withdrawal have been described in which postmortem examination ultimately revealed pathological changes consistent with PD (Rajput et al. 1982). Reduced putaminal ^{18}F-dopa uptake on positron emission tomography has been reported in two out of seven individuals with DIP (Brooks 1991). Four of the five patients with normal PET scans recovered fully with cessation of drug therapy. The two patients with abnormal scans had persistent evidence of parkinsonism requiring levodopa therapy, suggesting underlying PD.

The relationship of DIP to other neuroleptic-induced extrapyramidal syndromes is intriguing. Like DIP, tardive dyskinesia is reported to occur more frequently in the elderly (Jus et al. 1976, Pineau et al. 1976, Crane and Smeets 1974, Jeste and Wyatt 1982, Woerner et al. 1991). In a study of 215 patients over the age of 55 years after the initiation of neuroleptic therapy evidence of parkinsonism was found in 103 patients by week 43 of drug therapy (Saltz et al. 1991). Tardive dyskinesia developed in 40% of the parkinsonian patients compared to 12% of nonparkinsonian subjects. The coexistence of DIP and tardive dyskinesia has been reported by others (Fann and Lake 1974, De Fraites et al. 1977, Rao et al. 1987). The occurrence of both hypokinetic and hyperkinetic drug-induced side effects in a common patient population is difficult to explain. A possible explanation may be that presynaptic receptor blockade is related to the development of both DIP and tardive dyskinesia (Seeman et al. 1974). Differential effects of neuroleptics on dopamine receptor subtypes may also play a part. Elderly subjects may be especially vulnerable to DIP and tardive dyskinesia due to diminished drug metabolism, dopaminergic neuronal loss, or alterations in dopamine receptors (Finch 1973, Glazer et al. 1983, Goetz et al. 1982).

Treatment of neuroleptic-induced parkinsonism

The first line treatment of DIP is, whenever possible, the withdrawal of the offending drug. The underlying condition for which the drug was initially prescribed may subsequently worsen, which is a particular difficulty in the instance of psychosis associated with schizophrenia. It is prudent to weigh the benefits that the patient derives from the drug against the severity and disability of DIP. Mild nondisabling DIP occurring in individuals who have achieved good control of psychotic symptoms on a stable dose of neuroleptic may require only observation and no intervention. Alternatively, the patient can be switched to an atypical neuroleptic with less potential for extrapyramidal motor side effects such as olanzapine or risperidone.

Domperidone and betahistine can be substituted for neuroleptic drugs used to control nausea and dizziness (Parkes 1986). Domperidone is not commercially available in the US. Drug-induced movement disorders have occasionally been associated with the use of domperidone (Debontridder 1980). Antiemetics, which do not act via dopamine blockade, such as ondansetron and benzquinamide hydrochloride, can also be used in some instances.

Standard antiparkinsonian drugs can be used to treat DIP. Anticholinergic drugs reportedly decrease the signs and symptoms of neuroleptic-induced parkinsonism to a greater degree than in PD. This drug action has been suggested to be of use as a means of distinguishing between DIP and PD (Hornykiewicz 1975). Dopaminergic drugs may provoke the very symptoms for which the neuroleptic drug was first prescribed (Hauser 1980). In a double-blind crossover study, the effects of levodopa and the dopaminergic agonist apomorphine were assessed in 12 schizophrenic patients with DIP (Merello et al. 1996). No clear benefit from antiparkinsonian drug treatment was detected, though no acute exacerbation of psychiatric symptoms occurred. This seeming lack of effect may be explained by the robust and relatively persistent dopamine receptor blockade of neuroleptic drugs. Propranolol does not benefit tremor in DIP (Metzer et al. 1993). In a single case report, pyridoxine was reported to improve DIP and tardive dyskinesia in an individual with neuroleptic treated schizophrenia (Sandyk and Pardeshi 1990). While electroconvulsive shock therapy is usually considered to be safe in PD, it reportedly caused worsening of immobility in a psychiatric patient with DIP and tardive dystonia (Hanin et al. 1995).

Dopamine storage and transport inhibitors causing parkinsonism

Reserpine, an antihypertensive that is now rarely prescribed, depletes brain dopamine and other biogenic amines by interfering with presynaptic vesicular storage mechanisms. It can produce both clinical and experimental parkinsonism (Carlsson et al. 1957). Reserpine is still sometimes used to treat tardive dyskinesia (Fahn 1983, Klawans et al. 1983). Since individuals with tardive dyskinesia may have an increased risk of developing DIP, close monitoring of these patients is warranted if treatment with reserpine is employed. Tetrabenazine, a synthetic analogue of reserpine, also depletes amines and may also block postsynaptic dopamine receptors (Reches et al. 1983). Not currently marketed in the US, tetrabenazine appears to be useful in the treatment of hyperkinetic disorders (Jankovic 1983). Parkinsonism has been reported as the most common side effect of tetrabenazine exposure, affecting 53 of 217 patients receiving the drug for hyperkinesia (Jankovic and Orman 1988).

Alpha-methyldopa, a false neurotransmitter for dopamine, has been reported to cause DIP and to exacerbate existing PD (Rosenblum and Montgomery 1980,

Gillman and Sandyk 1984). Alpha-methyldopa has been used as an antihypertensive drug and has even been employed in the treatment of PD (Fermaglich and Chase 1973). The significance of the few reported cases of DIP with this drug is unclear.

Calcium channel blockers causing parkinsonism

Available in Europe and Latin America, the piperazine derivatives, flunarizine and cinnarizine, act as calcium entry blockers and have been prescribed for various disorders including vertigo, migraine, and tinnitus (Godfraind et al. 1982, Holmes et al. 1984). Extrapyramidal reactions including DIP and exacerbation of PD have been associated with their use (Marti Masso et al. 1987, Micheli et al. 1989). A primate model of cinnarizine-induced parkinsonism has also been described (Fadda et al. 1989). Parkinsonism is thought to be due to the antidopaminergic effects of these compounds at pre or postsynaptic sites (De Vries and Beart 1984). The persistence of parkinsonian signs, particularly in the aged, many months after the cessation of the offending drug has been reported (Garcia-Ruiz et al.1992). DIP due to calcium channel blockers may have a genetic component as a relatively higher occurrence of other movement disorders among relatives of affected individuals has been found (Negrotti et al. 1992). Calcium channel blockers available in the US are rarely associated with clinical parkinsonism (Dick and Barold 1989). The antidopaminergic effect of one such agent, nimodipine, has been demonstrated experimentally (Pileblad and Carlsson 1986).

Other drugs reported to cause parkinsonism

Other drugs of various classes have occasionally been associated with parkinsonism, though a causal relationship is often difficult to establish (see Table 4.3). Amiodarone can cause several neurological side effects including a tremor resembling essential tremor. However, DIP has also been described (LeMaire et al. 1982, Palakurthy et al. 1987, Werner and Olanow 1989).

In single case reports, parkinsonism has been ascribed to cholinergic drugs including bethanechol and the cholinesterase inhibitor pyridostigmine that does not penetrate the blood–brain barrier (Iwasaki et al. 1988, Fox et al. 1989). In the case of bethanacol, parkinsonism may result from cholinergic overactivity in the striatum, although in one case a postmortem demonstrated pathological changes consistent with PD (Fox et al. 1989). Lithium commonly produces a postural tremor but it is unclear as to whether it can cause DIP. Cogwheel rigidity has been found on examination in a small percentage of patients taking lithium (Kane et al. 1978). Two patients were reported to develop parkinsonian symptoms after

Table 4.3 Miscellaneous drugs causing parkinsonism

Reserpine
Tetrabenzaine
Alpha-methyldopa
Calcium channel blockers e.g., cinnarizine, flunarizine
Amiodarone
Bethamechol
Pyridostigmine
Lithium
Diazepam
Fluoxetine
Phenelzine
Procaine
Meperidine
Amphotericin B
Cephaloridine
5-fluorouracil
Vincristine–adriamycin

lithium therapy but both had prior exposure to neuroleptic drugs (Tyrer et al. 1980).

DIP was reported in four patients on high dose (≥ 100 mg daily) diazepam being used in the treatment of schizophrenia (Suranyi-Cadotte et al. 1985). The selective serotonin reuptake inhibitor antidepressants fluoxetine (Bouchard et al. 1989, Tate 1989, Gernaat et al. 1991, Steur 1993), and paroxetine (Jiminez-Jiminez et al. 1994) have been associated with parkinsonism. Isolated instances of parkinsonism have also been ascribed to other agents including phenelzine (Teusink et al. 1984), procaine (Gjerris 1971), meperidine (Lieberman and Goldstein 1985), amphotericin B (Fisher and Dewald 1983), cephaloridine (Mintz et al. 1971), 5-fluorouracil (Bergevin et al. 1975), and vincristine combined with adriamycin (Boranic and Raci 1979).

Summary

DIP is common, particularly in the elderly. Dopamine receptor blockers, used primarily as antipsychotics and antiemetics, are most frequently responsible for this condition. Other pharmacological classes of medications have also been implicated, although the mechanism of DIP in such instances is unclear. The susceptibility of the individual to develop DIP has not been established, but may, in some cases, represent latent PD or a heritable trait. Further scrutiny of the occurrence and characteristics of DIP would provide a better understanding of this phenomenon and may also give a greater insight into the cause and pathogenesis of PD.

REFERENCES

Albanese A, Colosimo C, Bentivoglio AR, Bergonzi P (1992) Unsuspected, surreptitious drug-induced parkinsonism. *Neurology*, 42, 459.

Anton-Stephens D (1954) Preliminary observations on the psychiatric uses of chlorpromazine (Largactil). *Journal of Mental Science*, 100, 543–57.

Ayd FJ (1961) A survey of drug-induced extrapyramidal reactions. *Journal of the American Medical Association*, 175, 1054–60.

Baldessarini RJ, Frankenburg FR (1991) Clozapine. A novel antipsychotic agent. *New England Journal of Medicine*, 324, 746–54.

Bateman DN, Darling WM, Boys R, Rawlins MD (1989) Extrapyramidal reactions to metoclopramide and prochlorperazine. *Quarterly Journal of Medicine*, 71, 307–11.

Bateman DN, Rawlins MC, Simpson JM (1986) Extrapyramidal reactions to prochlorperazine and haloperidol in the United Kingdom. *Quarterly Journal of Medicine*, 59, 549–56.

Bennett JP, Landow ER, Schuh LA (1993) Suppression of dyskinesias in advanced Parkinson's disease. II. Increasing daily clozapine doses suppress dyskinesias and improve parkinsonism symptoms. *Neurology*, 43, 1551–5.

Bergevin PR, Patwardhan VC, Weissman J, Lee SM (1975) Neurotoxicity of 5-fluorouracil. *Lancet*, 1, 410.

Boranic M, Raci F (1979) A parkinson-like syndrome as side effect of chemotherapy with vincristine and adriamycin in a child with acute leukaemia. *Biomedicine*, 31, 124–5.

Bouchard RH, Pourcher E, Vincent P (1989) Fluoxetine and extrapyramidal side effects. *American Journal of Psychiatry*, 146, 1352–3.

Brooks DJ (1991) Detection of preclinical Parkinson's disease with PET. *Neurology*, 41, Suppl. 2, 24–7.

Carlsson A, Lindquist M, Magnusson T (1957) 3,4–Dihydroxyphenylalanine and 6-hydroxytryptophan as reserpine antagonists. *Nature*, 180, 1200–1.

Crane GE, Smeets RA (1974) Tardive dyskinesia and drug therapy in geriatric patients. *Archives of General Psychiatry*, 30, 341–3.

Crowley TJ, Hoehn MM, Rutledge CO Stallings MA, Heaton RK, Sundell S, Stilson D (1978) Dopamine excretion and vulnerability to drug-induced parkinsonism. Schizophrenic patients. *Archives of General Psychiatry*, 35, 97–104.

Crowley TJ, Rutledge CO, Hoehn MM, Stallings MA, Sundell S (1976) Low urinary dopamine and prediction of phenothiazine-induced parkinsonism: A preliminary report. *American Journal of Psychiatry*, 133, 703–6.

De Vries DJ, Beart PM (1984) Competitive inhibition of [^{3}H]spiperone binding to D-2 dopamine receptors in striatal homogenates by organic calcium channel antagonists and polyvalent cations. *European Journal of Pharmacology*, 106, 133–9.

De Fraites EG Jr, Davis KL, Berger PA (1977) Coexisting tardive dyskinesia and parkinsonism: a case report. *Biological Psychiatry*, 12, 267–72.

Debontridder O (1980) Dystonic reactions after domperidone. *Lancet*, 2, 1259.

Delay J, Deniker P (1968) Drug-induced extrapyramidal syndromes. In: *Handbook of Clinical Neurology*, Vol. 6, *Diseases of the Basal Ganglia*, eds. Vinken PJ, Bruyn GW. Amsterdam: North-Holland Publishing Company. New York: Wiley Interscience Division, John Wiley & Sons Inc.

Dick RS, Barold SS (1989) Diltiazem-induced parkinsonism. *American Journal of Medicine*, 87, 95–6.

Duvoisin RC (1977) Problems in the treatment of parkinsonism. *Advances in Experimental Medicine and Biology*, 90, 131–55.

Ehringer H, Hornykiewicz O (1960) Verteilung von noradrenalin und dopamin (3-hydroxytyramin) im Gehirn des Menschen und ihr Verhalten bei Erkrankungen des extrapyramidalen Systems. *Klinische Wochenschrift*, 38, 1236–9.

Fadda F, Gessa GL, Mosca E, Stefanini E (1989) Different effects of the calcium antagonists nimodipine and flunarizine on dopamine metabolism in the rat brain. *Journal of Neural Transmission*, 75, 195–200.

Fahn S (1983) Treatment of tardive dyskinesia: Use of dopamine-depleting agents. *Clinical Neuropharmacology*, 6, 151–8.

Fann WE, Lake CR (1974) On the coexistence of parkinsonism and tardive dyskinesia. *Diseases of the Nervous System*, 35, 324–6.

Fermaglich J, Chase TN (1973) Methyldopa or methyldopahydrazine as levodopa synergists. *Lancet*, 1, 1261–2.

Finch CE (1973) Catecholamine metabolism in the brains of ageing male mice. *Brain Research*, 52, 261–76.

Fisher JF, Dewald J (1983) Parkinsonism associated with intraventricular amphotericin B. *Journal of Antimicrobial Chemotherapy*, 12, 97–9.

Fox JH, Bennett DA, Goetz CG, Penn RD, Savoy S, Clasen R, Wilson RS (1989) Induction of parkinsonism by intraventricular bethanechol in a patient with Alzheimer's disease. *Neurology*, 39, 1265.

Friedman JH, Lannon MC (1989) Clozapine in the treatment of psychosis in Parkinson's disease. *Neurology*, 39, 1219–21.

Friedman JH, Lannon MC (1990) Clozapine-responsive tremor in Parkinson's disease. *Movement Disorders*, 5, Suppl. 3, 225–9.

Garcia-Ruiz PJ, de Yebenes JG, Jimenez-Jimenez FJ, Vazquez A, Urra DG, Morales B (1992) Parkinsonism associated with calcium channel blockers: a prospective follow-up study. *Clinical Neuropharmacology*, 15, 19–26.

Gernaat HB, Van de Woude J, Touw DJ (1991) Fluoxetine and parkinsonism in patients taking carbamazepine (letter). *American Journal of Psychiatry*, 148, 1604–5.

Gershanik OS (1994) Drug-induced parkinsonism in the aged. Recognition and prevention. *Drugs and Aging*, 5, 127–32.

Giladi N, Kao R, Fahn S (1997) Freezing phenomenon in patients with parkinsonian syndromes. *Movement Disorders*, 12, 302–5.

Gillman MA, Sandyk R (1984) Parkinsonism induced by methyldopa. *South African Medical Journal*, 65, 194.

Gjerris F (1971) Transitory procaine-induced parkinsonism. *Journal of Neurology, Neurosurgery, and Psychiatry*, 34, 20–2.

Glazer WM, Naftolin F, Moore DC, Bowers MB, MacLusky NJ (1983) The relationship of circulating estradiol to tardive dyskinesia in men and postmenopausal women. *Psychoneuroendocrinology*, 8, 429–34.

Godfraind T, Towse G, Van Nueten JM (1982) Cinnarizine: A selective calcium entry blocker. *Drugs of Today (Medicamentos de Actualidad)*, 18, 27–42.

Goetz CG (1983) Drug-induced parkinsonism and idiopathic Parkinson's disease. *Archives of Neurology*, 40, 325–6.

Goetz CG, Weiner WJ, Nausieda PA, Klawans HL (1982) Tardive dyskinesia: pharmacology and clinical implications. *Clinical Neuropharmacology*, 5, 3–22.

Goldman D (1955) Treatment of psychotic states with chlorpromazine. *Journal of the American Medical Association*, 157, 1274–7.

Grimes D, Hassan MN, Preston DN (1982) Adverse neurologic effects of metoclopramide. *Canadian Medical Association Journal*, 126, 23–5.

Hall RA, Jackson RB, Swain JM (1956) Neurotoxic reactions resulting from chlorpromazine administration. *Journal of the American Medical Association*, 161, 214–18.

Hanin B, Lerner Y, Srour N (1995) An unusual effect of ECT on drug-induced parkinsonism and tardive dystonia. *Convulsive Therapy*, 11, 271–4.

Hansen TE, Brown WL, Weigel RM, Casey DE (1992) Underrecognition of tardive dyskinesia and drug-induced parkinsonism by psychiatric residents. *General Hospital Psychiatry*, 14, 340–4.

Hardie RJ, Lees AJ (1988) Neuroleptic-induced Parkinson's syndrome: clinical features and results of treatment with levodopa. *Journal of Neurology, Neurosurgery and Psychiatry*, 6, 850–4.

Hauser RS (1980) Amantadine-associated recurrence of psychosis. *American Journal of Psychiatry*, 137, 240–2.

Hershey LA, Gift T, Rivera-Calminlin L (1982) Not Parkinson's disease. *Lancet*, 2, 49.

Holmes B, Brogden RN, Heel RC, Speight TM, Avery GS (1984) Flunarizine. A review of its pharmacodynamic and pharmacokinetic properties and therapeutic use. *Drugs*, 27, 6–44.

Hornykiewicz O (1975) Parkinsonism induced by dopaminergic antagonists. *Advances in Neurology*, 9, 155–64.

Hubble JP (1993) Drug-induced parkinsonism. In: *Parkinsonian Syndromes*, eds. Koller WC, Stern M, pp. 111–22. New York: Marcel–Dekker.

Hubble JP (1997) Drug-induced parkinsonian syndromes. In: *Movement Disorders: Neurologic Principles and Practice*, eds. Watts RL, Koller WC, pp. 325–30. New York: McGraw-Hill.

Indo T, Ando K (1982) Metoclopramide-induced parkinsonism: clinical characteristics of ten cases. *Archives of Neurology*, 39, 494–6.

Iwasaki Y, Wakata N, Kinoshita M (1988) Parkinsonism induced by pyridostigmine. *Acta Neurologica Scandinavica*, 78, 236.

Jankovic J (1983) Tetrabenazine in the treatment of hyperkinetic movement disorders. *Advances in Neurology*, 37, 277–89.

Jankovic J, Orman J (1988) Tetrabenazine therapy of dystonia, chorea, tics, and other dyskinesias. *Neurology*, 38, 391–4.

Jeste DV, Wyatt RJ (1982) Understanding and treating tardive dyskinesia. New York: Guilford Press.

Jiminez-Jiminez FJ, Tejeiro J, Martinez-Junquera G, Cabrera-Valdivia F, Alarcon J, Garcia-Albea E (1994) Parkinsonism exacerbated by paroxetine. *Neurology*, 44, 2406.

Jus A, Peneau R, Lachance R, Pelchat G, Jus K, Pires P, Villeneuve R (1976) Epidemiology of tardive dyskinesia. Part II. *Diseases of the Nervous System*, 37, 257–61.

Kane J, Honigfeld G, Singer J, Meltzer H (1988) Clozapine for the treatment-resistant schizophrenic: A double-blind comparison with chlorpromazine. *Archives of General Psychiatry*, 45, 789–96.

Kane J, Rifkin A, Quitkin F, Klein DF (1978) Extrapyramidal side effects with lithium treatment. *American Journal of Psychiatry*, 135, 851–3.

Kane J, Smith JM (1982) Tardive dyskinesia: prevalence and risk factors, 1959–1979. *Archives of General Psychiatry*, 39, 473–81.

Kennedy PF, Hershon HI, McGuire RJ (1971) Extrapyramidal disorders after prolonged phenothiazine therapy. *British Journal of Psychiatry*, 118, 509–18.

Kerwin R, Taylor D (1996) New antipsychotics: a review of their current status and clinical potential. *CNS Drugs*, 6, 71–2.

Kinross-Wright V (1954) Chlorpromazine – a major advance in psychiatric treatment. *Postgraduate Medicine*, 16, 297.

Klawans HL Jr, Bergen D, Bruyn GW (1973) Prolonged drug-induced parkinsonism. *Confinia Neurologica*, 35, 368–77.

Klawans HL, Tanner CM, Barr A (1983) The reversibility of 'permanent' tardive dyskinesia. *Clinical Neuropharmacology*, 7, Suppl. 2, 153–9.

Korczyn AD, Goldberg GJ (1976) Extrapyramidal effects of neuroleptics. *Journal of Neurology, Neurosurgery, and Psychiatry*, 39, 866–9.

Lehmann HE, Hanrahan GE (1954) Chlorpromazine: new inhibiting agent for psychomotor excitement and manic states. *Archives of Neurology and Psychiatry*, 71, 227.

LeMaire JF, Autret A, Biziere K, Romet-Lemone JL, Gray F (1982) Amiodarone neuropathy: further arguments for human drug-induced neurolipidosis. *European Neurology*, 21, 65–8.

Lieberman AN, Goldstein M (1985) Reversible parkinsonism related to meperidine. *New England Journal of Medicine*, 312, 509.

Marsden CD, Tarsy D, Baldessarini RJ (1975) Spontaneous and drug-induced movement disorders. In: *Psychiatric Aspects of Neurologic Disease*, eds. Benson DF, Blumer D. New York: Grune and Stratton.

Marti-Masso JF, Obeso JA, Carrera N, Martinez-Lage JM (1987) Aggravation of Parkinson's disease by cinnarizine. *Journal of Neurology, Neurosurgery and Psychiatry*, 50, 804–5.

Marti-Masso JF, Poza JJ, Lopez de Munain A (1996) Drugs inducing or aggravating parkinsonism: A review. *Therapie*, 51, 568–77.

McClelland HA (1976) Assessment of drugs in schizophrenia. Discussion on assessment of drug-induced extrapyramidal reactions. *British Journal of Clinical Pharmacology*, 3, 401–3.

Merello M, Starkstein S, Petracca G, Cataneo EA, Manes F, Leiguarda R (1996) Drug-induced parkinsonism in schizophrenic patients: Motor response and psychiatric changes after acute challenge with L-Dopa and apomorphine. *Clinical Neuropharmacology*, 19, 439–43.

Metzer WS, Newton JE, Steele RW, Claybrook M, Paige SR, McMillan DE, Hays S (1989) HLA antigens in drug-induced parkinsonism. *Movement Disorders*, 4, 121–8.

Metzer WS, Paige SR, Newton JEO (1993) Inefficacy of propranolol in attenuation of drug-induced parkinsonian tremor. *Movement Disorders*, 8, 43–6.

Micheli FE, Fernandez Pardal MM, Giannaula R, Gatto M, Casas Parera I, Paradiso G, Torres M, Pikielny R, Fernandex Pardal J (1989) Movement disorders and depression due to flunarizine and cinnarizine. *Movement Disorders*, 4, 139–46.

Miller LG, Jankovic J (1989) Metoclopramide-induced movement disorders. *Archives of Internal Medicine*, 149, 2486–92.

Mintz U, Liberman UA, Vries A de (1971) Parkinsonism syndrome due to cephaloridine. *Journal of the American Medical Association*, 216, 1200.

Moleman P, Janzen G, von Bargen BA, Kappers EJ, Pepplinkhuizen L, Schmitz PI (1986) Relationship between age and incidence of parkinsonism in psychiatric patients treated with haloperidol. *American Journal of Psychiatry*, 143, 232–4.

Moleman P, Schmitz PJM, Ladee GA (1982) Extrapyramidal side effects and oral haloperidol: An analysis of explanatory patient and treatment characteristics. *Journal of Clinical Psychiatry*, 43, 492–6.

Montastruc JL, Llau ME, Rascol O, Senard JM (1994) Drug-induced parkinsonism. *Fundamental and Clinical Pharmacology*, 8, 293–306.

Negrotti A, Calzetti S, Sasso E (1992) Calcium-entry blockers-induced parkinsonism: possible role of inherited susceptibility. *Neurotoxicology*, 13, 261–4.

Palakurthy PR, Iyer V, Meckler RJ (1987) Unusual neurotoxicity associated with amiodarone therapy. *Archives of Internal Medicine*, 147, 881–4.

Parkes JD (1986) Domperidone and Parkinson's disease. *Clinical Neuropharmacology*, 9, 517–32.

Perez Gilabert Y, Mateo D, Gimenez-Roldan S (1994) Patient care in a hospital-based unit for treating Parkinson's disease and movement disorders: a 3 year prospective study. *Neurologica*, 9, 317–23.

Pileblad E, Carlsson A (1986) In vivo effects of the Ca^{2+}-antagonist nimodipine on dopamine metabolism in mouse brain. *Journal of Neural Transmission*, 66, 171–87.

Pineau R, Lachance R, Pelchat G, Jus K, Pires P, Pires P, Villenueve R (1976) Epidemiology of tardive dyskinesia. Part I. *Diseases of the Nervous System*, 37, 210–14.

Rajput AH, Rozdilsky B, Hornykiewicz O, Shannak K, Lee T, Seeman P (1982) Reversible drug-induced parkinsonism: clinicopathologic study of two cases. *Archives of Neurology*, 39, 644–6.

Rao JM, Cowie VA, Mathew B (1987) Tardive dyskinesia in neuroleptic medicated mentally handicapped subjects. *Acta Psychiatrica Sandinavica*, 76, 507–13.

Reches A, Burke RE, Kuhn CM, Hassan MN, Jackson VR, Fahn S (1983) Tetrabenazine, an amine-depleting drug, also blocks dopamine receptors in rat brain. *Journal of Pharmacology and Experimental Therapeutics*, 225, 515–21.

Rosenblum AM, Montgomery EB (1980) Exacerbation of parkinsonism by methyldopa. *Journal of the American Medical Association*, 244, 2727–8.

Saltz BL, Woerner MG, Kane JM, Leiberman JA, Alvir JM, Bergmann KJ, Blank K, Koblenzer J,

Kahaner K (1991) Prospective study of tardive dyskinesia incidence in the elderly. *Journal of the American Medical Association*, 266, 2402–6.

Sandyk R, Pardeshi R (1990) Pyridoxine improves drug-induced parkinsonism and psychosis in a schizophrenic patient. *International Journal of Neuroscience*, 52, 225–30.

Scholz E, Dichgans J (1985) Treatment of drug-induced exogenous psychosis in parkinsonism with clozapine and fluperlapine. *European Archives of Psychiatry and Neurological Sciences*, 235, 60–4.

Seeman P, Staiman A, Lee T (1974) The membrane action of tranquilizers in relation to neuroleptic-induced parkinsonism and tardive dyskinesia. In: *Advances in Biochemical Psychopharmacology, The Phenothiazines and Structurally Related Drugs*, eds. Forrest IS, Carr CJ, Usdin E, pp. 137–48. New York: Raven Press.

Sethi KD, Patel B, Meador KJ (1989) Metoclopramide-induced parkinsonism. *Southern Medical Journal*, 82, 1581–2.

Steck H (1954) Le syndrome extrapyramidal et diencephalique au cours des traitements au forgactil au Serpasil. *Annales Medico-Psychologiques*, 737–43.

Stephen PJ, Williamson J (1984) Drug-induced parkinsonism in the elderly. *Lancet*, 2, 1082–3.

Steur EN (1993) Increase of Parkinson disability after fluoxetine medication. *Neurology*, 43, 211–13.

Suranyi-Cadotte BE, Nestoros JN, Nair NP, Lal S, Gauthier S (1985) Parkinsonism induced by high doses of diazepam. *Biological Psychiatry*, 20, 455–7.

Tate JL (1989) Extrapyramidal symptoms in a patient taking haloperidol and fluoxetine (letter). *American Journal of Psychiatry*, 146, 399–400.

Teusink JP, Alexopoulos GS, Shamoian CA (1984) Parkinsonian side effects induced by a monoamine oxidase inhibitor. *American Journal of Psychiatry*, 141,118–19.

Tyrer P, Alexander MS, Regan A, Lee I (1980) An extrapyramidal syndrome after lithium therapy. *British Journal of Psychiatry*, 136, 191–4.

Weiden PJ, Mann JJ, Haas G, Mattson M, Frances A (1987) Clinical nonrecognition of neuroleptic-induced movement disorders: a cautionary study. *American Journal of Psychiatry*, 144, 1148–53.

Werner EG, Olanow CW (1989) Parkinsonism and amiodarone therapy. *Annals of Neurology*, 25, 630–2.

Woerner MG, Kane JM, Lieberman JA, Alvir J, Bergmann KJ, Borenstein M, Schooler NR, Mukherjee S, Rotrosen J, Rubinstein M (1991) The prevalence of tardive dyskinesia. *Journal of Clinical Psychopharmacology*, 11, 34–42.

Wolters EC, Hurwitz TA, Mak E, Teal P, Peppard FR, Remick R, Calne S, Calne DB (1990) Clozapine in the treatment of parkinsonian patients with dopaminomimetic psychosis. *Neurology*, 40, 832–4.

Yamamoto M, Ujike H, Ogawa N (1987) Metoclopramide-induced parkinsonism. *Clinical Neuropharmacology*, 10, 287–9.

5

Essential tremor in the elderly

Rajesh Pahwa and William C Koller

Introduction

Essential tremor (ET) is the most common movement disorder in the elderly. Senile tremor, familial tremor and benign tremor are some of the other terms used to describe ET. Although ET could be a trivial disorder, in some individuals it can be disabling and progressive and could be confused with other neurodegenerative diseases. In this chapter, we will discuss the epidemiology, clinical features and therapy of ET.

Epidemiology

ET is reported from all the regions of the world, indicating a global occurrence (Hornabrook and Nagurney 1976, Haerer et al. 1982, Rautakorpi et al. 1982, Moretti et al. 1983, Aiyesiloju et al. 1984, Rajput et al. 1984, Bharucha et al. 1988, Salemi et al. 1994). Depending on the study methods, prevalence estimates vary widely. The incidence and prevalence of ET increases with advancing age. Hornabrook and Nagurney (1976) examined a region in New Guinea for characteristics and prevalence of ET. They reported no cases of ET under 30 years old, but in the 50–59 year old age group there were 17 cases per 1000, which increased to 41 cases per 1000 over the age of 60 years. Louis et al. (1995) studied a randomized sample of 2117 Medicare recipients (older than 65 years) in the Washington Heights Inwood area in Manhattan, New York. They reported a crude prevalence of 39.2 per 1000 subjects over the age of 65 years. Age is a risk factor for ET. Data from multiple studies show a dramatic increase in the prevalence of ET with aging (see Fig. 5.1).

Genetics

The tendency of ET to run in families has been recognized for many years. Family history positivity varies by report from 17 to 96% (Marshall 1962, Hornabrook and

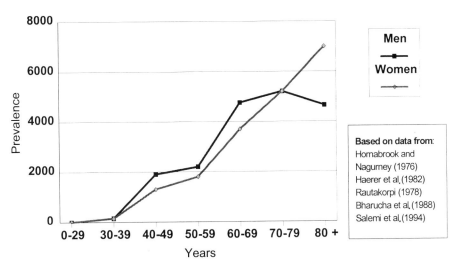

Fig. 5.1   Crude age specific prevalence of ET per 100 000 population.

Nagurney 1976, Rautakorpi 1978, Rajput et al. 1984, Aiyesiloju et al. 1984). The genealogical reports published to date support the assumption that familial ET is inherited in an autosomal dominant manner (Dana 1887, Buckley 1938, Jager and King 1955, Bain et al. 1994). Genetic anticipation, defined as an earlier age of disease onset in successive family generations, is recognized in some families with ET (Critchley 1949, Larsson and Sjogren 1960, Bain et al. 1994, Jankovic et al. 1997). Kaneko et al. (1993) reported an increased number of CAG repeats in the androgen receptor gene in a subject with late onset ET. A tremor indistinguishable from ET may be observed in patients with autosomal dominant idiopathic torsion dystonia (Ozelius et al. 1989). Similarly, individuals with other genetic disorders such as X-linked spino bulbar muscular atrophy (SBMA) (LaSpada et al. 1993) and familial parkinsonism linked to chromosome 4q21–q23 (Polymeropoulos et al. 1996) have tremor similar to ET. Recently, Higgins et al. (1997) reported the results of linkage analysis in a large American family of Czech descent with dominantly inherited ET and genetic anticipation. Genetic loci on chromosome 2p22-p25 established linkage to this region. Their finding suggested that a single highly penetrant gene is sufficient to cause at least one form of ET. Their results suggest that X-linked SBMA and ET may share a similar tremorgenic mechanism.

Gulcher et al. (1997) performed a genome wide scan for familial ET in Iceland. The scan revealed one locus on chromosome 3q13 when the data were analysed either parametrically, assuming an autosomal dominant model, or non parametrically. This gene appears to account for ET in about 80% of the Icelandic families they studied. A more definite assessment on how the linked gene affects these families may be possible only after cloning of the gene.

Clinical manifestations

Tremor is usually the sole manifestation of ET. Tremor is defined as an involuntary oscillation of a body part produced by alternating or synchronous contractions of reciprocally innervated antagonistic muscles (Jankovic and Fahn 1980). Although mild abnormalities of tone and gait may be present, neurological examination is usually otherwise unremarkable (Larsson and Sjogren 1960). Essential tremor is usually postural; that is the tremor is best seen with maintenance of a fixed posture (Koller 1984a). The tremor is attenuated with movement of the limbs towards a target (Critchley 1949, Larsen and Calne 1983, Elble 1986). However, a recent community-based study has emphasized the presence of kinetic tremor in otherwise untreated and previously unknown cases of ET (Louis et al. 1998). Resting tremor is rare but may be more common in elderly subjects.

The most frequent body parts affected by ET are the hands (Bain et al. 1994; Borges et al. 1994; Koller et al. 1994). Usually the tremor is unilateral at the onset, but with time both hands develop tremor (Critchley 1949, Larsson and Sjogren 1960, Longe 1985). Tremor usually causes an adduction–abduction movement of the fingers and a flexion–extension movement of the hands (Critchley 1949, Koller 1984a). Handwriting deteriorates, but true parkinsonian micrographia, when on attempting to write handwriting progressively decreases in size to almost a single line, does not occur. The head is the next most frequently affected body part. Head tremor is usually associated with hand tremor (Longe 1985, Herskovits et al. 1988). The other body parts associated with hand tremor include voice, legs, trunk and chin (Larsson and Sjogren 1960, Rautakorpi 1978, Findley and Gresty 1981, Gerstenbrand et al. 1982, Longe 1985, Massey and Paulson 1985, Herskovits et al. 1988 and see Fig. 5.2).

Tremor progression

Over time tremor amplitude can slowly increase and tremor can spread to unaffected body parts. Critchley (1949) suggested that for the first couple of years there is slow progression of tremor followed by little or no change for several years. Finally, with advancing age tremor may suddenly worsen.

Factors influencing ET

Age influences the expression of ET. The tremor frequency usually declines and amplitude increases with age (Marshall 1962, Herskovits et al. 1988). There is also increasing involvement of multiple body areas with age. Since functional disability in ET is mainly related to tremor amplitude, elderly subjects with ET are more disabled compared to younger subjects (Rajput et al. 1993, Elble 1986). Other factors that influence tremor severity include fatigue, temperature extremes, emotional

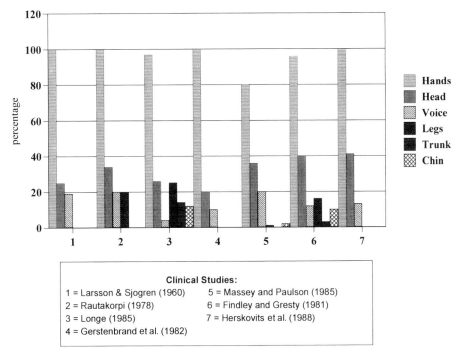

Fig. 5.2   Percentage of body parts affected by ET.

upset, sexual arousal, central nervous system stimulants and diurnal fluctuations in catecholamine levels (Critchley 1949, Wake et al. 1974, Larsen and Calne 1983).

Disability

ET was once known as 'benign essential tremor' because life expectancy is normal (Rajput et al. 1984). However, it is well known that ET can cause significant psychological and functional disability (Rajput et al. 1984, Busenbark et al. 1991, Bain et al. 1994). In fact, approximately 15% of patients with ET referred to a university clinic retired from work due to tremor (Rautakorpi 1978). Busenbark et al. (1991) compared quality of life measured by the Sickness Impact Profile in 753 patients with ET, 145 patients with PD and 87 control subjects. Quality of life was impaired in patients with ET compared to controls, but to a lesser degree than that found in patients with PD. Communication, work, emotional behaviour, home management, recreation and pastimes were particularly impaired in ET (Busenbark et al. 1991). Patients with hand tremors have major functional disability that includes impaired writing, drinking from a cup, feeding and manipulating fine objects (Rajput et al. 1975, Rajput et al. 1984, Busenbark et al. 1991, Bain et al. 1994). Severe voice tremor can make speech very difficult to understand, especially in elderly patients. Although embarrassment is the major disability in patients with head tremor (Pahwa et al. 1995), Rajput (1997) described a patient with head tremor who could not get a haircut at a barber shop!

Differential diagnosis

ET is most commonly misdiagnosed as PD (Koller 1984a), especially in elderly subjects with gait abnormality and bradykinesia related to aging. Resting tremor can occur in ET though its significance is unknown. One autopsy study of nine cases of ET reported resting tremor in six cases in life. Despite the presence of resting tremor Lewy bodies were not found in any of these cases in the substantia nigra (Rajput et al. 1993). All the patients with resting tremor had a clinical history of ET of more than 10 years, all were over 60 years old when the resting tremor developed, and in all the subjects resting tremor was preceded by postural and kinetic tremor (Rajput et al. 1993). Cerebellar degenerative diseases in early stages can also be mistaken for ET in the elderly. Drug-induced tremor, due to lithium, valproic acid and neuroleptics, can also be confused with ET.

Clinical variants

In ET the degree of postural and kinetic tremor may vary. In cases of kinetic predominant tremor a marked dissociation occurs with the postural component being minimal or absent (Biary and Koller 1987). Although cerebellar signs are not found, disability may be severe due to the marked degree of intention tremor.

Task specific tremor (see Table 5.1) is produced mainly by the act of performing certain specific motor activities. The most common task specific tremor is primary writing tremor. Pronation of the arm while writing produces a pronation/supination tremor that is not seen during other movements of the arm (Rothwell et al. 1979, Klawans et al. 1982, Ravits et al. 1985). Other activities involving pronation also result in tremor, though impaired writing is the major source of disability. It is not associated with other neurological abnormalities. Other task specific tremors include those associated with golf club swinging, fist clenching, shaving, combing, using a screwdriver, sewing, cutting with scissors, holding a glass or cup and protruding the tongue (Rothwell et al. 1979, Kachi et al. 1985, Ravits et al. 1985, Rosenbaum and Jankovic 1988). Patients with task specific tremor usually manifest tremor during a specific task involving repetitive and frequently performed movements. Some investigators believe task specific tremor may be a variant of ET, whereas others have suggested it may be a form of dystonia. Primary writing tremor has some characteristics similar to ET because it shares some of the electrophysiologic and clinical characteristics (Kachi et al. 1985, Koller and Martyn 1986). However, there are other investigators (Ravits et al. 1985, Elble et al. 1990) who regard primary writing tremor as a manifestation of writer's cramp.

Table 5.1 Specific tasks associated with tremors

Writing
Golf club swinging
Cutting with scissors
Holding cup or glass
Protruding tongue
Shaving
Combing
Using a screwdriver
Sewing

ET can be restricted to one body part. Isolated tremors of the tongue, chin and voice may occur. Tongue tremor is found if the tongue is tested in the postural position. Often patients are unaware of any difficulty with the tongue tremor. Rarely, tongue tremor can affect speaking and eating. An isolated chin tremor not involving the lips may also occur. An isolated chin tremor, which is stimulus sensitive, has been described in families (Grossman 1957, Lawrence et al. 1968). It may begin at birth and it usually improves with age. Speech involvement can be the predominant or sole symptom in ET (Brown and Simonson 1967, Hachinski et al. 1975). Truncal tremor occurring as a presenting symptom of ET is rare. Heilman (1984) described three patients with the sole symptom of orthostatic tremor of the trunk and the proximal legs. Tremor is present after standing for several seconds, increases with time and can lead to falling (Koller et al. 1986).

Treatment

Although there is no cure for ET, pharmacological and surgical therapies presently available can help control tremor in the majority of patients (see Table 5.2). Tremor of different body parts and various tremor variants may have different levels of pharmacological responsiveness and some patients might not respond to the currently available therapies.

Alcohol

A majority of patients with ET report a dramatic but short term improvement of tremor with alcohol (Growdon et al. 1975, Koller and Biary 1984). However, tolerance to alcohol and fear of addiction make many clinicians avoid the routine use of ethanol in the treatment of ET. Schroeder and Nasrallah (1982) in a retrospective survey of records reported that alcohol abuse was present in 67% of patients with ET. However, Koller (1983) conducted a prospective study and found that the

Table 5.2 Therapies for ET

Medications: definite benefit
Beta adrenergic blockers
Primidone
Alcohol

Medications: possible benefit
Benzodiazepines
Phenobarbital
Carbonic anhydrase inhibitors
Gabapentin

Medications: questionable benefit
Levodopa
Anticholinergics
Amantadine
Clonidine
Trazadone
Verapamil
Nicardipine
Flunarizine
Surgical procedures
Thalamotomy
Thalamic stimulation

prevalence of pathological drinking in ET did not differ from that of patients with other tremor disorders or chronic neurological disease without tremor.

The mechanism of action of ethanol is unknown. Growdon et al. (1975) found that orally administered ethanol produced a dramatic reduction in essential tremor but intra arterial infusion had no effect. They concluded that tremor is reduced by a central mechanism. Boecker et al. (1996) used PET scans to investigate the effect of ethanol on regional cerebral blood flow in six patients with alcohol-responsive ET and age matched controls. Ethanol ingestion led to bilateral decreases of cerebellar blood flow in both patient and control groups. In the patient group additional increase of regional cerebral blood flow was observed in inferior olivary nuclei. They concluded that alcohol suppressed tremor via a reduction of afferent input to the inferior olivary nuclei caused by abnormal cerebellar input. It can be concluded that the occasional use of alcohol before meals is not contraindicated and the risk of alcoholism is low.

Beta adrenergic blockers

Marshall (1968) was among the first investigators to suggest that beta adrenergic blockers might be helpful in the treatment of ET. This was supported by some (Sevitt 1971, Winkler and Young 1974), but not all studies (Foster et al. 1973, Sweet et al. 1974). Numerous investigations have since confirmed the efficacy of propranolol in treating ET (Murray 1972, Tolosa and Loewenson 1975). It is generally estimated that 50–70% of patients with ET involving the hands gain symptomatic benefit from treatment with propranolol. It is not known why some patients do not respond to this treatment. Some reports suggest that chronic propranolol treatment is better in younger patients and those with short duration of disease, though other reports suggest that propranolol is more effective in older patients.

The mechanism of action of beta adrenergic blockers in ET is unknown. Young (1982) proposed a central site of action because he noticed no effect of intravenous or intra arterial propranolol and a delay in the effect of chronic oral therapy. However, other investigators have proposed a peripheral site of action (Jefferson et al. 1979, Huttunen et al. 1984). ET can also be helped by beta-blockers that do not readily penetrate the blood–brain barrier, such as atenolol and sotalol. However, the concentration of atenolol in the cerebrospinal fluid has been noted to be higher than that of propranolol (Taylor et al. 1981). Specific $beta_2$ antagonists (ICI 118551 and LI 32–468) which predominantly act peripherally are effective in decreasing tremor, which further supports a peripheral $beta_2$ mechanism of action (Jefferson et al. 1979, Huttunen et al. 1984).

Although propranolol has the greatest effect on upper extremity tremor, it also suppresses head, voice and tongue tremor (Koller 1984b, Koller 1985, Biary and Koller 1987). In dose response studies of propranolol, 240–320 mg/day was found to be the upper limit of the optimal dose range. However, older patients will not be able to tolerate such high doses. In some subjects sustained release preparations of propranolol can be more effective than normal formulations (Koller 1985).

Other orally active beta-adrenergic blocking drugs such as metoprolol, nadolol, atenolol, timolol and pindolol have also been shown to be beneficial in ET. A comparison study of timolol (5 mg twice daily) and atenolol (100 mg daily) demonstrated that atenolol, unlike timolol, was not effective at the dose employed (Dietrichson and Espen 1981). A double-blind study with metoprolol (150 mg daily) and propranolol (120 mg daily) revealed that both were effective in the treatment of tremor (Calzetti et al. 1981). Another study with the use of metoprolol, atenolol and sotalol found that only sotalol was superior to placebo (Leigh et al. 1983). In general, $beta_1$ antagonists are better than placebo in the treatment of ET but are not as effective as $beta_2$ antagonists (Calzetti et al. 1981, Leigh et al. 1981, Larsen and Teravainen 1981).

Beta-blockers should be used with caution in elderly subjects and in all patients with bronchospastic disease. Relative contraindications include heart failure, second or third degree heart block, asthma or other bronchospastic disease and insulin dependent diabetes. Most of the adverse effects are related to beta-adrenergic blockage. Common adverse effects in elderly subjects include fatigue, weight gain, nausea, diarrhoea, rash, impotence and mental status changes. If a side effect such as impotence occurs with propranolol, changing to a different beta-blocker may result in disappearance of the adverse effect without loss of benefit.

Primidone

When primidone was administered to an epileptic patient with ET, tremor was noticeably reduced (O'Brien et al. 1981). This led to a study with primidone in 20 patients with ET at an initial dose of 125 mg/day, increasing to 750 mg/day (O'Brien et al. 1981). Twelve patients had a good clinical response, but six patients did not tolerate the drug even at the starting dose. Findley and Calzetti (1982) studied 11 patients with ET and reported that tremor was reduced by 66% and over 90% in two patients at a mean dose of 590 mg/day. In a placebo-controlled study using accelerometry, Koller and Royse (1986) reported that primidone (50–1000 mg/day) reduced the amplitude of tremor in both untreated and propranolol treated patients. Primidone decreased tremor more than propranolol. Control of tremor was lost when primidone was replaced by phenobarbital. The most dramatic response frequently occurs during the first week of primidone therapy (Dietrichson and Espen 1987). Although the long-term effect of primidone on ET has not been studied, a few studies suggest that tolerance to primidone may develop (Crystal 1986, Shale and Fahn 1987). However, other investigators found that the antitremor effect of primidone was maintained for a one year period (Koller and Vetere-Overfield 1989, Sasso et al. 1990). Primidone should be used in small doses in the elderly, starting at 25 mg at bedtime and very gradually increasing to 250 mg. In elderly subjects primidone can cause nausea and impaired balance.

The mechanism of action of primidone is unknown. Primidone is converted to two active metabolites: phenyethylmalonamide (PEMA) and phenobarbital. The administration of high doses of PEMA had no effect on tremor (Calzetti et al. 1981) and phenobarbital has only minimal antitremor action (Koller and Royse 1986). Primidone itself, or an unrecognized metabolite, appears to be the responsible agent.

Benzodiazepines

Although there have been very few studies of benzodiazepines in ET, they have been used clinically for a long time in the mistaken belief that tremor was due to anxiety. Thompson et al. (1984) studied the effect of clonazepam in ET and found no improvement in tremor, though sedation was a common side effect. However, subsequently clonazepam has been found to be effective in kinetic predominant tremor (Biary and Koller 1987) and in orthostatic tremor (Heilman 1984, Papa and Gershanik 1988). Huber and Paulson (1988) studied alprazolam in a double-blind, placebo-controlled study in 24 patients with ET. Significant improvement occurred, though half the patients in the study complained of fatigue and sedation. The antitremor effect of benzodiazepines is likely to be due to a secondary reduction in anxiety. In animal models of tremor, diazepam probably suppresses tremor through enhancement of GABAergic neurotransmission (Rappaport et al. 1984).

Benzodiazepines commonly cause confusion and falls in elderly subjects and need to be used with great caution. Unfortunately low doses are unlikely to improve tremor.

Phenobarbital

Phenobarbital has been used for many years for ET, though there have been conflicting reports regarding benefit. Some studies have reported that phenobarbital is more effective than placebo (Baruzzi et al. 1983, Findley and Cleeves 1985). However, Koller and Royse (1986) found no effect of phenobarbital (90 mg/day) in 12 patients with ET. In a double-blind comparison of primidone and phenobarbital, Sasso et al. (1988) found primidone superior to both placebo and phenobarbital in reducing tremor in 13 patients. The effectiveness of phenobarbital in ET is controversial and drowsiness often limits its use in elderly subjects.

Carbonic anhydrase inhibitors

The carbonic anhydrase inhibitor methazolamide has been reported to be highly effective in ET, based on the results of an open label trial involving 28 patients (Muenter et al. 1991). A total of 12 patients reported marked improvement, four reported moderate improvement, four reported mild improvement and eight patients reported no improvement. Head and voice tremor responded particularly well. Although Busenbark et al. (1992) also found in an open label trial that the carbonic anhydrase inhibitor acetazolamide decreased tremor, patients did not report improvement in functional disability. A later double-blind placebo-controlled study (Busenbark et al. 1993) failed to demonstrate any superiority of methazolamide over placebo in any of the measures tested. Only two patients continued the drug. Methazolamide appears to have limited efficacy in the treatment of ET.

Other drugs

Although antiparkinsonian medications such as levodopa and anticholinergic treatment have been used in ET there have been no formal studies. Similarly, Critchley (1972) reported amantadine to be helpful for ET. Other studies have confirmed that an occasional patient with ET may respond to this drug (Manyam 1981, Obeso et al. 1986, Koller 1984a). Other drugs that have been reported to have questionable benefit in ET include clonidine (Caccia and Mangoni 1985, Koller et al. 1986), thymoxamine (Mai and Olsen 1981), trazadone (McLeod and White 1986), mephenesin (Critchley 1972), nifedipine (Topaktas et al 1987), verapamil (Topaktas et al. 1987), nicardipine (Jimenez-Jimenez et al. 1994), flunarizine (Curran and Lang 1993) and gabapentin (Pahwa et al. 1998).

Botulinum toxin injections

Botulinum toxin intramuscular injection, which is mainly used for focal dystonias, has been used for the treatment of ET. Botulinum toxin causes muscle paresis by acting on the peripheral nerve endings to block release of acetylcholine. In an open label trial, Jankovic and Schwartz (1991) reported that botulinum toxin injections reduced various body tremors in 67% of treated patients. Pahwa et al. (1995) studied botulinum toxin in a double-blind study in head tremor and found that 40% of the patients had improvement of their tremor.

Thalamotomy

Stereotaxic thalamotomy is an effective procedure for the treatment of ET. Improvement in technical aspects and advances in neurophysiological location of the lesion site have renewed the interest in thalamotomy. The ventralis oralis posterior (VOP) and the ventralis intermedius (VIM) thalamic nuclei receive cerebellar afferents and are the most common targets for the treatment of tremor (Bertrand et al. 1969, Narabayashi and Ohye 1980). Stereotaxic thalamotomy is performed with the use of mild sedation and local anaesthesia (Goldman and Kelly 1992). The stereotaxic coordinates are generated by use of the computerized tomographic scanning and computerized programs. Goldman and Kelly (1992) reported outcome after thalamotomy in seven patients who underwent unilateral thalamotomy and in one patient who underwent bilateral thalamotomy. At follow-up (mean 17.3 months) all patients had marked improvement of the targeted tremor. Jankovic et al. (1995) reported that after a mean follow-up of 53.4 months, 83% of ET patients had cessation of or moderate to marked improvement in their contralateral tremor with a concomitant improvement in function. Shahzadi et al. (1995) reported that 86% of the ET patients had significant postoperative improvement in tremor, though 42% of the patients had recurrence of tremor after five years. Unilateral thalamotomy in ET has a mortality rate of less than 0.3%, mostly related to postoperative complications. Confusion, contralateral hemiparesis, dysarthria and seizures can occur in the postoperative period, but usually resolve rapidly. Bilateral thalamotomy is associated with more severe and long lasting complications such as severe dysarthria and permanent cognitive impairment.

Thalamic stimulation

It had long been observed that during a thalamotomy procedure stimulation of the target site had the same effects as its destruction. This paradoxical effect is related to stimulus frequency and cannot be induced under 100 Hz stimulation. The main advantages of stimulation compared to thalamotomy include reversibility, the ability to change stimulus parameters to increase efficacy or reduce side effects, and the fact that bilateral operations can be performed without causing permanent dysarthria (Benabid et al. 1989). The mechanics of lead placement are similar to thalamotomy, though the lead is internalized under the skin and connected to an implantable pulse generator, which is placed under the clavicle. The disadvantages of stimulation include the cost of the system, the presence of foreign material and the future need to replace the energy source. Thalamic stimulation results in a significant reduction in tremor and a marked reduction in global disability (Benabid et al. 1991, 1993, Koller et al. 1997). Complications related to stimulation are usually minor and include paraesthesia, headache, disequilibrium, gait disorder, dysarthria and localized pain (Benabid et al. 1991, 1993, Koller et al. 1997). Thalamotomy and thalamic stimulation should be reserved for patients with severe drug resistant tremor causing marked functional disability.

REFERENCES

Aiyesiloju AB, Osuntodum BO, Bademosi O, Adeuja AO (1984) Hereditary neurodegenerative disorders in Nigerian Africans. *Neurology* 34, 361–2.

Bain PG, Findley LJ, Thompson PD (1994) A study of hereditary essential tremor. *Brain* 117, 805–24.

Baruzzi A, Procaccianti G, Martinelli, P (1983) Phenobarbital and propranolol in essential tremor: a double-blind controlled clinical trial. *Neurology* 33, 3, 296–300.

Benabid AL, Pollak P, Gervason C (1991) Long-term suppression of tremor by chronic stimulation of the ventral intermediate thalamic nucleus. *Lancet*, 337, 403–6.

Benabid AL, Pollak P, Hommel M (1989) Treatment of Parkinson tremor by chronic stimulation of the ventral intermediate nucleus of the thalamus. *Revue Neurologique*, 145, 4, 320–3.

Benabid AL, Pollack P, Seigneuret E (1993) Chronic VIM thalamic stimulation in Parkinson's disease, essential tremor and extrapyramidal dyskinesias. *Acta Neurochirurgica. Supplementum (Wien)*, 58, 39–44.

Bertrand C, Hardy J, Molina-Negro P, Martinez SN (1969) Tremor of attitude. *Confinia Neurologica*, 31, 37–41.

Bharucha NE, Bharucha EP, Bharucha AE, Bhise AV, Schoenberg BS (1988) Prevalence of essential tremor in the Parsi community of Bombay, India. *Archives of Neurology*, 45, 907–8.

Biary N, Koller W (1987) Kinetic predominant essential tremor: successful treatment with clonazepam. *Neurology* 37, 3, 471–4.

Boecker H, Wills AJ, Ceballos-Baumann A, Samuel M, Thompson PD, Findley LJ, Brooks DJ (1996) The effect of ethanol on alcohol-responsive essential tremor: a positron emission tomography study. *Annals of Neurology*, 39, 5, 650–8.

Borges V, Ferraz HB, De-Andrade LA (1994) Essential tremor: clinical characterization in a sample of 176 patients. *Arquivos De Neuro-psiquiatria*, 52, 2,161–5.

Brown JR, Simonson J (1967) Organic voice tremor. *Neurology*, 17, 520–7.

Buckley P (1938) Familial tremor. *Proceedings of the Royal Society of Medicine*, 31, 297.

Busenbark KL, Nash J, Nash S, Hubble JP, Koller WC (1991) Is essential tremor benign? *Neurology*, 41, 12, 1982–3.

Busenbark KL, Pahwa R, Hubble J, Hopfensperger K, Koller WC, Pogrebra K (1993) Double-blind controlled study of methazolamide in the treatment of essential tremor. *Neurology* 43, 1045–7 (published erratum *Neurology* 1993, 43, 1910).

Busenbark KL, Pahwa R, Hubble J, Koller WC (1992) The effect of acetazolamide on essential tremor: an open label trial. *Neurology*, 42, 1394–5.

Caccia MR, Mangoni A (1985) Clonidine in essential tremor: preliminary observations from an open trial. *Journal of Neurology*, 232, 55–7.

Calzetti S, Findley LJ, Gresty MA, Perucca E, Richens A (1981) Metoprolol and propranolol in essential tremor: a double-blind, controlled study. *Journal of Neurology, Neurosurgery, and Psychiatry*, 44, 814–19.

Critchley E (1972) Clinical manifestations of essential tremor. *Journal of Neurology, Neurosurgery, and Psychiatry*, 35, 365–72.

Critchley M (1949) Observations on essential (heredofamilial) tremor. *Brain* 72, 113–39.

Crystal HA (1986) Duration of effectiveness of primidone in essential tremor [letter]. *Neurology*, 36, 11, 1543.

Curran T, Lang AE (1993) Flunarizine in essential tremor. *Clinical Neuropharmacology*, 16, 460–3.

Dana CL (1887) Hereditary tremor, a hitherto undescribed form of motor neurosis. *American Journal of Medical Science*, 94, 386–93.

Dietrichson P, Espen E (1981) Effects of timolol and atenolol on benign essential tremor: placebo-controlled studies based on quantitative tremor recording. *Journal of Neurology, Neurosurgery, and Psychiatry*, 44, 8, 677–83.

Dietrichson P, Espen E (1987) Primidone and propranolol in essential tremor: a study based on quantitative tremor recording and plasma anticonvulsant levels. *Acta Neurologica Scandinavica*, 75, 5, 332–40.

Elble RJ (1986) Physiologic and essential tremor. *Neurology*, 36, 2, 225–31.

Elble RJ, Moody C, Higgins C (1990) Primary writing tremor. A form of focal dystonia? *Movement Disorders*, 5, 2, 118–26.

Findley LJ, Calzetti S (1982) Double-blind controlled study of primidone in essential tremor: preliminary results. *British Medical Journal*, 285, 608.

Findley LJ, Cleeves L (1985) Phenobarbital in essential tremor. *Neurology*, 35, 1784–7.

Findley LJ, Gresty MA (1981) Tremor. *British Journal of Hospital Medicine*, 26, 16–32.

Foster JB, Longley BP, Stewart W (1973) Propranolol in essential tremor. *Lancet* 1, 817, 1455.

Gerstenbrand F, Klingler D, Pfeiffer B (1982) Essential tremor: phenomenology and epidemiology. *Nervenarzt*, 53, 1, 46–53.

Goldman MS, Kelly PJ (1992) Stereotactic thalamotomy for medically intractable essential tremor. *Stereotactic and Functional Neurosurgery*, 58, 22–5.

Grossman BJ (1957) Trembling of the chin – an inheritable dominant character. *Pediatrics*, 19, 4535.

Growdon JH, Shahani BT, Young RR (1975) The effect of alcohol on essential tremor. *Neurology*, 28, 259–62.

Gulcher JR, Jonsson P, Kong A, Kristjansson K, Frigge ML, Karason A (1997) Mapping of familial essential tremor gene FET1 to chromosome 3q13. *Nature Genetics*, 17, 84–7.

Hachinski VC, Thomsen IV, Buch NH (1975) The nature of primary vocal tremor. *Canadian Journal of Neurological Sciences*, 2, 195–7.

Haerer AF, Anderson DW, Schoenberg BS (1982) Prevalence of essential tremor: Results from the Copiah County study. *Archives of Neurology*, 39, 750–1.

Heilman KM (1984) Orthostatic tremor. *Archives of Neurology*, 4, 880–1.

Herskovits E, Figueroa E, Mangone C (1988) Hereditary essential tremor in Buenos Aires (Argentina). *Arquivos de Neuro-psiquiatria*, 46, 3, 238–47.

Higgins JJ, Pho Lt, Nee LE (1997) A gene (ETM) for essential tremor maps to chromosome 2p22-p25. *Movement Disorders*, 12, 859–64.

Hornabrook RW, Nagurney JP (1976) Essential tremor in Papua New Guinea. *Brain*, 99, 659–72.

Huber SJ, Paulson GW (1988) Efficacy of alprazolam for essential tremor. *Neurology*, 38, 241–3.

Huttunen J, Teravainen H, Larsen TA (1984) Beta-adrenoreceptor antagonists in essential tremor. *Lancet*, 1, 857.

Jager BV, King T (1955) Hereditary tremor. *Archives of Internal Medicine*, 95, 788–93.

Jankovic J, Beach J, Pandolfo M, Patel PI (1997) Familial essential tremor in four kindreds. Prospects for genetic mapping. *Archives of Neurology*, 54, 289–94.

Jankovic J, Cardoso F, Grossman RG, Hamilton WJ (1995) Outcome after stereotactic thalamotomy for parkinsonian, essential, and other types of tremor. *Neurosurgery*, 37, 680–6, Discussion 686–7.

Jankovic J, Fahn S (1980) Physiologic and pathologic tremors: Diagnosis, mechanism and management. *Annals of Internal Medicine*, 93, 460–5.

Jankovic J, Schwartz K (1991) Botulinum toxin treatment of tremors. *Neurology*, 41, 1185–8.

Jefferson D, Jenner P, Marsden CD (1979) Relationship between plasma propranolol concentration and relief of essential tremor. *Journal of Neurology, Neurosurgery, and Psychiatry*, 42, 831–7.

Jiminez-Jiminez FJ, Garcia-Ruiz PJ, Cabrera-Valdivia F (1994) Nicardipine versus propranolol in essential tremor. *Acta Neurologica (Napoli)*, 16, 184–8.

Kachi T, Rothwell JC, Cowan JM, Marsden CD (1985) Primary writing tremor: its relationship to benign essential tremor. *Journal of Neurology, Neurosurgery, and Psychiatry*, 48, 545–50.

Kaneko K, Igarashi S, Miyatake T, Tsuji S (1993) Essential tremor and CAG repeats in the androgen receptor gene. *Neurology*, 43, 1618–19.

Klawans HL, Glantz R, Tanner CM, Goetz CG (1982) Primary writing tremor: a selective action tremor. *Neurology*, 32, 2, 203–6.

Koller WC (1983) Alcoholism in essential tremor. *Neurology*, 33, 8, 1074–6.

Koller WC (1984a) Diagnosis and treatment of tremor. *Neurologic Clinics*, 2, 499–514.

Koller WC (1984b) Propranolol therapy for essential tremor of the head. *Neurology*, 34, 8, 1077–9.

Koller WC (1985) Long-acting propranolol in essential tremor. *Neurology*, 35, 1, 108–10.

Koller WC, Biary N (1984) Effect of alcohol on tremors: comparison with propranolol. *Neurology*, 34, 2, 221–2.

Koller WC, Busenbark K, Miner K (1994) The relationship of essential tremor to other movement disorders: report on 678 patients. Essential Tremor Study Group. *Annals of Neurology*, 35, 6, 717–23.

Koller WC, Glatt S, Biary N, Rubino FA (1987) Essential tremor variants: Effect of treatment. *Clinical Neuropharmacology*, 10, 342–50.

Koller WC, Herbster G, Cone S (1986) Clonidine in the treatment of essential tremor. *Movement Disorders*, 1, 4, 235–7.

Koller WC, Martyn B (1986) Writing tremor: its relationship to essential tremor. *Journal of Neurology, Neurosurgery, and Psychiatry*, 49, 2, 220.

Koller W, Pahwa R, Busenbark K, Hubble J, Wilkinson S, Lang A, Tuite P, Sime E, Lazano A, Hauser R, Malapira T, Smith D, Tarsy D, Miyawaki E, Norregaard T, Kormos T, Olanow CW (1997) High frequency unilateral thalamic stimulation in the treatment of essential and parkinsonian tremor. *Annals of Neurology*, 42, 3, 292–9.

Koller WC, Royse VL (1986) Efficacy of primidone in essential tremor. *Neurology*, 36, 1, 121–4.

Koller WC, Vetere-Overfield B (1989) Acute and chronic effects of propranolol and primidone in essential tremor. *Neurology*, 39, 12, 1587–8.

Larsen TA, Calne DB (1983) Essential tremor. *Clinical Neuropharmacology*, 6, 3, 185–206.

Larsen TA, Teravainen H (1981) Beta-blockers in essential tremor [letter]. *Lancet*, 2, 533.

Larsson T, Sjogren T (1960) Essential tremor: A clinical and genetic population study. *Acta Psychiatrica et Neurologica Scandinavica*, 36, Suppl. 144, 1–176.

LaSpada AR, Wilson EM, Lubahn DB, Harding AE, Fischbeck KH (1993) Meiotic instability and genotype-phenotype correlation of trinucleotide repeat in X-linked spinal and bulbar muscular atrophy. *Nature Genetics*, 4, 301–4.

Lawrence BM, Matthews W, Diggle JA (1968) Hereditary quivering of the chin. *Archives of Disease in Childhood*, 43, 249–54.

Leigh PN, Jefferson D, Twomey A, Marsden CD (1983) Beta-adrenoreceptor mechanisms in essential tremor; a double-blind placebo-controlled trial of metoprolol, sotalol and atenolol. *Journal of Neurology, Neurosurgery, and Psychiatry*, 46, 8, 710–15.

Leigh PN, Marsden CD, Twomey A, Jefferson D (1981) Beta-adrenoceptor antagonists and essential tremor. *Lancet*, 1, 1106.

Longe AC (1985) Essential tremor in Nigerians: a prospective study of 35 cases. *East African Medical Journal*, 62, 9, 672–6.

Louis ED, Ford B, Wendt KJ, Cameron G (1998) Clinical characteristics of essential tremor: data from a community-based study. *Movement Disorders*, 13, 803–8.

Louis ED, Marder K, Cote L, Pullman S, Ford B, Wilder D, Tang MX, Lantigua R, Gurland B, Mayeux R (1995) Differences in the prevalence of essential tremor among elderly African

Americans, whites, and Hispanics in northern Manhattan, NY. *Archives of Neurology*, 52, 12, 1201–5.

Mai J, Olsen RB (1981) Depression of essential tremor by alpha-adrenergic blockade. *Journal of Neurology, Neurosurgery, and Psychiatry*, 44, 1171.

Manyam BV (1981) Amantadine in essential tremor. *Annals of Neurology*, 9, 198–9.

Marshall J (1962) Observations on essential tremor. *Journal of Neurology, Neurosurgery, and Psychiatry*, 25, 122–5.

Marshall J (1968) Handbook of Clinical Neurology. Amsterdam: North-Holland Publishing Company.

Massey EW, Paulson GW (1985) Essential vocal tremor: clinical characteristics and response to therapy. *Southern Medical Journal*, 78, 3, 316–17.

McLeod NA, White LE (1986) Trazodone in essential tremor. *Journal of the American Medical Association*, 256, 2675–6.

Moretti G, Calzetti S, Quartucci G, Gallo A, Scoditti U, Nalati T, Rizzi C, D'Ambrosio E (1983) Epidemiological study on tremor in the aged [Article in Italian]. *Minerva Medica*, 74, 1701–5.

Muenter MD, Daube JR, Caviness JN, Miller PM (1991) Treatment of essential tremor with methazolamide. *Mayo Clinic Proceedings*, 66, 991–7.

Murray TJ (1972) Treatment of essential tremor with propranolol. *Canadian Medical Association Journal*, 107, 10, 984–6.

Narabayashi H, Ohye C (1980) Importance of microstereoencephalotomy for tremor alleviation. *Applied Neurophysiology*, 43, 222–7.

O'Brien MD, Upton AR, Toseland PA. (1981) Benign familial tremor treated with Primidone. *British Medical Journal*, 282, 178–80.

Obeso JA, Luquin MR, Artieda J, Martinez-Lage JM (1986) Amantadine may be useful in essential tremor. *Annals of Neurology*, 19, 99–100.

Ozelius L, Kramer PL, Moskowitz CB, Kwiatkowski DJ, Brin MF, Bressman SB, Schuback DE, Falk CT, Risch N, de Leon D (1989) Human gene for torsion dystonia located on chromosome 9q32–q34. *Neuron*, 2, 1427–34

Pahwa R, Busenbark K, Swanson-Hyland EF, Dubinsky RM, Hubble JP, Gray C, Koller WC (1995) Botulinum toxin treatment of essential head tremor. *Neurology*, 45, 822–4.

Pahwa R, Lyons K, Hubble JP, Busenbark KL, Rienerth JD, Pahwa A, Koller WC (1998) Double-blind controlled trial of gabapentin in essential tremor. *Movement Disorders*, 13, 465–7.

Papa SM, Gershanik OS (1988) Orthostatic tremor: an essential tremor variant? *Movement Disorders*, 3, 97–108.

Polymeropolous MH, Higgins JJ, Golbe LI, Johnson WG, Ide SE, Di Iorio G, Sanges G, Stenroos ES, Pho LT, Schaffer AA, Lazzarini AM, Nussbaum RL, Duvoisin RC (1996) Mapping of a gene for Parkinson's disease to chromosome 4q21–q23. *Science*, 274, 1197–9.

Rajput AH (1997) *Movement Disorders: Neurologic Principles and Practice*, New York: McGraw-Hill. pp. 673–86.

Rajput AH, Jamieson H, Hirsch S, Quraishi A (1975) Relative efficacy of alcohol and propranolol in action tremor. *Canadian Journal of Neurological Sciences*, 2, 31–5.

Rajput AH, Offord KP, Beard CM, Kurland LT (1984) Essential tremor in Rochester, Minnesota: a 45 year study. *Journal of Neurology, Neurosurgery, and Psychiatry*, 47, 5, 466–70.

Rajput AH, Rozdilsky B, Ang L, Rajput A (1993) Significance of parkinsonian manifestations in essential tremor. *Canadian Journal of Neurological Sciences*, 20, 2114–17.

Rappaport MS, Gentry RT, Schneider DR, Dole VP (1984) Ethanol effects on harmaline-induced tremor and increase of cerebellar cyclic GMP. *Life Sciences*, 34, 49–56.

Rautakorpi I (1978) Essential tremor: An epidemiological, clinical, and genetic study. Dissertation, Turku, Finland.

Rautakorpi I, Takala J, Marttila RJ, Sievers K, Rinne UK (1982) Essential tremor in a Finnish population. *Acta Neurologica Scandinavica*, 66, 58–67.

Ravits J, Hallet M, Baker M, Wilkins D (1985) Primary writing tremor and myoclonic writer's cramp. *Neurology*, 35, 1387–91.

Rosenbaum F, Jankovic J (1988) Focal task-specific tremor and dystonia: categorization of occupational movement disorders. *Neurology*, 38, 522–7.

Rothwell JC, Traub MM, Marsden CD (1979) Primary writing tremor. *Journal of Neurology, Neurosurgery, and Psychiatry*, 42, 1106–14.

Salemi G, Savettieri G, Rocca WA, Meneghini F, Saporito V, Morgante L, Reggio A, Grigoletto F, Di Perri R (1994) Prevalence of essential tremor: a door-to-door survey in Terrasini, Sicily. Sicilian Neuro-Epidemiologic Study Group. *Neurology*, 44, 61–4.

Sasso E, Perucca E, Calzetti S (1988) Double-blind comparison of primidone and phenobarbital in essential tremor. *Neurology*, 38, 5, 808–10.

Sasso E, Perucca E, Fava N, Calzetti S (1990) Primidone in the long-term treatment of essential tremor: A prospective study with computerized quantitative analysis. *Clinical Neuropharmacology*, 67, 76.

Schroeder D, Nasrallah HA (1982) High alcoholism rate in patients with essential tremor. *American Journal of Psychiatry*, 139, 11, 1471–3.

Sevitt I (1971) The effect of adrenergic beta-receptor blocking drugs on tremor. *Practitioner*, 207, 677–8.

Shahzadi S, Tasker RR, Lozano A (1995) Thalamotomy for essential and cerebellar tremor. *Stereotactic and Functional Neurosurgery*, 65, 11–17.

Shale H, Fahn S (1987) Response of essential tremor to treatment with primidone. *Neurology*, 37, 123.

Sweet RD, Blumberg J, Lee JE, Mcdowell FH (1974) Propranolol treatment of essential tremor. *Neurology*, 24, 64–7.

Taylor EA, Jefferson D, Carroll JD, Turner P (1981) Cerebrospinal fluid concentrations of propranolol, pindolol and atenolol in man: evidence for central actions of beta-adrenoceptor antagonists. *British Journal of Clinical Pharmacology*, 12, 549–59.

Thompson C, Lang A, Parkes JD, Marsden CD (1984) A double-blind trial of clonazepam in benign essential tremor. *Clinical Neuropharmacology*, 7, 83–8.

Tolosa ES, Loewenson RB (1975) Essential tremor: treatment with propranolol. *Neurology*, 25, 11, 1041–4.

Topaktas S, Onur R, Dalkara T (1987) Calcium channel blockers and essential tremor. *European Neurology*, 27, 114–19.

Wake A, Takahashi Y, Onishi T, Nakashima T, Yasumoto I (1974) Treatment of essential tremor by behaviour therapy. Use of Jacobson's progressive relaxation method. *Seishin Shinkeigaku Zasshi, Psychiatrica et Neurologia Japonica (Tokyo)*, 76, 7, 509–17.

Winkler GF, Young RR (1974) Efficacy of chronic propranolol therapy in action tremors of the familial, senile or essential varieties. *New England Journal of Medicine*, 290, 984–8.

Young RR (1982) Essential–familial tremor and other action tremors. *Seminars in Neurology*, 2, 386–91.

6

Gait apraxia and multi-infarct states

Richard Liston and Raymond C Tallis

Introduction

There is an extensive literature on gait apraxia or 'higher-level gait disorders' as they have recently been called (Nutt et al. 1993). The term encompasses walking difficulties that are out of proportion to those that would be expected on the basis of the bedside neurological examination and that are best explained by disorders of integration of cerebral activity. There have been few attempts to formulate unifying theories regarding these gait disorders and this is borne out by the large number of synonyms used to describe what are essentially the same or very similar gait disorders (see Table 6.1). In this chapter, we shall attempt to unravel the conceptual muddle that surrounds these gait disorders. Firstly, we shall review the historical accounts of such disorders in the literature. Secondly, we shall describe a recent, though unsatisfactory classification. Thirdly, we shall propose our own classification based on neuroanatomical and neurophysiological correlations drawn largely from the existing literature on gait initiation, especially in relation to Parkinson's disease (PD). Finally, we will suggest how a clearer understanding of the disease processes may aid in developing rational approaches to therapeutic interventions. Throughout this chapter we shall focus particularly on the higher-level gait disorders associated with cerebral multi-infarct states (CMIS) and refer to these as vascular higher-level gait disorders (vascular HLGDs). It must however be remembered that, along with CMIS, many other disease processes can lead to these gait disorders: many of the original descriptions were of frontal lobe tumours.

Gait apraxia and the frontal lobes

It has been recognized for well over a century that frontal lobe lesions can cause gait impairment, particularly in elderly patients. Bruns (1892) described impairment of gait secondary to such lesions and named this condition 'ataxia of gait'. He described two patients with frontal lobe tumours, and two patients with frontal lobe damage as part of a more diffuse disease process. Originally many authors

Table 6.1 Synonyms for HLGDs

Gait apraxia
Frontal ataxia
Frontal disequilibrium
Frontal ataxia and disequilibrium
Frontal gait disorder
Subcortical disequilibrium
Marche à petit pas
Vascular pseudoparkinsonism
Lower body parkinsonism
Arteriosclerotic parkinsonism
Gait disorder of Binswanger's disease
Cautious gait
Isolated gait ignition failure

thought that these 'ataxic gaits' were secondary to cerebellar lesions, the precise location of direct or indirect damage to the cerebellum being unknown. Bruns himself thought that the 'cerebellar' signs were due to compression of the cerebellum from frontal tumours or disruption of the fronto-ponto-cerebellar tract. Gerstmann and Schilder (1926) described two similar cases, one of whom had a frontal glioma, and they first used the term 'gait apraxia'. Van Bogaert and Martin (1929) subsequently used the term 'frontal disequilibrium' and described the gait disorder in one patient with a frontal lobe abscess and in another with a frontal lobe glioma. Austregesilo and Fortes (1936) suggested that the cumbersome term 'frontal ataxia and disequilibrium' be used, suggesting two distinct components of the disorder. Earlier, Gordon (1917) had concluded that the frontal lobe is the centre for equilibrium and orientation. In their seminal descriptions, Meyer and Barron (1960) subsequently described seven cases using the term 'apraxia of gait', which they preferred to 'frontal ataxia'. Their aim was to describe the deterioration in gait that occurs from cerebral damage particularly in the region of the frontal lobes, although they did concede that some of their cases suffered from diffuse cerebral damage. The authors clearly documented that the disease process was not cerebellar in nature. They defined 'apraxia of gait' as an inability to use the lower limbs in the act of walking, which could not be accounted for by demonstrable sensory weakness or motor impairment. They speculated that any lesion such as tumour, abscess or arteriosclerosis, which involved mesial aspects of the frontal and parietal lobes, could produce the syndrome. They argued that the primary difficulty appeared to be in the initiation of movement, particularly in the abstract performance of motor movement such as taking the first step, kicking an imaginary ball or writing numbers with the feet. They concluded that apraxia of gait is a 'trans-cortical innervatory paralysis': the disturbance of gait initiation being at a cortical level with the motor mechanism for movement of the legs, at lower levels, remaining intact.

From the above historical descriptions, it is clear that frontal lobe damage can cause a syndrome with two distinct components. The first is difficulty with movement initiation involving varying combinations of gait ignition failure, shuffling, freezing and difficulty making turns. The second component common to these descriptions is disequilibrium or poor balance. In virtually all the above accounts, the descriptions of disordered gait patterns include these two basic clinical findings.

Vascular parkinsonism and cerebral multi-infarct states

Critchley (1929) gave wider currency to the idea of 'arteriosclerotic (vascular) parkinsonism' and described rigidity and slowness of movements in the syndrome along with the absence of tremor. He stated that the characteristics of these gaits were essentially the same as those described by Marie (1901) as 'marche à petit pas', which occurred in état lacunaire. Some of the patients he described, however, may have had multiple system atrophy, progressive supranuclear palsy or corticobasal ganglionic degeneration, which limits our ability to interpret his findings. Nonetheless, the characteristic gait was one with short steps, shuffling, difficulty initiating movements, difficulty with turning, vertigo, giddiness and poor balance. This description is clearly similar to that described occurring secondary to frontal lobe damage. Critchley's description of the gaits as being due to a weakness of walking out of proportion to the relative strength of the individual movements of the limbs is also very similar to Meyer and Barron's description of gait apraxia.

Fitzgerald and Jankovic (1989) subsequently studied 10 patients with marked gait difficulty and minimal upper limb involvement and compared them to 100 patients with typical PD. They used the phrase 'lower body parkinsonism' to describe patients in the former group who, compared to PD patients, had a lower mean duration of symptoms, more initial complaints of disordered gait and were more likely to have hypertension. Of this group 20% responded to levodopa compared to 96% of the patients with PD. They also stated that gait disturbance and postural instability were the dominant motor features, similar to Critchley's patients. Clinically the gait disturbances manifested as slowness, shuffling, intermittent freezing, initiation failure, turning difficulties and response to visual cues. They speculated that the ability to overcome freezing by visual cues (discussed later) suggests that in patients with lower body parkinsonism and PD, the programme for the learned movement (gait) is preserved but there is an inability to access it. They proposed that chronic subcortical ischaemia secondary to hypertensive vascular disease might be responsible for the disorder resulting in disconnection between basal ganglia (BG) and the supplementary motor area. We will elaborate further on these neuro-anatomical and neuro-physiological correlations later in this chapter.

Chang et al. (1992) investigated 250 patients with parkinsonism and performed magnetic resonance imaging (MRI) on 13 patients who did not respond or showed a poor response to levodopa. Of this group 11/13 (85%) had ischaemic lesions that were thought to account for their parkinsonism. Bradykinesia, rigidity and gait disturbance was prominent but resting tremor was absent. They did not comment on the presence or absence of disequilibrium. Three types of lesions were common: frontal lobe infarcts, basal ganglia lacunar infarcts and periventricular and deep subcortical white matter lesions. They concluded that parkinsonian patients who show poor or no response to levodopa therapy should be investigated for a vascular aetiology.

Thompson and Marsden (1987) described 12 patients with Binswanger's disease or subcortical vascular states, all of whom had longstanding hypertension and who presented with walking difficulty. They described the gait as combining 'bradykinesia' and 'ataxia'. Gait abnormality was described as being out of proportion to the observed clinical findings on bedside testing and gait ignition failure, shuffling and disequilibrium were again described. With the patient either seated or lying, upper limb mobility and facial expressions were relatively well preserved. Patients presented with insidious decline in mobility, difficulty walking and falls. Diagnosis was made based on CT scan evidence of bilateral low attenuation white matter lesions throughout the frontal and parietal lobes. Four patients also had lacunar infarcts. The authors suggested that the disorder was similar to that seen in frontal lobe lesions, hydrocephalus and 'senile disorders of gait'. They proposed that the syndrome is due to damage to afferent and efferent interconnections of the leg areas between the motor cortex, the supplementary motor cortex, the basal ganglia, and the cerebellum. As already suggested, there is obvious and significant overlap between the gait disorders associated with frontal lobe damage from either vascular or nonvascular causes, vascular parkinsonism and Binswanger's disease. In addition, different disease processes, including frontal lesions, diffuse cerebral disease, multiple lacunar infarcts, basal ganglia infarcts and subcortical ischaemia, may lead to very similar gait disorders. The similarity of all these disorders raises the question as to whether they can be understood in terms of a unifying theory.

Current classifications

Nutt et al. (1993) have aimed to do just that. In an attempt at clarification, they group these gait disorders together as 'higher-level gait disorders' on the basis that the abnormal gaits are due to disorders of the highest sensorimotor systems and cannot be accounted for by the neurological signs, if any, that are elicited by standard bedside examination. Basic motor functions such as power and coordination should be intact, as should sensory function with no visual, labyrinthine impairment. Nutt et al. (1993) divided these gait disorders into five groups: cautious gait, isolated gait ignition failure, subcortical disequilibrium, frontal disequilibrium, and frontal gait disorder. However, this classification is confusing in that some types of gaits are classified according to presumed location (frontal gait disorder), others according to clinical phenomenology (isolated gait ignition failure, cautious gait) and others according to a mixture of the two (frontal disequilibrium, subcortical disequilibrium). In the next section we shall develop this classification, attempting to relate the clinical phenomena to presumed sites of lesions.

Gait ignition – the interaction between the basal ganglia and the frontal lobes

As these gait disorders probably represent types of motor programming failure similar to those seen in PD, we shall propose possible locations of infarcts within the pathways controlling the motor programming of normal gait. But first we need to understand how this system works normally, how it can malfunction in PD and how this can give us insights into what is happening in vascular HLGDs.

The motor cortex contains several distinct areas in the frontal lobes, which receive inputs from sensory pathways, motor control structures and modulatory pathways, including the thalamus and BG. This cluster of distinct frontal fields is fundamentally involved in movement planning and performance (Donoghue and Sanes 1994). The most widely recognized fields are:

1 the primary motor cortex (M1), which probably controls muscle force and the direction of movement;
2 the premotor area (PMA), which is probably involved in coupling environmental cues to motor acts and may be responsible for the motor response to *external* stimuli (Chen et al. 1995 and see Fig. 6.1)
3 the supplementary motor area (SMA), which is possibly involved in the preparation and execution of complex voluntary movements, especially if these movements are learned, and may thus be responsible for the *internal* cueing and guidance of acquired, skilled motor acts of the limbs (Roland et al. 1980, Chen et al. 1995, Thaler et al. 1995 and see Fig. 6.1).

In the case of normal walking – an internally cued, well learned motor act – it has been suggested that the SMA fires just prior to gait ignition. This probably reflects preparatory activity for each subcomponent of a movement sequence (Georgiou et al. 1993). This preparatory activity may represent submovement programme selection, i.e. a complex set of instructions for each submovement, which

Externally cued movement

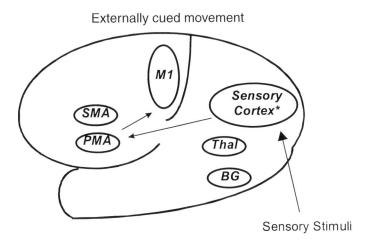

Sensory Stimuli

Internally cued movement

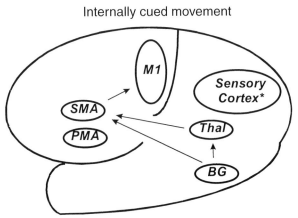

Fig. 6.1   Mechanism of gait ignition. BG, basal ganglia; M1, primary motor cortex; PMA, premotor area; SMA, supplementary motor area; Thal, ventro-lateral nucleus of the thalamus. *Visual, vestibular and proprioceptive inputs.

is subsequently sent to the M1. Activity in the SMA is switched off by phasic activity generated by the BG. This probably provides a nonspecific cue both to trigger the submovement (i.e. SMA sends the instructions to the M1) and to instruct the SMA to prepare for the next (Phillips et al. 1994). This allows the submovement to be executed normally and on time (Georgiou et al. 1993). It is this interaction, between phasic activity from the BG and premotor activity in the SMA, which is responsible for the smooth running of predictable, learned, automatic movement sequences that depend on *internal cues*. The sequence of activation is different when movements occur in response to *external cues*. In this situation the BG/SMA pathways could, according to this theory, be bypassed: sensory information from the environment feeds directly into the PMA through visual, auditory and proprioceptive pathways and the PMA subsequently activates the M1 (Marsden 1989).

Motor programming failure in PD and the response to external cues

In pathological situations such as PD it has been argued that there is disordered cueing from the BG: a disturbance in internal rhythm formation in the BG means that the SMA is not switched off on time (Georgiou et al. 1993, Freeman et al. 1993). Submovements are therefore not triggered and no new preparatory activity occurs in the SMA. This causes some of the classical clinical features of PD including gait ignition failure, bradykinesia and freezing. Furthermore, PD patients seem to be greatly disadvantaged by the absence of external cues from the environment and it is likely that in the presence of damage to the BG/SMA pathways, patients rely heavily on intact sensory/PMA pathways to initiate submovements (Georgiou et al. 1993). This view is supported by the existing PD literature, which shows that a variety of tasks, including finger tapping, drawing movements, learning strategies, set shifting, and walking, improve in response to external cues (Georgiou et al. 1993, Buytenhuijs et al. 1994, Fimm et al. 1994, Martin et al. 1994, Morris et al. 1994, Phillips et al. 1994).

New concepts of vascular HLGDs

It is probable that an analogous situation may exist in other higher-level gait disorders, especially in those patients with 'parkinsonian' type gait disorders in cerebral multi-infarct states (CMIS). It is possible that this is caused by infarction in the SMA or its connections via the periventricular white matter to the BG or indeed in the BG itself. This supports Meyer and Barron's (1960) original concept of gait apraxia being caused by any mesial frontal lesion, which is the anatomical site of the SMA. Further support is gained from current evidence suggesting that damage (periventricular white matter lesions or leucoaraiosis detected on magnetic resonance scanning) to critical pathways linking the BG to the ventrolateral nucleus of the thalamus and to the SMA leads to abnormal gait in early vascular dementia (Hennerici et al. 1994). Chang et al. (1992) also found an association between vascular pseudoparkinsonism and frontal or BG infarcts or leucoaraiosis. These critically placed infarcts presumably disrupt the timing cues from the BG as happens in PD and may therefore be expected to cause similar gait abnormalities. Some patients with vascular HLGDs find walking easier when responding to external cues, e.g. stepping over objects or coloured patterns on the ground (Wright 1979, Jantra et al. 1992), as is commonly seen in PD (Bagley et al. 1991, Weissenborn 1993). It may be relevant, therefore, in the context of CMIS, that virtual reality images simulating 'obstacles' in the patients' physical world have been shown to be an effective form of rehabilitation in PD (Weghorst et al. 1995). Marsden (1989) has hypothesized that the success of these treatments involving external cues may be due to input feeding directly into the PMA from the sensory cortex, bypassing the damaged or deafferented SMA, as already stated above.

However, a significant number of patients with vascular HLGDs do not have movement ignition and timing problems, but present with disequilibrium as their primary complaint. This is clearly consistent with both the original descriptions of gait apraxia and of vascular parkinsonism and is reflected in the classification of Nutt et al. (1993), where disequilibrium is a prominent feature in three of the five patterns of disordered gait described: frontal gait disorder, frontal disequilibrium and subcortical disequilibrium. It is possible that these patients have a primary disorder in their sensory/PMA pathways and while they have no difficulties with automatic internally cued movements, since the BG/SMA pathways are intact, they are unable fully to utilize sensory information from the environment, including proprioceptive, auditory, vestibular and visual information to help initiate and control submovements. They are to some extent 'walking around in the dark', having difficulty integrating external information into their movement sequences; hence their disequilibrium. The dependency of equilibrium on visual cues is supported by studies in normal individuals that show that vision influences the amplitude and velocity of body sway during quiet stance (Day et al. 1993). In contrast with patients whose predominant feature is gait ignition failure, these patients would not be expected to benefit from environmental cues.

Classification based on the above hypotheses

We would suggest the following classification of vascular HLGDs, which would link the clinical features with the putative mechanisms of normal gait and the location of pathological damage in a transparent and meaningful way (see Table 6.2).

Ignition apraxia

Patients with vascular HLGDs with movement ignition difficulties, such as gait ignition failure, shuffling, and difficulty with turns and freezing have infarcts in the BG/thalamus/SMA pathways and/or ischaemic lesions in their connections in the periventricular white matter (Fitzgerald and Jankovic 1989). These patients have difficulties with internally driven automatic movements. We further hypothesize that these patients' gait characteristics should improve when externally cued. We suggest this gait disorder be named ignition apraxia. This group will include isolated impairment of gait ignition and possibly some cases of 'cautious gait' from the classification of Nutt et al. (1993). However, the latter is a very wide and probably

Table 6.2 Classification of vascular HLGDs

	Clinical features	Response to visual cues	Ability to alter cadence in response to auditory cues	Site of lesion
Ignition apraxia	Gait ignition failure, shuffling, freezing	Yes	Yes	SMA, BG or connections
Equilibrium apraxia	Poor balance and falls	No	No	PMA or connections
Mixed gait apraxia	Gait ignition failure, shuffling, freezing. Poor balance and falls	Yes	Yes	PMA or connections *and* SMA, BG or connections

unhelpful category and encompasses patients whose gaits are hesitant for a wide variety of reasons including visual impairment, falls and loss of confidence.

Equilibrium apraxia

We hypothesize that patients with vascular HLGDs causing disequilibrium have infarcts in the sensory/PMA pathways and/or ischaemic lesions in their connections in the periventricular white matter. These patients will have difficulties primarily with externally cued movements; the automatic internal cueing mechanism is normal. The patients' gait should not improve when externally cued. We suggest that this gait disorder be named equilibrium apraxia. This group includes subcortical disequilibrium and frontal disequilibrium in the classification of Nutt et al. (1993).

Mixed gait apraxia

Clearly lesions may affect the connections of both the SMA and PMA and it is to be expected that there will be patients with both disequilibrium and gait ignition difficulties. We suggest that this gait disorder be named mixed gait apraxia. The clinical features seem to correspond to frontal gait disorder in the classification of Nutt et al. (1993).

Reduction of the classification of vascular HLGDs to two types (plus a mixed type) makes it possible to relate the problem to putative underlying physiological mechanisms, in turn related to damage at anatomically distinct sites. The validity of this anatomically underpinned classification will need to be tested with blind interpretation of neuroimaging of patients with vascular HLGDs, with particular attention to SMA, PMA and periventricular white matter. Further correlations may be sought with the responsiveness (or lack of responsiveness) of the gait to external cues. The outcomes of these studies will not only be of theoretical interest: a clearer understanding of the underlying pathophysiology of the different types of vascular HLGDs will create a better framework for rational therapeutic interventions (Mickelborough et al. 1997).

Towards a rational therapy

The standard treatment for these gait disorders centres on physiotherapist administered gait retraining. The elements of such treatment, however, have not been clearly documented, nor have their relationship to the underlying pathophysiological mechanisms been clearly defined. Edwards et al. (1990) have emphasized that such a process is an essential precursor to developing and evaluating therapies. Using similar thinking to that used above in describing our classification of HLGDs, we have designed a comprehensive treatment schedule for these gait disorders, with a total of 31 possible interventions (Mickelborough et al. 1997). In developing the schedule we have drawn on recognized interventions for the gait initiation failure seen in PD and the disequilibrium seen in stroke and also on the approaches recommended by Edwards et al. (1990) in standardizing physiotherapy schedules for research. Essentially, we have postulated that vascular HLGDs will be amenable to physiotherapeutic interventions under three broad headings and we call these the 'modules of intervention'. The treatment schedule modules are:

1 Physiotherapeutic interventions to treat gait initiation and turning difficulties (5 exercises)
2 Physiotherapeutic interventions to improve postural alignment and enhance balance reactions (16 exercises)
3 Physiotherapeutic interventions aimed at the other components of vascular HLGDs (10 exercises)

Using the schedule

The specific interventions an individual patient requires will depend on the pattern of their disordered gait and should be tailored to it. It is envisaged that all patients should initially be assessed and treated within each module. The choice of subsequent exercises will then depend on evaluation and continuing assessment. The reason for this is that most cases of vascular HLGDs are mixed to some extent: even patients with 'pure' ignition or equilibrium apraxias may well have elements of subclinical balance or ignition problems respectively.

The efficacy of this schedule will require objective evaluation, using simple clinical outcome measures as well as more complex measures, which might include gait analysis using footprint data from an inked walkway, three dimensional video analysis, electrogoniometry and accelerometry (Holden et al. 1984, Waagfjord et al.

1990, Wilkinson et al.1995). These latter are not yet widely available (Bell et al. 1996). It is important to determine whether improvements seen on more sophisticated tests translate into functional improvement. We are currently using such methods to evaluate this schedule, specifically comparing it to treadmill retraining.

Conclusion

There is an increasing awareness that higher-level gait disorders, typically seen in PD, may also be associated with other conditions, in particular cerebral multi-infarct states.

In this chapter, we set out the evolution of understanding of these gait disorders. We have suggested that the observed clinical features may be related to putative underlying anatomical damage in accordance with what is currently understood about the initiation and maintenance of gait. We have proposed a classification of the main types of vascular HLGDs into ignition apraxia, equilibrium apraxia, and mixed apraxia. This is a simplification of the classification of Nutt et al. (1993) and builds on current explanations of the gait disorder seen in PD. It is postulated that ignition apraxia is due predominantly to damage to the supplementary motor area or to its connections with the basal ganglia and that equilibrium apraxia is due to damage to the sensory/premotor area pathways. The correlative of this is that the former will respond well to external cues (as the major problem is the difficulty in internal cueing), and that the latter will not respond to external cues as the pathways that utilize such cues are damaged.

We suggest that this classification of the elements of apraxia may have implications for the more precise targeting and tailoring of physiotherapy and other interventions for patients with vascular HLGDs. The hypothesis and the therapeutic implications arising from it remains speculative at present and needs to be supported by future research.

REFERENCES

Austregesilo A, Borges Fortes A (1936) Syndrome du déséquilibre et ataxie frontale (pseudo-manifestations cérébello-vestibulaires) étude experimentale. *Encephale*, 31, 1–14.

Bagley S, Kelly B, Tunnicliffe N, Turnbull GI, Walker JM (1991) The effect of visual cues on the gait of independently mobile Parkinson's disease patients. *Physiotherapy*, 77, 415–20.

Bell F, Shaw LM, Rafferty D, Rennie J, Richards JD (1996) Movement analysis technology in clinical practice. *Physical Therapy Review*, 1, 13–22.

Bruns L (1892) Uber storengen des gleichgewichtes bei stirnhirntumoren. *Deutsche Medizinische Wochenschrift*, 18, 138–3.

Buytenhuijs EL, Berger HJC, Van Spaendonck KPM, Horstink MWIM, Borm GF, Cools AR (1994) Memory and learning strategies in patients with Parkinson's disease. *Neuropsychologia*, 32, 335–2.

Chang CM, Yu YL, Ng HK, Fong KY (1992) Vascular pseudoparkinsonism. *Acta Neurologica Scandinavica*, 86, 588–2.

Chen YC, Thaler D, Nixon PD, Stern CE, Passingham RE (1995) The function of the medial premotor cortex. 2. The timing and selection of learned movements. *Experimental Brain Research*, 102, 461–3.

Critchley M (1929) Arteriosclerotic parkinsonism. *Brain*, 52, 23–83.

Day BL, Steiger MJ, Thompson PD, Marsden CD (1993) Effect of vision and stance width on human body motion when standing: implications for afferent control of lateral sway. *Journal of Physiology*, 469, 479–99.

Donoghue JP, Sanes JN (1994) Motor areas of the motor cortex. *Journal of Clinical Neurophysiology*, 11, 382–96.

Edwards S, Partridge C, Mee R (1990) Treatment schedules for research: a model for physiotherapy. *Physiotherapy*, 76, 605–7.

Fimm B, Bartl G, Zimmerman P, Wallesch C-W (1994) Different mechanisms underly shifting set on external and internal cues in Parkinson's. *Brain and Cognition*, 25, 287–304.

Fitzgerald PM, Jankovic J (1989) Lower body parkinsonism: Evidence for vascular aetiology. *Movement Disorders*, 4, 249–60.

Freeman JS, Cody FWJ, Schady W (1993) The influence of external timing cues upon the rhythm of voluntary movements in Parkinson's disease. *Journal of Neurology, Neurosurgery, and Psychiatry*, 56, 1078–84.

Georgiou N, lansek R, Bradshaw JL, Phillips JG, Mattingley JB, Bradshaw JA (1993) An evaluation of the role of internal cues in the pathogenesis of parkinsonian hypokinesia. *Brain*, 116, 1575–87.

Gerstmann J, Schilder P (1926) Uber eine besondere gangstorung bei stirnhirnerkrankung. *Weiner Medizinische Wochenschrift*, 76, 97–107.

Gordon A (1917) Lesions of the frontal lobe simulating cerebellar involvement. Differential diagnosis. *Journal of Nervous and Mental Diseases*, 46, 261–75.

Hennerici MG, Oster M, Cohen S, Schwartz A, Motsch L, Daffertshofer M (1994) Are gait disturbances and white matter degeneration early indicators of vascular dementia? *Dementia*, 5, 197–202.

Holden MK, Gill KM, Magliozzi ME, Nathan J, Piehl-Baker L (1984) Clinical gait assessment in the neurologically impaired. *Physical Therapy*, 64, 35–40.

Jantra P, Monga TN, Press JM, Gervais BJ (1992) Management of apraxic gait in a stroke patient. *Archives of Physical Medicine and Rehabilitation*, 73, 95–7.

Marie P (1901) Des foyers lacunaires de désintégration et de différentes autres états cavitaires du cerveau. *Revue Neurologique*, 21, 281–98.

Marsden CD (1989) Slowness of movement in Parkinson's disease. In: *Movement Disorders*, Vol. 4, Suppl. 1, eds. Fahn S and Marsden CD, pp. 26–37. New York: Raven Press.

Martin KE, Phillips JG, lansek R, Bradshaw JL (1994) Inaccuracy and instability of sequential movements in Parkinson's disease. *Experimental Brain Research*, 102, 131–40.

Meyer JS, Barron DW (1960) Apraxia of gait: a clinico-physiological study. *Brain*, 83, 261–84.

Mickelborough J, Liston R, Harris B, Pomeroy V, Tallis RC (1997) Conventional physiotherapy of higher-level gait disorders in patients with cerebral multi-infarct states. *Physiotherapy Theory and Practice*, 13, 127–38.

Morris ME, lansek R, Matyas TA, Summers 0JJ (1994) The pathogenesis of gait hypokinesia in Parkinson's disease. *Brain*, 117, 1169–81.

Nutt JG, Marsden CD, Thompson PD (1993) Human walking and higher-level gait disorders, particularly in the elderly. *Neurology*, 43, 268–79.

Phillips JG, Martin KE, Bradshaw JL, lansek R (1994) Could bradykinesia in Parkinson's disease simply be overcompensation. *Journal of Neurology*, 241, 439–47.

Roland PE, Larsen B, Larsen NA, Skinhoj E (1980) Supplementary motor area and other cortical areas in organization of voluntary movement in man. *Journal of Clinical Neurophysiology*, 43, 118–36.

Thaler D, Chen YC, Nixon PD, Stern CE, Passingham RE (1995) The function of the medial pre-motor cortex. 1. Simple learned movements. *Experimental Brain Research*, 102, 445–6.

Thompson PD, Marsden CD (1987) Gait disorders of subcortical arteriosclerotic encephalopathy: Binswangers disease. *Movement Disorders*, 2, 1–8.

Van Bogaert L, Martin P (1929) Sur deux signes due syndrome de desquilibration frontale: l'apraxie de la marche et l'atonie statique. *Encephale*, 24, 11–18.

Waagfjörd J, Levangie PD, Certo CME (1990) Effects of treadmill training on gait in a hemiparetic patient. *Physical Therapy*, 70, 549–58.

Weghorst SJ, Prothero J, Furness T, Anson D, Riess T (1995) Virtual images in the treatment of Parkinson's disease akinesia. *Medicine Meets Virtual Reality Conference* 11, 30, 242–3.

Weissenborn S (1993) The effect of using a two-step verbal cue to a visual target above eye level on the Parkinsonian gait: A case study. *Physiotherapy*, 79, 26–31.

Wilkinson MJ, Menz HB, Raspovic A (1995) The measurement of gait parameters from footprints. *The Foot*, 5, 84–90.

Wright WB (1979) Stammering gait. *Age and Ageing*, 8, 8–12.

7

The epidemiology of Parkinson's disease and parkinsonism in elderly subjects

Jolyon Meara and Peter Hobson

Introduction

The study of Parkinson's disease (PD) in populations – the epidemiology of PD – is an arduous and difficult undertaking. Descriptive epidemiology of a disease provides a picture of the *prevalence* – the amount of disease present in a given population; the *incidence* – how frequently new cases develop in a given population over time; the *mortality* – the risk of death associated with the disease; and the *natural history* of the disease. The risk of disease is best measured by incidence as prevalence figures can be distorted by differential survival between study populations. Analytical epidemiology investigates the associations, exposures, risk factors, and comorbidities of a disease in an effort to determine the aetiology. There are also increasing attempts to describe the disability, handicap, quality of life and health and social service provision resulting from specific diseases (see Chapter 8).

The major causes of neurodegenerative disease, Alzheimer's disease (AD), PD and motor neurone disease (MND) all share a strong age associated risk and are likely to be an issue of increasing public health concern as a result of the worldwide aging of populations. Certified deaths from AD, PD and MND have been projected to overtake cancer as the second commonest cause of death in the USA by the year 2040 (Lilienfield et al. 1990).

A major difficulty in interpreting the many and varied epidemiological studies of PD is that PD is a relatively rare disorder, the diagnosis of which, for practical purposes, relies solely on the clinical skills of history taking and bedside examination. Diagnostic accuracy for PD, particularly in older subjects, is poor (Hughes et al. 1992). There is also debate on whether PD is strictly a single *disease* or is better termed a *syndrome* caused by several diseases (Duvoisin 1989). The studies of autosomal dominant familial parkinsonism indicate that differing neuropathology can cause identical clinical pictures between pedigrees and that identical pathology can cause varied clinical presentations within a single family. Disagreement even exists as to what constitutes the typical pathology of PD and there is a pressing need for more detailed and extensive prospective clinicopathological cohort studies. These

Table 7.1 Key areas to address in the evaluation of epidemiological studies in parkinsonism

- The criteria used for the diagnosis of parkinsonism and the method of establishing diagnosis (case note review, screening questionnaire, or bedside examination)
- The characteristics of the population studied
- The methods of case ascertainment used (medical records, drug prescription, recall by physicians, total census approach). Many prevalent cases of PD will be medically undiagnosed at the time of the study and some medically known cases will not be on drug treatment or be under medical review
- The inclusion or exclusion of cases of vascular parkinsonism, and drug-induced parkinsonism
- The inclusion or exclusion of elderly subjects in residential homes, nursing homes or other long-term care institutions
- The inclusion or exclusion of elderly subjects with dementia

factors can considerably complicate the interpretation of epidemiological studies in PD. Certain aspects of such studies need to be critically evaluated (see Table 7.1).

Prevalence

PD affects all racial groups and has a fairly uniform worldwide distribution, though the prevalence in Africa, China and Japan is reduced (Zhang and Roman 1993). Differences in prevalence between racial groups may reflect differing environmental rather than genetic factors (Schoenberg et al. 1988, Jendroska et al. 1994). Prevalence differences between studies, even after adjusting to a standard population, may be artefacts of diagnosis and survival. Despite differences in absolute prevalence between countries, disease risk may be similar if mortality rates also vary. Prevalence rates for PD in subjects over the age of 65 years appear to be similar across several European countries (de Rijk et al. 1997). This study, based on 14 636 individuals over the age of 65 years in four countries using a total census approach or stratified random samples, reported a prevalence of 2.3% for parkinsonism and 1.6% for PD, age adjusted to the 1991 European standard population. Studies around the world based on all ages suggest a prevalence for PD of around 120/100 000 population. PD shows a strong exponential age associated risk that appears to be maintained even in extreme old age (Ben-Shlomo 1996). PD is slightly more common in men than in women, which may reflect differences in occupational exposure to environmental agents causing PD.

In prevalence studies using a total census approach, up to a third or more of subjects ascertained as having PD were medically undiagnosed before the study, even in countries with well developed health services (Schoenberg et al. 1985, Morgante et al. 1992, de Rijk et al. 1997). A study of all residents over the age of 65 years in a US retirement town revealed a prevalence of known PD of 2% and medically undiagnosed PD of 5% (Khatter et al. 1996). Undiagnosed, but clinically symptomatic, parkinsonism was found in 1% of older subjects in general practice in the UK (Meara et al. 1997). Drug prescription for PD appears to be an unreliable method of case ascertainment used alone, as many subjects in receipt of medication will not have PD or even parkinsonism (Meara et al. 1999) and a proportion of known cases of PD, likely to be elderly and frail or with minimal symptoms, will not be on active drug treatment (Morgante et al. 1992).

Incidence

Changes in disease incidence provide a powerful tool to investigate disease risk, disease associations and disease aetiology. Unfortunately, incidence studies of diseases that are relatively infrequent require long-term follow-up of populations and must achieve high levels of disease ascertainment. In PD the best long-term data on incidence has come from the longitudinal study from Rochester, Minnesota (Rajput et al. 1984). These studies indicate a relatively unchanging age adjusted incidence for PD of around 20/100 000 population between the years 1967–1979. However, despite a constant overall incidence, an increasing incidence for disease in older subjects and a falling incidence in younger subjects may have occurred over this time (Ben-Shlomo 1996).

Mortality

Several studies from around the world seem to indicate that mortality is still at least doubled in PD despite drug treatment (Hoehn and Yahr 1967, Ebmeier et al. 1990, Bennett et al. 1996) and that age specific mortality rates appear to be increasing in those over 75 years old and falling in younger patients (Lilienfeld et al. 1990, Clarke 1993, for detailed review see Ben-Shlomo 1996). One reason for this finding, and there are several competing explanations, is that the incidence of PD/parkinsonism in older subjects may be increasing.

Long-term care

Parkinsonism is likely to be particularly prevalent in long-term care institutions such as hospitals, nursing homes and residential/retirement homes (Moghal et al. 1995). Few studies have been specifically targeted at this population group. A study in the United States of over 5000 nursing home residents over the age of 55 years reported a prevalence for medically diagnosed PD of nearly 7% (Mitchell et al. 1996). In this study nursing home residents with PD tended to be more disorientated, more depressed, more functionally disabled and to deteriorate faster over an 18 month period than residents without PD. Hallucinations and dementia appear to be two major factors increasing the risk of admission to nursing homes of elderly people with PD (Goetz and Stebbins 1993, 1995). Nursing home residents who develop parkinsonism after admission to the nursing home are less likely to be diagnosed, assessed and treated. One study in France found that 42% of cases of PD in elderly subjects living in institutions were medically undiagnosed (Tison et al. 1994). In this study, out of a sample group of 357 people living in institutions 63 subjects (18%) were found to have parkinsonism with 36 of this group (57%) being diagnosed as PD. We have approached the problem by asking nursing officers in nursing homes to report residents with known PD and also residents with both tremor and shuffling gait. Out of a study group of 2005 nursing home residents, known PD was reported to be present in 6.8% and possible PD (tremor plus gait disturbance) was reported in 2% of residents (unpublished observations). Further data are required to define the extent of the problem of parkinsonism in nursing homes and the extent to which diagnosis, assessment and treatment can reduce handicap and improve quality of life in this frail and vulnerable group (Larsen et al. 1991).

Risk factors for PD

The contribution of epidemiology to our understanding of risk factors for PD has been disappointing. The existence of autosomal dominant familial parkinsonism clearly indicates that Lewy-body type pathology can have a completely genetic basis (Golbe et al. 1993). However, the balance of environmental and genetic factors determining the risk of sporadic PD is unclear (see Fig. 7.1). Molecular biology is likely to make an important contribution to this area through the study of regulatory gene products (Bandmann et al. 1998). Exploring the contribution of environment and genetic inheritance may be helped by the study of migrant populations (Schoenberg et al. 1988).

Aging and the risk of PD

Prevalence studies have clearly shown that the risk of PD is powerfully associated with age, though this risk appears to fall in advanced age. This may be explained by the difficulty detecting and diagnosing PD in very elderly subjects and, given the small absolute numbers, confidence intervals are wide at this extreme of age. Studies using population methodology that have included elderly subjects in institutional care have shown that the risk of PD increases continually with age (Tison et al. 1994). The link between aging and PD may be explained by age related cell death, intrinsic aging processes in the brain increasing the susceptibility to PD, or

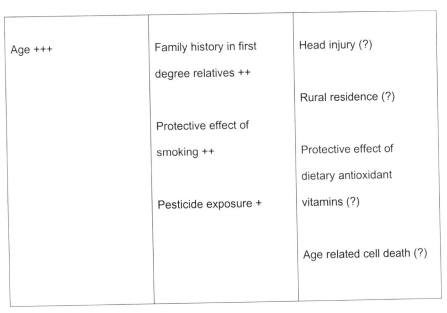

Age +++	Family history in first degree relatives ++	Head injury (?)
		Rural residence (?)
	Protective effect of smoking ++	Protective effect of dietary antioxidant vitamins (?)
	Pesticide exposure +	
		Age related cell death (?)

Fig. 7.1   Risk factors for Parkinson's disease.

by increasing the length of exposure to exogenous or endogenous causative agents. Most prevalence and case-control studies indicate the risk of PD to be slightly increased for the male sex.

Environmental, lifestyle and life event risk factors for PD

Environmental factors, associated comorbidities and lifestyle have been implicated in the aetiology of PD and can be examined by epidemiological techniques. Large scale cohort population studies can investigate risk factors with the greatest degree of certainty, but are time consuming and expensive to execute, particularly given the relative rarity of PD in most age groups. Case-control studies, where individuals with the index disease are matched with one or two control cases without the disease, are easier to mount and can more quickly investigate hypotheses of disease causation. Case-control studies can be subject to many sources of bias and confounding that can make interpretation of results quite difficult. Problems include the definition of cases, the selection of controls, the degree of matching that takes place and most importantly, recall bias of patients with a disease compared to subjects without a disease. The diagnosis of PD will make an individual peer back anxiously into the past to try to find some explanation and will increase the recollection of exposures to chemicals and other events. The manner in which interviews with cases and controls are conducted in order to obtain information can also bias the results if the interviewer is aware of the aetiological hypotheses being tested by the study. Theories of disease aetiology such as infection, head injury, and toxin exposure can be examined in matched groupings of cases and controls. Cell death in the substantia nigra in PD appears to develop rapidly over the six years or so before clinical signs of disease, indicating that exposures at or before this time might be particularly relevant as risk factors. However, the length of the latent period between a 'permissive' exposure and disease development is unknown.

The most robust epidemiological finding, replicated in several population and case-control studies, has been that people who smoke are less likely to develop PD (Doll et al. 1994). Whether this is due to a protective effect of smoking, or to the existence of a premorbid PD personality that makes smoking less likely, is unclear. The description of neurotoxin induced MPTP parkinsonism (Langston et al. 1983), coupled with the free radical theory of cell death in PD, resulted in several studies examining environmental risk factors for PD. The best case-control studies (Semchuk et al. 1991, 1992) suggest a link between the risk of PD and a positive family history of PD, past significant head injury and occupational pesticide use. However, such factors may explain only about a third of sporadic cases of PD. Apart from a general link to rural living, other case-control studies have reported variable findings and have not defined risk factors any more precisely.

Cohort studies avoid much of the bias of case-control studies, though the relative rarity of PD and the fact that it develops late in life requires the long-term follow-up of large groups of subjects. The incidence rate of PD can be measured in groups with and without some exposure felt to be relevant to the risk of developing PD. One small cohort study of head injury did not detect an increased risk of subsequent PD (Williams et al. 1991) and a further large study of dietary antioxidant vitamins indicated a protective effect of vitamin C, though not of vitamin E (Cerhan et al. 1994). Further hypotheses generated by basic medical science need to be developed concerning the aetiology of PD that can be tested in appropriate cohort and case-control epidemiological studies. At present the analytical epidemiology of PD awaits new theories to test.

Genetic risk of PD

Considerable advances have recently been made in genetic studies of parkinsonism, particularly in relation to defining the genetic basis of familial parkinsonism (Golbe et al. 1993) and the re-analysis of concordance rates for PD in monozygotic and dizygotic twin studies (Johnson et al. 1990). The balance between genetic predisposing and causative factors and environmental exposure in sporadic PD remains to be determined (Hawkes 1997, Bandmann et al. 1998). Considerable interest exists in the genetic basis of neurodegenerative mechanisms that could account for PD (Fahn et al. 1998). Studies of familial parkinsonism in the large Contursi kindred led to the detection of a gene defect segregating to chromosome

4q21–22 that encodes for a cytoplasmic protein called alpha-synuclein (Polymeropoulos et al. 1996).

The epidemiology of parkinsonism not due to PD

The prevalence of parkinsonism in elderly subjects may be much higher than previously thought and although overall PD accounts for around 70% of all cases of medically diagnosed parkinsonism, this figure will be lower in older populations in whom other causes of parkinsonism are more common. How much lower has never been determined. One retrospective case note study has reported that up to a third of all subjects over the age of 65 years may have evidence of parkinsonism, though a definite diagnosis of PD could be made in only around 10% of this group (Bennett et al. 1996). The diagnosis of parkinsonism was based on the finding of two or more of the following: bradykinesia, gait disturbance, rigidity and tremor. A possible reason for such a high prevalence of parkinsonism in this study may have been because of the frequency of postural tremor in elderly subjects. Although the likeliest cause of such tremor would be essential tremor, the study methodology would have counted such tremor as a parkinsonian sign. A community total census 'door-to-door' study of elderly subjects reported finding tremor in 43% of the study group and half of these individuals were diagnosed as having essential tremor (Khatter et al. 1996). We have studied the prevalence of medically undiagnosed tremor in general practice in the UK based on the use of a screening questionnaire to subjects over the age of 65 years and found that tremor was reported by 12% of the study group (Meara et al. 1997). Essential tremor was diagnosed in half of this group.

Very little is known of the epidemiology of parkinsonism not due to PD in elderly people. Multisystem degenerative diseases, such as multiple system atrophy (MSA) and progressive supranuclear palsy (PSP), that can present as parkinsonism, are much rarer disorders than PD. Furthermore, the onset of MSA is uncommon after the age of 70 years, though this may reflect the poor prognosis of patients with late onset disease (Wenning et al. 1994). The epidemiological study of PSP is made difficult by the fact that possibly half the course of the disease may pass before it becomes possible to distinguish this disorder clinically from rapidly progressive PD. The epidemiology of vascular parkinsonism is also poorly understood and has not been studied systematically in elderly populations (Critchley 1981, Fitzgerald and Jankovic 1989, Fenelon et al. 1995). Elderly people appear to be more susceptible to drug-induced parkinsonism (see Chapter 4) and are also much more likely than younger people to be prescribed neuroleptic drugs. The relationship between AD and extrapyramidal signs is intriguing and some cases of parkinsonism in elderly subjects may result from AD (Hamill et al. 1988, Hulette et al. 1995).

Interestingly, elderly subjects with extrapyramidal signs appear to have higher mortality and to be at greater risk of developing cognitive impairment than subjects without such signs (Richards et al. 1993, Bennett et al. 1996).

Conclusion

The increasing number of descriptive epidemiological studies of PD in various populations indicate that the prevalence of PD is remarkably similar worldwide with the exception of certain racial groups in whom the risk of developing PD appears reduced. Apparent differences in reported prevalence rates tend to disappear once allowance for differing methodologies and population structure are made.

The risk of developing PD is strongly related to age. It is unlikely that age related cell death in the brain is sufficient alone to result in PD and the effect of age more likely reflects the impact of disease, genetic factors, and exogenous and endogenous environmental agents. The most powerful risk factor for PD after age itself is a positive family history of the disease. Exciting recent developments in genetic studies of familial parkinsonism may in time help elucidate the pathophysiological genetic mechanisms behind some cases of sporadic PD. A multifactorial basis for most cases of sporadic PD seems likely, based on the findings of analytical epidemiological studies using cohort and case-control designs.

Parkinsonism as a syndrome appears to be far more common in elderly people than previously thought and results in considerable misdiagnosis, inappropriate treatment and missed therapeutic opportunities. In elderly subjects there appears to be considerable overlap between PD, AD, MND and dementia with Lewy bodies that suggests common genetic and environmental factors.

REFERENCES

Bandmann O, Marsden CD, Wood NW (1998) Genetic aspects of Parkinson's disease. *Movement Disorders*, 13, 2, 203–11.

Bennett DA, Beckett LA, Murray AM, Shannon KM, Goetz CG, Pilgrim DM, Evans DA (1996) Prevalence of parkinsonian signs and associated mortality in a community population of older people. *New England Journal of Medicine*, 334, 71–6.

Ben-Shlomo Y (1996) How far are we in understanding the cause of Parkinson's disease? *Journal of Neurology, Neurosurgery, and Psychiatry*, 61, 4–16.

Cerhan JR, Wallaxe RB, Folsom AR (1994) Antioxidant intake and risk of Parkinson's disease. *American Journal of Epidemiology*, 139, S65.

Clarke CE (1993) Mortality from Parkinson's disease in England and Wales 1921–1989. *Journal of Neurology, Neurosurgery, and Psychiatry*, 48, 690–3.

Critchley M (1981) Arteriosclerotic pseudoparkinsonism. In: *Research Progress in Parkinson's Disease*, eds. F Clifford Rose and R Capildeo, pp. 40–2. London: Pitman Medical.

de Rijk MC, Tzourio C, Breteler MMB, Dartigues JF, Amaducci L, Lopez-Pousa S, Manubens-Bertran JM, Alperovitch A, Rocca WA (1997) Prevalence of parkinsonism and Parkinson's disease in Europe: the EUROPARKINSON collaborative study. *Journal of Neurology, Neurosurgery, and Psychiatry*, 62,10–15.

Doll R, Peto R, Wheatley K, Gray R, Sutherland I (1994) Mortality in relation to smoking: 40 years' observations on male British doctors. *British Medical Journal*, 309, 901–11.

Duvoisin RC (1989) Is there a Parkinson's disease? In: *Disorders of Movement: Clinical, Pharmacological and Physiological Aspects*, pp. 1–10. Academic Press Ltd.

Ebmeier KP, Calder SA, Crawford JR, Stewart L, Beeson JAO, Mutch WJ (1990) Parkinson's disease in Aberdeen: survival after 3.5 years. *Acta Neurologica Scandinavica*, 81, 294–9.

Fahn S, Clarence-Smith KE, Chase TN (1998) Parkinson's disease: neurodegenerative mechanisms and neuroprotective interventions – report of a workshop. *Movement Disorders*, 13, 759–67.

Fenelon G, Gray F, Wallays C (1995) Parkinsonism and dilatation of the perivascular spaces (etat crible) of the striatum: a clinical, magnetic resonance imaging and pathological study. *Movement Disorders*, 10, 754–60.

Fitzgerald PM, Jankovic J (1989) Lower body parkinsonism: evidence for a vascular etiology. *Movement Disorders*, 4, 249–60.

Goetz CG, Stebbins GT (1993) Risk factors for nursing home placement in advanced Parkinson's disease. *Neurology*, 43, 2227–9.

Goetz CG, Stebbins GT (1995) Mortality and hallucinations in nursing home patients with advanced Parkinson's disease. *Neurology*, 45, 669–71.

Golbe LI, Lazzarini AM, Schwarz KO, Mark MH, Dickson DW, Duvoisin RC (1993) Autosomal dominant parkinsonism with benign course and typical Lewy-body pathology. *Neurology*, 43, 2222–7.

Hamill RW, Caine E, Eskin T, Lapham L, Shoulson I, McNeill TH (1988) Neurodegenerative disorders and ageing. Alzheimer's disease and Parkinson's disease – common ground. *Annals of the New York Academy of Sciences*, 515, 411–20.

Hawkes CH (1997) Is Parkinson's disease inherited? *British Journal of Hospital Medicine*, 57,4, 130–3.

Hoehn MM, Yahr MD (1967) Parkinsonism: onset, progression, and mortality. *Neurology*, 17, 427–42.

Hughes AJ, Daniel SE, Kilford L, Lees A (1992) Accuracy of clinical diagnosis of idiopathic Parkinson's disease: a clinico-pathological study of 100 cases. *Journal of Neurology, Neurosurgery, and Psychiatry*, 55, 181–4.

Hulette C, Mirra S, Wilkinson W, Heyman A, Fillenbaum G, Clark C (1995) The consortium to establish a registry for Alzheimer's disease (CERAD). Part IX. A prospective cliniconeuropathologic study of Parkinson's features in Alzheimer's disease. *Neurology*, 45, 1991–5.

Jendroska K, Olasode BJ, Daniel SE, Elliott L, Ogunniyi AO, Aghadiuno PU, Osuntokun BO, Lees AJ (1994) Incidental Lewy-body disease in black Africans. *Lancet*, 344, 882–3.

Johnson WG, Hodge SE, Duvoisin RC (1990) Twin studies and the genetics of Parkinson's disease: a reappraisal. *Movement Disorders*, 5, 187–94.

Khatter AS, Kurth MC, Brewer MA, Crinnian CT, Drazkowski JF, Flitman SS, Imke S, Spector SA, Wood KL, Lieberman AN (1996) Prevalence of tremor and Parkinson's disease. *Parkinsonism and Related Disorders*, 2, 4, 205–8.

Langston JW, Ballard P, Tetrud JW, Irwin I (1983) Chronic parkinsonism in humans due to a product of meperidine-analog synthesis. *Science*, 219, 970–80.

Larsen JP and the Norwegian Study Group of Parkinson's disease in the elderly (1991) Parkinson's disease as community health problem: study in Norwegian nursing homes. *British Medical Journal*, 303, 741–3.

Lilienfeld DE, Chan E, Ehland J, Godbold J, Landrigan PJ, Marsh G, Perl D (1990) Two decades of increasing mortality from Parkinson's disease among the US elderly. *Archives of Neurology*, 47, 731–4.

Meara RJ, Bhowmick BK, Hobson JP (1999) Accuracy of diagnosis in patients with presumed Parkinson's disease in a community-based disease register. *Age and Ageing*, 28, 99–102.

Meara RJ, Bisarya S, Hobson JP (1997) Screening in primary health care for undiagnosed tremor in an elderly population in Wales. *Journal of Epidemiology and Community Health*, 51, 574–5.

Mitchell SL, Kiely DK, Kiel DP, Lipsitz LA (1996) The epidemiology, clinical characteristics and natural history of older nursing home residents with a diagnosis of Parkinson's disease. *Journal of the American Geriatrics Society*, 44, 394–9.

Moghal S, Rajput AH, Meleth R, D'Arcy C, Rajput R (1995) Prevalence of movement disorders in institutionalized elderly. *Neuroepidemiology*, 14, 297–300.

Morgante L, Rocca WA, Di Rosa AE, De Dominico P, Grigoletto F, Meneghini F, Reggio A, Savettieri G, Castiglione MG, Patti F, Di Perri R (1992) Prevalence of Parkinson's disease and other types of parkinsonism: a door-to-door survey in three Sicilian municipalities. *Neurology*, 42, 1901–7.

Mutch WJ, Dingwall-Fordyce I, Downie AW, Paterson JG, Roy SK (1986) Parkinson's disease in a Scottish city. *British Medical Journal*, 292, 534–6.

Polymeropoulos MH, Higgins JJ, Golbe LI, Johnson WG, Ide SE, Di Iorio G, Sanges G, Stenroos ES, Pho LT, Schaffer AA, Lazzarini AM, Nussbaum RL, Duvoisin RC (1996) Mapping of a gene for Parkinson's disease to chromosome 4q21–q23. *Science*, 274, 1197–9.

Rajput AH, Offord KP, Beard C, Kurland LT (1984) Epidemiology of parkinsonism: incidence, classification and mortality. *Annals of Neurology*, 16, 278–82.

Richards M, Stern Y, Marder K, Cote L, Mayeux R (1993) Relationships between extrapyramidal signs and cognitive function in a community dwelling cohort of patients with Parkinson's disease and normal elderly individuals. *Annals of Neurology*, 33, 267–74.

Schoenberg BS, Anderson DW, Haerer AF (1985) Prevalence of Parkinson's disease in the bi-racial population of Copiah County, Mississippi. *Neurology*, 35, 841–5.

Schoenberg BS, Osuntokun BO, Adeuja AOG, Bademosi O, Nottidge V, Anderson DW, Haerer AF (1988) Comparison of the prevalence of Parkinson's disease in black populations in the rural United States and in rural Nigeria: door-to-door community studies. *Neurology*, 38, 645–6.

Semchuk KM, Love EJ, Lee RG (1991) Parkinson's disease and exposure to rural environmental factors: a population-based case-control study. *Canadian Journal of Neurological Sciences*, 18, 279–86.

Semchuk KM, Love EJ, Lee RG (1992) Parkinson's disease and exposure to agricultural work and pesticide chemicals. *Neurology*, 42,1328–35.

Tison F, Dartigues JF, Dubes L, Zuber M, Alperovitch A, Henry P (1994) Prevalence of Parkinson's disease in the elderly: a population study in Gironde, France. *Acta Neurologica Scandinavica*, 90, 111–15.

Wenning GK, Ben-Shlomo Y, Magalhaes M (1994) Clinical features and natural history of multiple system atrophy. An analysis of 100 cases. *Brain*, 117, 835–45.

Williams DB, Annegers JF, Kokmen E, O'Brien PC, Kurland LT (1991) Brain injury and neurologic sequelae: a cohort study of dementia, parkinsonism, and amyotrophic sclerosis. *Neurology*, 41, 1554–7.

Zhang Z-X, Roman GC (1993) Worldwide occurrence of Parkinson's disease: an updated review. *Neuroepidemiology*, 12, 195–208.

8

Health and social needs of people with Parkinson's disease and the worldwide organization of their care

Peter Hobson

Introduction

Trying to unravel the complex health needs of elderly people is a major task faced by health care systems throughout the world, made all the more important by the fact that this group is a disproportionately high consumer of health care resources. Not only industrialized societies, but also developing countries, are facing a demographic challenge as life expectancy increases. The health needs of this group are complex and variable, reflecting the extreme heterogeneity of elderly people. However, all too often care tends to be fragmented and haphazard, reflecting and reinforcing ageist values.

The health and social needs of elderly patients with Parkinson's disease (PD) can be analysed in terms of specific needs related to PD and also in terms of general needs arising from any chronic illness in an elderly person. This chapter will not attempt to give definitive answers to what is needed to meet the health and social needs of patients with PD. It will instead try to give a brief description of the way in which services have developed for patients with PD and how research might best address the future development of such services.

Demographic changes

The proportion of populations throughout the world aged 65 and over is estimated to increase substantially into the next century. This change results from a slowing down of mortality rates, a decline in fertility rates and from advances in medical care and public health. By the year 2025 around 59 countries are likely to have more than 2 million elderly people in their population (Kinsella and Taeuber 1993). The United States population will have the greatest proportion of elderly in the world by the year 2000. These demographic changes are not a phenomenon exclusive to the industrialized European and North American nations. Developing nations are also experiencing similar changes. China's elderly population in the next quarter of a century is expected to double and Japan has already experienced an increase of 7–14% in their elderly population between 1970–1996 (Kinsella 1996). The impact of demographic changes will be especially important for diseases that demonstrate a strong age associated risk such as PD and Alzheimer's disease. The burden of such neurodegenerative diseases will significantly increase into the next century (Lilienfeld et al. 1990, Zhang and Roman 1992).

Health care systems throughout the world are presented with the problems of how to deliver services and finance healthcare for elderly people with finite resources. Developing countries often have to meet this challenge, handicapped by political and economic instability (Gibson 1992). Within developing nations there is often a lack of adequate state support or privately financed health care and as a result health services, if they exist, are likely to be basic and difficult to access. Because of the differing health care systems in place throughout the world it is difficult, if not impossible, to draw international comparisons of optimal care for patients with PD. However, it is still possible to draw together guidelines of what is considered to be best practice in the provision of services for PD patients and their carers.

The organization and provision of services for PD – a global view

A review of the organization of services for PD and how these services are financed in a selected number of countries is presented in Table 8.1. The major differences seen in the organization and delivery of care reflect socio-economic policies pursued by the various countries. The information for this chapter has been drawn from a number of sources. The vast majority of published work was sourced from electronic databases such as Medline. The Internet also provided a useful source of information for contact addresses of the various PD societies throughout the world. PD discussion groups on the Internet were also contacted for their assistance.

The organization and provision of services for PD

The main medical contact for patients with PD is the family doctor, or general practitioner (GP). A typical GP practice in the UK will have no more than five patients with PD. It is unlikely therefore that a GP will be able to develop sufficient expertise to deal with the complex medical and psychosocial problems encountered by PD patients throughout the course of their illness (Mutch 1992). The GP acts as the gatekeeper for access to more specialist services for PD where they exist.

The complex needs of PD patients may be best met through a multidisciplinary team (MDT) of health and social work professionals. In a number of countries

Table 8.1 Organization of services for Parkinson's disease patients in selected countries

United States of America	In the United States private physicians manage the majority of patients with PD. More specialist neurological management in the form of movement disorder clinics is restricted to university departments and large urban hospitals. Geriatricians are not reimbursed for the care of elderly patients with PD.
	Patients through direct payments or private health insurance finance most medical services. For patients who are disabled or over the age of 65 years the federal government Medicare meets healthcare costs. The Medicaid programme covers some of the poor.
Canada	The services for Parkinson's disease patients can be organized differently from province to province and sometimes region to region depending on local funding arrangements. Some of the large cities have multidisciplinary movement disorder clinics. Some elderly patients are managed by geriatricians, with younger patients managed by neurologists. Those living in remote or rural areas depend upon the family doctor for support.
	The Canadian national health care system (Medicare) is based on a universal coverage for all of the population. The Medicare system is funded from the federal income tax. The cost for drug treatment is usually restricted to those over the age of 65 years.
United Kingdom	Routine care for patients with PD is managed by the GP. The GP can refer the patient for specialist assessment by a geriatrician or neurologist. Specialist clinics are increasingly being developed nationwide. A number of PD nurse specialists, initially supported by the UK Parkinson's Disease Society and pharmaceutical industry, have been appointed. Health care is provided through the National Health Service (NHS), which is free and covers the entire population. Funding for the NHS comes from a number of sources: national health insurance levied on both employers and employees; a small proportion of funding also comes through prescription charges (4%); the vast majority of funding for the NHS comes from general taxation. Private health care insurance is available in the UK although this tends to offer limited coverage.
Denmark	In Denmark there are an estimated 6000 patients with PD. Services are provided mainly from neurologists either in university departments, specialist clinics or in private practice. In more remote areas patients are managed by their general practitioners. The health care system in Denmark is very comprehensive and is financed through taxation (85%) and patient payments (15%). Partial payment for drugs is met by the health service, however some groups such as the elderly are exempt from payments.

Table 8.1 (*cont.*)

Finland	Services for patients with PD are generally provided through general practitioners and neurology clinics. There is one movement disorder clinic (Helsinki University Hospital) and a rehabilitation centre funded by The Finnish Parkinson's Disease Society. The Social Insurance Institution of Finland (KELA), which has been in existence for 60 years, is financed by employers (20%), employees (18%), the state (48%) and other means (15%). The KELA provides partial funding of fees charged by physicians, clinics, medication costs and transportation. This has to be applied for annually by patients. Some costs are financed by state sponsored gambling (the Slot Machine Association). The laws and statutes of social welfare are another source of funding for patients.
Estonia	Neurologists at local general hospitals manage patients with PD. There is also a University clinic at Tartu (south Estonia) and a multidisciplinary clinic at Tallinn (capital of Estonia). The Estonian Parkinson's Society has helped to develop more access to specialists and specialist physiotherapy groups. The health care system in Estonia is funded wholly by the state.
Japan	Access to specialist help for PD patients is mostly through neurology clinics.
	The Japanese healthcare system is financed through private health insurance with patients paying for approximately 20% of medical costs. In common with other chronic illnesses when patients with PD reach a certain level of disability all medical charges are financed.
South Africa	In urban areas there are a number of hospital-based movement disorder clinics. Neurologists also treat patients privately at a number of clinics. Those living in the more remote or rural areas of South Africa often do not receive any form of medical assistance. The state finances health services in the provincial areas of South Africa. However, the amount the state contributes to an individual's health care is means tested. Those patients with private medical health insurance tend to have access to better services.
New Zealand	Patients in urban areas are managed in specialist clinics by neurologists or geriatricians with a specialist interest in movement disorders. The Parkinsonism Society of New Zealand also provides a number of field officers (usually registered nurses) who assist in the support and management of patients. New Zealand was the first country in the world, in 1938, to offer free public hospitals. The revenues for health care are raised through taxation in a similar way to that of the UK. Interestingly, in terms of total health expenditure as a percentage of GDP, New Zealand appears to be a modest spender compared to other countries.

specialist movement disorder clinics have been established, usually in large cities and academic settings, and can provide a focus for the activity of a MDT (Mutch 1992). Medical input to specialist clinics is usually from trained neurologists or geriatricians. Clinics can provide accurate diagnosis, assessment, referral to other disciplines, therapy interventions and regular review (Meara and Hobson 1998a, Meara et al. 1999a). Physical therapy plays an important part in the treatment of all stages in PD, though limited formal evidence exists for its effectiveness (Gibberd et al. 1981, Scott and Caird 1983, Robertson and Thompson 1984, Formisano et al. 1992, Comella et al. 1994). Psychological and educational programmes coupled with MDT interventions and intensive group therapy are increasingly being proposed as useful additions to medical therapy (Gauthier et al. 1987, Ellgring et al. 1990, Montgomery et al. 1994). The clinical effectiveness of specialist clinics has received little attention, though one study in the UK has shown some long-term benefits (Meara and Hobson 1998b). A vital link between the GP and secondary care could be provided by the introduction of specialist PD nurses to promote better organization of shared care. This type of specialist service is currently being evaluated in the UK. A nurse with skills in comprehensive geriatric assessment is likely to most ably meet the demands of the PD specialist nurse role (see Table 8.2).

In the UK several studies have shown a high level of unmet need in patients with PD and carers in terms of the provision and uptake of services (Oxtoby 1982, Mutch et al. 1986, Peto et al. 1997, Meara and Hobson 1997). Less than one-third of patients with PD undergo assessment by a MDT (see Table 8.3). The improvements in the uptake of physiotherapy and speech and language therapy services reported in later studies (Peto et al. 1997, Meara and Hobson 1997) may be accounted for by the recent increase in movement disorder clinics (see Table 8.4). Peto et al. 1997 found that service use increased with longer duration of disease, but even when a local specialist service exists a high proportion of patients are still not referred for specialist assessment (Meara and Hobson 1997). More research is needed to determine if new or existing services for PD are effective and efficient.

Social networks and support in PD

Social relationships and support networks have in a number of studies been found to be factors predictive of health outcomes and service utilization (Walliston et al. 1983, House et al. 1988, Sugisawa et al. 1994, Bosworth and Schaie 1997). Social networks share common characteristics through their size, source and proximity of family or friends. Social networks can act as a means of emotional support, or conversely, as a barrier to adequate help. The ability of an elderly person with PD to remain independent will be clearly influenced by their access to support and help (Berkman et al. 1992, Wenger 1991). A small number of studies have investigated

Table 8.2 The potential roles of a PD specialist nurse

- Community outreach support from a movement disorder clinic
- Liaison with GPs and primary health care teams; PD specialists; therapy services; other community/hospital-based services; social services; private sector and voluntary groups
- Rapid assessment and follow-up for both acute and elective hospital admissions
- Drug therapy monitoring/advice
- Identifying the unmet needs of patients, carers and health professionals
- Education, support and advice for patients, carers and other health professionals
- Palliative care
- Assessment of elderly patients in residential/nursing home care

Table 8.3 Recent therapy service inputs for PD patients in the UK

Service	Oxtoby (1982) $n=261$	Mutch et al. (1986) $n=267$	Peto et al. (1997) $n=178$	Meara and Hobson (1997) $n=172$
Occupational therapy	13%	25%	24%	26%
Physiotherapy	17%	7%	39%	29%
Speech and language therapy	3%	4%	25%	30%

Table 8.4 Service receipt (%) in the previous year for patients attending a movement disorder clinic compared to those managed by their general practitioner

Service	Specialist clinic managed $n=102$ (%)	GP managed $n=70$ (%)
Occupational therapy	37	9 *
Physiotherapy	43	8 *
Speech therapy	46	6 *
GP contact	98	60 *
Social worker	17	5 *
Physiotherapist	43	5 *
District nurse	15	5 *

Note:
* $P<0.05$

Table 8.5 Service provision utilization frequencies (%) in 12 month period by support network type

Service	Family dependent (n = 16)	Locally integrated (n = 35)	Local self-contained (n = 33)	Wider community (n = 11)	Private (n = 15)
GP	16 (100%)	33 (94%)	30 (91%)	11 (100%)	11 (73%)
Consultant/Specialist	15 (94%)	19 (54%)	23 (70%)	7 (64%)	6 (40%)
Occupational therapist	8 (50%)	8 (23%)	9 (27%)	3 (27%)	4 (27%)
Physiotherapist	6 (37%)	11 (31%)	10 (30%)	2 (18%)	4 (27%)
Social worker	1 (6%)	3 (9%)	6 (18%)	1 (9%)	1 (7%)
Speech therapist	7 (44%)	11 (31%)	13 (39%)	3 (27%)	4 (27%)
Care assistant	1 (6%)	9 (26%)	3 (9%)	3 (27%)	4 (27%)
District nurse	6 (37%)	1 (3%)	4 (12%)	2 (18%)	5 (33%)

the social support of people with PD (McCarthy and Brown 1989, Ehmann et al. 1990, Miller et al. 1996). All these have shown that low self esteem, poor coping strategies and depressive symptomatology are associated with reduced social support. We have examined the support and help provided by social networks and the influence they have upon the management of PD patients living in the community using a network typology devised by Wenger (Wenger 1990, 1991). The results (see Table 8.5) indicate that the social network influences the delivery of appropriate services and interventions for patients with PD (unpublished observations). This has implications for health professionals, service providers and planners, who need to recognize and be made more aware of the importance and influence of social support and networks in chronic disease.

Meeting the needs of caregivers

Carers of patients with PD, usually a spouse, are likely to be similarly aged and may also suffer from chronic illness. Caring for an elderly spouse with PD can result in the deterioration of a marital relationship to that of nurse and patient (Pinder 1990). Estimates of the financial costs for informal care in the UK suggest an annual figure of around 24 billion pounds (Adams 1991). Stress, frustration, exhaustion, depression and physical illness are commonly reported by caregivers (Mui 1995). The burden of care in PD is reflected in the high levels of carer distress reported in several studies (Calder et al. 1991, Miller et al. 1996, O'Reilly et al. 1996, Herrmann et al. 1997, Meara et al. 1999b). The UK Parkinson's Disease Society discussion document *Meeting a need?* (1994) addresses the needs of patients and carers and recommends the provision of appropriate respite care, relevant and intelligible information on PD and how to obtain help and guidance. Arksey et al. (1998) evaluated the needs of carers of patients with physical disabilities who had been recently discharged from hospital and found that what they required was clear, unambiguous, practical and helpful information. Although the carer is likely to be the most important person in the provision of care for the patient, this vital role is often poorly recognized, ignored or undervalued. More research needs to be undertaken in this area in PD in order to find ways of reducing the distress that can be associated with caring.

Economic appraisals of the delivery of care for elderly patients with PD

Rationing of resources is a reality throughout all healthcare systems no matter how well funded. In the last 20 years there has been a rapid growth in the introduction of more effective, but also more expensive drug treatments for PD. New and expensive drug therapy that improves motor impairment in terms of reducing tremor or rigidity may have only marginal effects on handicap or disadvantage to the patient. More data are needed relating to the cost benefits of existing drugs compared with new drug therapies for PD in terms of improvements in disadvantage and health related quality of life. Appropriate evaluation of the impact of new treatments on health related quality of life would give patients, specialists and health care planners better information to make therapeutic and funding decisions. Some countries with state financed health care systems, such as the UK, place financial limits upon the introduction of new or existing treatments and evidence of the clinical effectiveness of treatment is increasingly being sought before funding will be given. This approach should be adopted in developing countries where high levels of economic and social deprivation already limit health care provision. In the absence of adequate state support or private insurance, many patients with PD are faced with difficult choices. In self-funding their treatment patients may elect to reduce medication or substitute expensive drugs for cheaper ones. Many drugs used in the treatment of PD such as combinations of levodopa and decarboxylase inhibitors, dopamine agonists and enzyme inhibitors, such as selegiline and tolcapone, are expensive and unaffordable in many areas of the world. Neurosurgical procedures, though not widely available, may be a cheaper long-term option than drug therapy in many countries.

Putting research into practice

The difficulty of collecting information that will inform not only health care professionals, but also patients and their carers cannot be underestimated. In the UK clinical audit is employed as a means to assess the quality of services and to develop effective interventions that will result in improvements in patient care. However, by its nature clinical audit tends to focus on clinical needs, failing to take into account the expectations of carers and patients. There is a need to work with the patients who actually make use of the particular service. Patients with PD who attend a specialist clinic may all appear to have the same service need, yet in reality individual needs are very dissimilar. Evidence of clinical effectiveness alone will not alter practice given the confounding effects of cultural, political, social and economic factors.

Epidemiological studies, clinical trials, observational studies and cost benefit studies are methods of ensuring representation of patient populations and measuring outcomes of interventions. Studies such as these should provide estimates of the size of specific illnesses and thereby allow health care planning to match need with resources. The assessment and evaluation of patients' experiences and their treatment is acknowledged as a vital component of health care. Elderly people tend to be underrepresented or excluded from a significant proportion of these studies. Furthermore, the methodologies used in outcome research may also be inappropriate for elderly people even when they have been included in studies. To illustrate this point the generic SF-36 (Ware and Sherbourne 1992), a health related quality of life instrument, has been used in a number of countries and has been demonstrated to have excellent psychometric qualities. However, the SF-36 may not be an appropriate instrument in elderly people with PD (Hill et al. 1996, Hobson and Meara 1997, Parker et al. 1998). All too often such generic measures are used inappropriately without the addition of disease specific or single domain measures from which more meaningful conclusions may be drawn. Hunter (1996) argues that there is not one definitive way to evaluate new or existing services and that a collaboration of varied research disciplines and research methodologies are the key to effective evaluation for the provision and organization of health services.

Palliative care in PD

There is a lack of any formal guidance on the management of palliative care in PD. In the UK patients with advanced PD who require nursing care are usually managed in nursing homes with routine medical care provided by the GP. Specialist involvement is unusual at this stage, often because of the inappropriateness of attendance at an outpatient clinic. However, at this stage in PD management there is still a very great need for close cooperation and effective communication between health professionals and the patient and family (Meara 1998). Most research in palliative care has concentrated on patients dying of cancer, who have tended to be younger and cared for in hospitals or hospices. One study found that elderly people with terminal illness do not receive the same professional medical interventions as younger patients (Seale and Cartwright 1994). Lindop et al. (1997) argue that the existing models of palliative care for cancer patients need to be broadened to encompass the needs for all patients with terminal illnesses and should include their families and carers.

Conclusion

The WHO and various PD working parties have suggested guidelines on what services are needed to meet the needs of patients with PD. However, the challenge is to implement these proposals within existing healthcare systems throughout the world. Greater emphasis should be placed upon collaboration between health and social care professionals, the voluntary sector and patients and their carers. Information technology can facilitate the dissemination of what is considered to be best practice in the management of PD. This technology is not available exclusively to health care professionals, and will be increasingly employed by patients, their carers and by pressure groups to demand better service and more effective interventions.

REFERENCES

Adams B (1991) Healthcare data briefing: Unpaid care. *Health Service Journal,* 100, 2, 26.

Arksey H, Heaton J, Sloper P (1998) Tell it like it is. *Health Service Journal,* 108, 5588, 32–3.

Berkman LF, Oxman TE, Seeman TE (1992) Social networks and social support among the Elderly: Assessment issues. In: *The Epidemiologic Study of the Elderly,* eds. Wallace RB, Woolson RF, pp. 196–212. Oxford: Oxford University Press.

Bosworth HB, Schaie W (1997) The relationship of social environment, social networks, and health outcomes in The Seattle Longitudinal Study: two analytical approaches. *Journal of Gerontology, Psychiatry and Science,* 52B, 5, 197–205.

Calder SA, Ebmeier KP, Stewart L, Crawford JR, Besson JAO (1991) The prediction of stress in carers: The role of behaviour, reported self-care and dementia in patients with idiopathic Parkinson's disease. *International Journal of Geriatric Psychiatry,* 6, 737–42.

Comella CL, Stebbins GT, Brown-Toms N, Goetz CG (1994) Physical therapy and Parkinson's disease: A controlled clinical trial. *Neurology,* 44, 376–8.

Ehmann TS, Beninger RJ, Gawel MJ, Riopelle RJ (1990) Coping, social support, and depressive symptoms in Parkinson's disease. *Journal of Geriatric Psychiatry and Neurology,* 3, 85–90.

Ellgring H, Seiler S, Nagel U, Perleth B, Gasser T, Oertel WH (1990) Psychosocial problems of Parkinson patients: approaches to assessment. *Advances in Neurology* 53, 349–53.

Gauthier L, Dalziel S, Gauthier S (1987) The benefits of group occupational therapy for patients with Parkinson's disease. *The American Journal of Occupational Therapy,* 41, 6, 360–5.

Formisano R, Pratesi L, Modarelli FT, Bonifati V, Meco G. (1992) Rehabilitation and Parkinson's disease. *Scandinavian Journal of Rehabilitation Medicine,* 24, 157–60.

Gibberd FB, Page NGR, Spencer KM (1981) Controlled trial of physiotherapy and occupational therapy for Parkinson's disease. *British Medical Journal*, 282, 1196.

Gibson MJ (1992) Public health and social policy. In: *Family Support for the Elderly: The International Experience*, eds. Kendig H, Hashimoto A, Coppard LC, pp. 88–114. Oxford: Oxford University Press.

Hill S, Harries U, Popay J (1996) Is the Short-Form 36 (SF-36) suitable for routine health outcomes assessment in health care for older people? Evidence from preliminary work in community-based health services in England. *Journal of Epidemiology and Community Health*, 50, 94–8.

Herrmann M, Freyholdt U, Fuchs G, Wallesch CW (1997) Coping with chronic neurological impairment: a contrastive analysis of Parkinson's disease and stroke. *Disability and Rehabilitation*, 19, 1, 6–12.

Hobson JP, Meara RJ (1997) Is the SF-36 Health Survey Questionnaire suitable as a self report measure of the health status of older adults with Parkinson's disease. *Quality of Life Research*, 3, 6, 213–16.

House JS, Landis HR, Umberson D (1988) Social relationships and health. *Science*, 241, 540–5.

Hunter DJ (1996) Evaluation of health services. In: *Epidemiology in Old Age*, eds. Ebrahim S, Kalache A, pp. 85–95. London: BMJ Publishing Group.

Kinsella K (1996) Demographic aspects. In: *Epidemiology in Old Age*, eds. Ebrahim S and Kalache A, pp. 32–40. London: BMJ Publishing Group.

Kinsella K, Taeuber C (1993) *An Ageing World II*. Washington: US Government Printing Office.

Lilienfeld DE, Chan E, Ehland J, Goldbold J, Landrigan PJ, Marsh G, Perl DP (1990) Two decades of increasing mortality from Parkinson's disease among the US elderly. *Archives of Neurology*, 7, 731–4.

Lindop E, Beach R, Read S (1997) A composite model of palliative care for the UK. *International Journal of Palliative Nursing*, 3, 5, 287–92.

McCarthy B, Brown R (1989) Psychosocial factors in Parkinson's disease. *British Journal of Clinical Psychology*, 28, 41–2.

Meara RJ (1998) Late stage Parkinson's disease. *Prescribers' Journal*, 38, 4, 233–42.

Meara RJ, Bhowmick BK, Hobson JP (1999a) Accuracy of diagnosis in patients with presumed Parkinson's disease in a community-based disease register. *Age and Ageing*, 28, 99–102.

Meara RJ, Hobson JP (1997) Levels of service provision for people with Parkinson's disease: A survey of community registered patient's perceptions. *The Journal of the British Association for Service to the Elderly*, 4, 3–10.

Meara RJ, Hobson JP (1998a) Comprehensive assessment of patients with Parkinson's disease. *Mature Medicine – Canada*, 1, 3, 15–18.

Meara RJ, Hobson JP (1998b) A longitudinal follow-up of patients with Parkinson's syndrome who attend a specialist movement disorder clinic. *Age and Ageing*, 27, Suppl. 1, 55.

Meara RJ, Mitchelmore E, Hobson JP (1999b) Use of the GDS-15 as a screening instrument for depressive symptomatology in patients with Parkinson's disease and their carers in the community. *Age and Ageing*, 28, 35–8.

Miller E, Berrios GE, Politynska BE (1996) Caring for someone with Parkinson's disease: factors that contribute to distress. *International Journal of Geriatric Psychiatry*, 11, 263–8.

Montgomery EB, Lieberman A, Singh G, Fries JF (1994) Patient education and health promotion can be effective in Parkinson's disease: A randomised controlled trial. *American Journal of Medicine*, 97, 429–35.

Mui AC (1995) Caring for the frail elderly parent. A comparison of adult sons and daughters. *Gerontologist*, 35, 86–93.

Mutch WJ (1992) Specialist clinics: A better way to care? *Journal of Neurology, Neurosurgery, and Psychiatry*, 55, Suppl. 41–4.

Mutch WJ, Strudwick A, Roy SK, Downie AW (1986) Parkinson's disease: disability, review and management. *British Medical Journal*, 282, 534–6.

O'Mahony PG, Rodgers H, Thomson RG, Dobson R, James OFW (1998) Is the SF-36 suitable for assessing health status of older stroke patients? *Age and Ageing*, 27, 19–22.

O'Reilly F, Finnan F, Allwright S, Smith GD, Ben-Shlomo Y (1996) The effects of caring for a spouse with Parkinson's disease on social, psychological and physical well-being. *British Journal of Clinical Practice*, 46, 507–12.

Oxtoby M (1982) *Parkinson's Disease Patients and their Social Needs*. London: Parkinson's Disease Society.

Parker SG, Peet SM, Jagger C, Farhan M, Castleden CM (1998) Measuring health status in older patients. The SF-36 in practice. *Age and Ageing*, 27, 13–18.

Parkinson's Disease Society (1994) *Discussion Document: Meeting a Need?* London: Parkinson's Disease Society.

Peto V, Fitzpatrick R, Jenkinson C (1997) Self-reported health status and access to health services in a community sample with Parkinson's disease. *Disability and Rehabilitation*, 19, 3, 97–103.

Pinder R (1990) *The Management of Chronic Illness: Patient and Doctor Perspectives on Parkinson's Disease*. London: MacMillan Press.

Robertson S, Thompson F (1984) Speech therapy in Parkinson's disease: a study of the efficacy and long-term effects of intensive treatment. *British Journal of Disorders of Communication*, 19, 213–24.

Scott S, Caird FI (1983) Speech therapy for Parkinson's disease. *Journal of Neurology, Neurosurgery, and Psychiatry*, 47, 302–4.

Seale C, Cartwright A (1994) *The Year Before Death*. Aldershot: Avebury Press.

Sugisawa H, Liang J, Liu X (1994) Social networks, social support and mortality among older people in Japan. *Journal of Gerontology: Social Sciences*, 49, S3–13.

Walliston BA, Alagna SW, De Villis BM, De Villis RF (1983) Social support with many aspects of health and illness. *Health Psychology*, 2, 367–91.

Ware JE, Sherbourne CD (1992) The MOS 36 item short form survey (SF-36): conceptual framework and item selection. *Medical Care*, 30, 473–83.

Wenger GC (1990) Change and adaptation in informal support networks of elderly people in Wales 1979–1987. *Journal of Ageing Studies*, 4, 4, 375–89.

Wenger, GC (1991). A network typology: From theory to practice. *Journal of Ageing Studies*, 5, 1, 147–62.

Zhang Z-X, Roman GC (1992) Worldwide occurrence of Parkinson's disease: an updated review. *Neuroepidemiology*, 12, 195–208.

9

The drug treatment of Parkinson's disease in elderly people

Theresa A Zesiewicz and Robert A Hauser

Introduction

The goal of medical management of Parkinson's disease (PD) is to control signs and symptoms for as long as possible while minimizing side effects. Medical therapy generally provides good control of symptoms for 4 to 6 years, though disability continues to progress despite best medical management, and many patients develop long-term complications. Such complications include motor fluctuations and dyskinesia associated with long-term levodopa therapy (Chase et al. 1993). Other common causes of disability in late stage disease include postural instability and dementia.

A key consideration in the treatment of elderly patients is that they are more susceptible to side effects from medication. Older people are more likely than younger individuals to be taking more prescribed and over the counter medication for a range of diseases. Medication prescribed for one condition can worsen another and side effects from medication can be mistaken as a new disease process and lead to further unnecessary prescribing (Williamson 1978). Cognitive impairment and delirium, both of which commonly develop as side effects of drug therapy, reduce compliance with drug treatment.

As people live longer the prevalence of PD will increase. PD is a significant risk factor for admission to nursing homes. Over 50% of prevalent cases of PD in one epidemiological study in France were living in nursing homes (Tison et al. 1994). Hallucinations are a particular factor that increases the risk of admission to nursing homes in PD and in many cases this will be related to the drug therapy prescribed for PD (Goetz and Stebbins 1995). Residents with PD make up around 5% of the nursing home population and there is evidence to suggest that optimal drug treatment in this group may have delayed or even prevented some admissions to nursing homes (Larsen et al. 1991).

The selection of drug therapy is often guided by information derived from clinical trials. Unfortunately, elderly people are under represented in drug trials and a post hoc analysis of elderly subgroups is rarely provided (Avorn 1990). Very few clinical trials have examined the best way to use available antiparkinsonian medication for different age groups, over either the short or long-term. Thus, until such information is available, a heavy reliance is placed on theoretical considerations, and anecdotal and personal experience. Not all drugs are available worldwide; in particular, apomorphine, domperidone and Madopar™ preparations are not currently licensed for use in the United States.

Drugs used in the treatment of PD in elderly patients

Levodopa

Levodopa combined with a peripheral decarboxylase inhibitor (PDI) is the gold standard of drug treatment for PD. It usually provides the greatest symptomatic improvement with the fewest side effects. Ehringer and Hornykiewicz (1960) demonstrated that PD is associated with decreased striatal dopamine concentration, but dopamine is not useful as a therapeutic agent because it does not cross the blood–brain barrier. Carlsson et al. (1957) had already reported that the administration of the dopamine precursor, levodopa, reversed reserpine induced parkinsonism in rats. Levodopa was subsequently demonstrated to improve signs and symptoms of PD (Cotzias et al. 1968).

Levodopa is a large neutral amino acid, with a serum half life of approximately one hour (Nutt and Fellman 1984). It is primarily absorbed in the proximal small bowel by a saturable, carrier mediated transport system. The stomach is capable of absorbing levodopa only to a limited extent (Cedarbaum 1987). Meals and anticholinergic medications slow gastric emptying and delay levodopa absorption (Cedarbaum 1987). In older patients, gastric stasis results in slower gastric emptying and increased duodenal levodopa absorption (Evans et al. 1980). In addition, first pass metabolic decarboxylation of levodopa in the gastrointestinal tract is reduced in older individuals. Because of these age associated changes, levodopa bioavailability is as much as 20% greater in the elderly (Evans et al. 1980).

Levodopa bioavailability is approximately 40% in young volunteers. Levodopa undergoes extensive peripheral metabolism, and less than 1% is excreted unchanged in the urine (Abrams et al. 1971). Nausea and vomiting are common side effects of levodopa due to the peripheral metabolism of levodopa to dopamine, which stimulates the area postrema of the medulla. Levodopa is usually administered with a PDI that does not penetrate the blood–brain barrier to reduce circulating peripheral dopamine, thereby minimizing the incidence of nausea and vomiting, and to increase the central bioavailability. Co-careldopa (Sinemet™) contains the PDI carbidopa; co-beneldopa (Madopar™) contains benserazide. Both carbidopa and benserazide reduce the amount of levodopa needed to achieve a clinical response by approximately 75%. Around 75–100 mg of carbidopa per day are usually sufficient to saturate peripheral decarboxylase, but some patients may require up to 200 mg (Rinne et al. 1973). The peripheral half life of levodopa when administered with a decarboxylase inhibitor is approximately two hours (Nutt et al. 1985). Levodopa absorption is facilitated by the administration of domperidone, a peripheral dopamine antagonist that promotes gastric emptying (Mearrick et al. 1974).

In older patients we introduce levodopa/PDI at a dose of 50 mg once each morning and increase to 50 mg levodopa three or four times daily, or 100 mg levodopa three times daily over a three to four week period. Further titration is based on clinical response. Most patients remain on 400–600 mg of levodopa/PDI for several years. Higher doses can and should be used if necessary to adequately control motor symptoms. Levodopa/PDI is usually administered one half hour before or one hour after meals to achieve the most consistent absorption.

Acute side effects of levodopa/PDI administration include nausea, postural hypotension, confusion and hallucinations. Nausea is the most common side effect of levodopa/PDI therapy. If nausea occurs, it can often be reduced by administering the dose immediately following meals or with a carbohydrate snack. If nausea persists, increasing the carbidopa dosage is usually quite helpful. Some patients require up to 200 mg of carbidopa per day. Domperidone can usually control this problem though other antiemetics such as metcloplamide and prochlorperazine should be avoided due to their central dopamine receptor blocking action. Uncommon side effects include anorexia, somnolence, increased serum transaminase levels and worsening of closed angle glaucoma. Levodopa/PDI can cause neuropsychiatric toxicity, ranging from delusions to delirium. Older patients are more vulnerable to these side effects. Postural hypotension is a potentially serious side effect of levodopa/PDI in older patients as it can lead to syncope, falls, and fractures. A review of all medications taken by the patient that may contribute to the problem should be undertaken. A reduction of the levodopa dosage may be necessary.

Levodopa/carbidopa controlled-release

The controlled (sustained) release (CR) preparation of co-careldopa is more slowly absorbed and provides more sustained serum levels than standard co-careldopa (Goetz et al. 1987). The bioavailability of levodopa in CR formulation is roughly 80% that of standard co-careldopa. Bioavailability is greater in the elderly, possibly owing to an age related decrease in gastric emptying. In addition, administering levodopa/carbidopa CR with food increases levodopa bioavailability by roughly 50%, and elevates peak plasma levels by 25% (Wilding et al. 1989). Co-careldopa controlled-release is available in a 200/50 mg and 100/25 mg strengths.

We introduce co-careldopa CR at a dose of one 100/25 mg tablet per day and increase to three tablets per day over several weeks. Another common dosing schedule is co-careldopa CR 200/50 twice daily. To convert a patient from standard levodopa/carbidopa to CR, the daily levodopa dosage is increased roughly 20% while the number of daily doses is decreased by 30–50% (Rodnitzky 1992). Further titration is undertaken as clinically indicated.

Co-careldopa CR is as effective as standard co-careldopa when dopamine replacement therapy is first required and may be more convenient (Block et al. 1997). Later in the disease, patients with motor fluctuations and no dyskinesia often experience less 'off' time following conversion from standard to CR formulation (Feldman et al. 1989). However, CR formulations tend to worsen peak dose dyskinesia, particularly later in the day when levodopa levels accumulate. Because co-careldopa CR takes longer than standard formulation to 'kick in' and provide clinical benefit, many patients with motor fluctuations take a combination of standard and CR co-careldopa as their first morning dose. Intake of subsequent CR doses is scheduled so that one dose takes effect before the previous dose wears off. A bedtime levodopa/carbidopa CR dose maintains therapeutic plasma concentrations longer into the night, resulting in greater mobility for patients who awaken within a few hours. However, this may lead to nightmares or hallucinations in some patients.

Co-beneldopa HBS

Co-beneldopa HBS (hydrodynamically balanced system) is a slowly dissolving preparation that floats on stomach contents for 5–12 hours, providing sustained release of levodopa proximal to its site of absorption. The bioavailability of co-beneldopa HBS is 50 to 60% that of standard formulation (Koller and Pahwa 1994). The pharmacokinetic profiles of co-careldopa CR and co-beneldopa HBS are similar.

Open label studies have found the HBS preparation to be effective in reducing motor fluctuations for patients on standard co-beneldopa. A randomised, double-blind, cross-over trial comparing standard and HBS preparations demonstrated significantly better clinical function while patients were taking co-beneldopa HBS, but no difference in 'off' time as measured by patient diaries (de Michele et al. 1989).

Dopamine agonists

There are five orally active dopamine agonist drugs available to treat PD: the ergot agonists – bromocriptine, pergolide, and cabergoline, and the non ergot agonists – pramipexole and ropinirole. An account of the parenterally administered agonist apomorphine, which is only available on a named patient basis in the US, is given in Chapter 3.

In contrast to levodopa, dopamine agonists do not undergo oxidative metabolism, and the long-acting dopamine agonists provide relatively sustained dopaminergic stimulation. Animal studies and preliminary clinical information suggest that dopamine agonists are associated with a lower incidence of motor fluctuations and dyskinesia than levodopa/PDI (see below). Long-acting dopamine agonists are effective as monotherapy in early disease and as adjunctive therapy in late stage disease for patients who are experiencing motor fluctuations on levodopa/PDI. In early disease, dopamine agonist monotherapy provides symptomatic benefit comparable to levodopa/PDI. Dopamine agonists reduce 'off' time, improve motor function, and allow levodopa dose reductions. When a dopamine agonist is added to levodopa/PDI, it may be necessary to reduce the levodopa dose if dopaminergic effects such as peak dose dyskinesia or hallucinations emerge or worsen.

However, as the disease progresses, dopamine agonists alone become insufficient to control symptoms and no longer provide as much symptomatic benefit as levodopa/PDI. Dopamine agonists are generally less well tolerated than levodopa/PDI. Side effects, such as postural hypotension, nausea and vomiting, and confusion can be minimized by introducing dopamine agonists at a low dose and slowly escalating, in order to identify most of those that do occur when they are mild. Rarely, an elderly patient will experience a dramatic side effect, such as syncope, with the first intake despite starting with the lowest dose. Although it is commonly stated that the elderly are more prone to side effects from dopamine agonists than levodopa/carbidopa, to our knowledge this has not been systematically evaluated. Patients with dementia are prone to hallucinations and increased confusion, and patients with low blood pressure or orthostasis may experience an exacerbation of hypotensive symptoms. Beyond these examples it is generally difficult to predict who will encounter side effects from a dopamine agonist. In our experience, many nondemented elderly patients tolerate dopamine agonists quite well and derive clinical benefit (Hindle et al. 1998).

Bromocriptine

Bromocriptine is an ergot alkaloid synthetic cyclic derivative of lysergic acid, with both pre and postsynaptic effects. It was originally developed as a prolactin inhibitor, but was also found to have antiparkinsonian activity (Calne et al. 1974). Bromocriptine is a strong D2 receptor agonist and a weak D2 receptor antagonist. It is rapidly absorbed from the gastrointestinal tract, strongly bound to plasma protein, and undergoes 90% first pass metabolism. Peak plasma levels are achieved in 30 to 210 minutes and its half life is approximately seven hours. Side effects include nausea, orthostatic hypotension, and psychiatric symptoms.

Bromocriptine monotherapy improves signs and symptoms of early PD (Bromocriptine Multicentre Trial Group 1990). However, it is less effective than levodopa over the long-term. Olanow (1988) found that bromocriptine monotherapy provided symptom reduction comparable to levodopa/PDI for six months but less benefit than levodopa/PDI after six months. One retrospective study that has been criticized on methodological grounds found that only one third of patients retained an adequate response on bromocriptine alone after three years. However, patients treated with bromocriptine were reported to have a lower incidence of motor fluctuations and peak dose dyskinesia than those treated with levodopa (Rinne 1987).

The most troublesome side effect of bromocriptine is postural hypotension. As many as 33% of patients will experience dizziness or lightheadedness when bromocriptine is first introduced. Nausea is also a common problem. Neuropsychiatric side effects include hallucinations, confusion, nightmares, agitation, and mood changes. Bromocriptine causes psychiatric disturbances more commonly than levodopa (Montastruc et al. 1993), which limits its use in elderly patients with pre-existing cognitive impairment. Other side effects include burning dysaesthesiae and livedo reticularis, a rash of the lower extremities. Rarely, pleural effusion, erythromelalgia, pulmonary and retroperitoneal fibrosis, and peripheral vascular disease have been described (LeWitt and Calne 1982).

We start bromocriptine at a dose of 1.25 mg per day and titrate up to 10 mg per day over one month. Further titration is based on clinical response and side effects. The usual maximum dose is 30–40 mg per day.

Pergolide

Pergolide is a semisynthetic clavine ergoline agonist that stimulates both D1 and D2 receptors (Goldstein et al. 1980). It is roughly 10 times more potent than bromocriptine on a mg for mg basis and is a strong D2 receptor agonist and a weak D1 receptor agonist. As with bromocriptine, pergolide is highly bound to plasma proteins and undergoes extensive first pass metabolism. Peak plasma levels are achieved in one to two hours, and its half life is 20–27 hours. For unexplained reasons, the half life of pergolide, derived from the suppression of prolactin secretion, is far longer than the therapeutic action of the drug in PD, which is at most around 6 hours.

Pergolide is effective as monotherapy in early disease and as an adjunct to levodopa/PDI in advanced disease (Mear et al. 1984, Olanow et al. 1994). Pergolide reduced 'off' time by 32% compared with 4% with placebo in a double-blind study comparing pergolide to placebo as an adjunct to levodopa in patients with motor fluctuations (Olanow et al. 1994). Motor function improved 35% in pergolide treated patients compared with 17% in placebo treated patients ($P<0.001$). Pergolide permitted a significant mean levodopa dose reduction of 24.7% compared with 4.9% in the placebo group. A single blind, crossover study found that pergolide provided significantly greater benefit than bromocriptine in PD patients experiencing a declining response to levodopa (Pezzoli et al. 1994). Side effects of pergolide are similar to those of bromocriptine. We introduce pergolide at a dose of 0.25 mg per day and slowly increase to approximately 0.25 mg three times daily over several weeks. Further titration is undertaken based on clinical response. The usual maximum dose is 3–4 mg per day.

Cabergoline

Cabergoline is an ergot dopamine agonist with strong D2 and weak D1 receptor affinity. Its plasma half life is approximately 65 hours, thereby allowing once a day dosing. Cabergoline is introduced at a dose of 0.5 mg/day and slowly escalated to a maximum dose of 4–5 mg/day. A one year comparison of cabergoline to levodopa as early monotherapy found that over 80% of patients in each group experienced >30% improvement in motor disability (Rinne et al. 1997). A total of 38% of cabergoline treated patients required levodopa supplementation by one year. Patients remaining on monotherapy exhibited clinical improvement comparable to those taking levodopa. As an adjunct to levodopa/carbidopa in suboptimally controlled patients, cabergoline provided significantly more 'on' time at six months in comparison to placebo and the cabergoline group was taking 18% less levodopa (Hutton et al. 1993).

Pramipexole

Pramipexole is a synthetic amino benzathiazol non-ergot agonist that binds with high affinity to the D2 family of dopamine receptors, especially the D3 receptor (Mieraau and Schingnitz 1992). It has little affinity for D1, 5HT, muscarinic, or adrenergic receptors. Pramipexole is rapidly absorbed, and reaches peak concentration in about two hours. It is 15% bound to plasma protein. The half life is approximately eight hours in young volunteers and 12 hours in elderly volunteers. Urinary excretion is the major route of elimination, and 90% of pramipexole is recovered in the urine unchanged. Renal insufficiency decreases elimination. Pramipexole clearance is about 75% lower in patients with severe renal impairment and 60% lower in patients with moderate renal insufficiency.

Pramipexole is effective as early monotherapy and as an adjunct to levodopa in advanced disease. In a large, prospective, double-blind trial comparing pramipexole to levodopa in early disease, pramipexole significantly improved motor scores compared with pretreatment values (Shannon et al. 1997). A six month trial comparing pramipexole to placebo as add on therapy in levodopa treated patients with motor fluctuations found that pramipexole reduced 'off' time by 31% compared with 7% in placebo treated patients (Lieberman et al. 1997). Motor function was improved by 25% in the pramipexole group compared to 12% in the placebo group. Pramipexole permitted a 27% reduction in levodopa dose compared to 5% in the placebo group.

Pramipexole is introduced at a dose of 0.125 mg/day and increased to 0.5 mg three times daily over one month. The usual maximum dose is 3 to 4.5 mg/day. Side effects include hallucinations, somnolence, nausea, constipation, and insomnia (Shannon 1996). As a non ergot dopamine agonist, pramipexole should not cause ergot related side effects such as erythromelalgia, and the rare but potentially serious complications of pleural and retroperitoneal fibrosis.

Ropinirole

Ropinirole is a nonergoline dopamine agonist that binds selectively to D2 receptors with little affinity for D1, 5HT, muscarinic, or adrenergic receptors (Eden et al. 1991). It is rapidly absorbed and extensively metabolized by the liver. The elimination half life of ropinirole is approximately six hours. Maximal plasma concentration is reached after approximately one and a half hours in fasting patients and after approximately four hours when taken with meals. Ropinirole clearance is reduced by 30% in elderly patients.

Ropinirole is effective as early monotherapy and as an adjunct to levodopa/PDI in advanced disease. In a six month study comparing ropinirole to placebo in early PD, motor function was significantly improved, by 24% at six months in ropinirole treated patients compared to a 3% worsening in placebo treated patients (Adler et al. 1997). Significantly fewer ropinirole treated patients required the introduction of levodopa/PDI (11% vs. 29%). A six month study (Ropinirole Study Group 1996), comparing ropinirole with bromocriptine as early monotherapy, found ropinirole alone provided significantly greater improvement than bromocriptine alone (34% vs. 20%). Another six month study (Rascol 1996) comparing ropinirole to levodopa in early disease found that a similar percentage of patients experienced >30% improvement (48% vs. 58%), although levodopa treated patients experienced significantly greater improvement overall (32% vs. 44%).

Ropinirole reduces 'off' time, improves clinical function and permits levodopa dose reductions in patients with fluctuating disease. In a comparison of ropinirole to placebo as adjunctive therapy to levodopa, 27.7% of ropinirole treated patients had at least a 20% reduction in levodopa dose *and* at least a 20% reduction in 'off' time at six months compared to 11% in the placebo arm (Kreider et al. 1996).

Ropinirole is introduced at a dose of 0.25 mg per day, with an initial target dose of 1 mg three times daily reached over one month. The usual maximum is 6–8 mg three times daily. Side effects are similar to those of the other currently available non-ergoline dopamine agonist pramipexole.

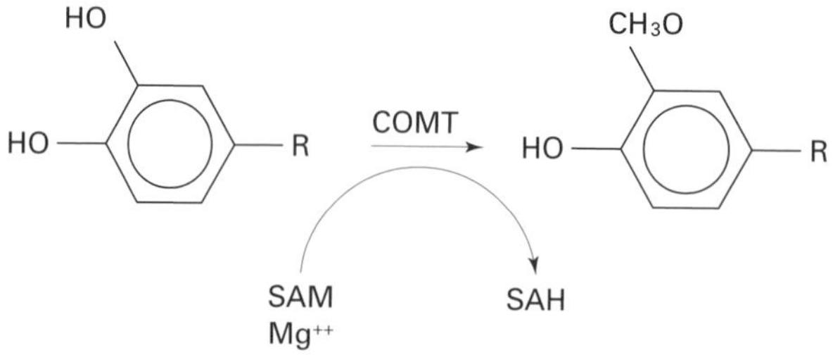

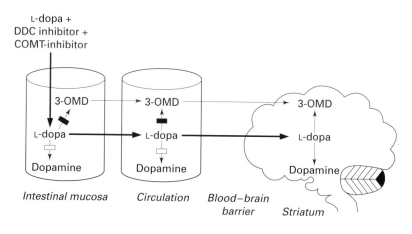

Fig. 9.1   Methylation of catechol substrate by COMT (catechol-*O*-methyltransferase). SAM, *S*-adenosyl-ʟ-methionine; SAH, *S*-methyl-L-homocysteine; R, side chain.

Fig. 9.2   Mechanism of peripheral COMT inhibition. Reprinted with permission from Kaakkola et al. (1996).

COMT inhibitors

Two inhibitors of catechol-O-methyltransferase (COMT), tolcapone and entacapone, have been developed and are available in some countries for clinical and trial use. COMT is one of the primary enzymes responsible for the catabolism of levodopa. COMT catalyses the transfer of a methyl group from *S*-adenosyl-ʟ-methionine (SAM) to the hydroxyl group of a catecholamine (see Fig. 9.1). When levodopa/PDI is administered, COMT metabolism of levodopa to 3–O-methyldopa (3–OMD) is prominent. 3–OMD has no antiparkinsonian activity and may marginally decrease levodopa absorption and transport across the blood–brain barrier (Nutt et al. 1987). Peripheral COMT inhibition blocks the peripheral metabolism of levodopa to 3–OMD, thereby extending the area under the time concentration curve and making more levodopa available for transport across the blood brain–barrier (see Fig. 9.2). When a COMT inhibitor is added to levodopa/PDI therapy, striatal dopamine levels are increased for longer. Central COMT inhibition might further maintain striatal dopamine levels by blocking the central metabolism of dopamine to homovanillic acid. COMT inhibitors reduce 'off' time, improve motor function, and allow levodopa dose reductions in advanced patients with motor fluctuations on levodopa.

Tolcapone

Tolcapone is a reversible COMT inhibitor, with both peripheral and central activity (Zurcher et al. 1990, Mannisto and Kaakkola 1990, Spencer and Benfield 1996). It is rapidly absorbed and has a half life of approximately two hours. Tolcapone has been demonstrated to improve motor function and allow levodopa dose reductions in patients on levodopa with either a stable or fluctuating response. A six month double-blind, placebo-controlled trial evaluating tolcapone in PD patients experiencing a stable response to levodopa/carbidopa found that tolcapone significantly improved motor function and decreased mean total daily levodopa doses compared to placebo (Waters et al. 1997). In patients with motor fluctuations on levodopa/PDI, a comparison of tolcapone (200 mg three times daily) to placebo found a significant mean reduction in 'off' time of 48% in the tolcapone group compared to 20% in the placebo group at three months (Rajput et al. 1997). Tolcapone allowed a 24% reduction in levodopa dose compared with a 1.6% increase in placebo treated patients. Another double-blind placebo-controlled study evaluating tolcapone in patients experiencing motor fluctuations on levodopa found tolcapone reduced 'off' time by 19% (Kurth et al. 1997). The central effects of tolcapone do not seem relevant to its actions in PD, as drug naïve patients do not improve on monotherapy with tolcapone (Hauser et al. 1998). The suggested possible antidepressant action of tolcapone needs to be confirmed.

Tolcapone is usually introduced at a dose of 100 mg three times daily. Side effects of tolcapone are mostly those related to increased dopaminergic stimulation and include dyskinesia, nausea, hallucinations and hypotension. Dopaminergic side effects can usually be improved by decreasing the levodopa dose. Patients with peak dose dyskinesia often experience a rapid and substantial increase in dyskinesia requiring a 25–50% reduction in levodopa dose. Other side effects include dizziness and urine discolouration. Of note, approximately 10% of patients experience diarrhoea and 3% discontinue tolcapone because of this side effect. Onset of diarrhoea usually occurs four to 12 weeks after initiation of therapy, but is uncommon after six months (Waters et al. 1997). There has been recent concern over the development of abnormal liver function tests in patients taking tolcapone and rare cases of fatal hepatic failure. In the US the recommendation has been made to monitor liver function tests regularly in patients on this drug and to use the drug only after other treatments have failed. In the European Union the product licence for tolcapone has been suspended and the drug withdrawn.

Entacapone

Entacapone is a reversible, peripheral COMT inhibitor that is less potent than tolcapone (McNeely and Davis 1997). Entacapone is rapidly absorbed and has an elimination half life of two to three hours (Mannisto et al. 1992, Myllyla et al. 1992, Nissinen et al. 1992). It is usually administered at a dose of 200 mg with each levodopa/PDI intake. Entacapone reduces 'off' time, improves clinical function, and allows levodopa dose reductions in patients with motor fluctuations on levodopa. In a six month study, entacapone significantly increased 'on' time. At the end of the six months, entacapone treated patients experienced a 1% improvement in motor function while taking 13% less levodopa, compared to placebo treated patients whose motor function had worsened by 9%, while taking 3% more levodopa (Kieburtz et al. 1996). The shorter duration of action of entacapone means that it must be administered with each dose of levodopa. This may be an advantage if fine adjustment of levodopa plasma levels is needed over the day. Side effects are very similar to those of tolcapone, though diarrhoea may be less of a problem. Studies thus far have not suggested that entacapone causes abnormal liver function (see tolcapone) and monitoring of liver function does not appear to be necessary in patients on this drug.

Monoamine oxidase-B inhibitors

Selegiline (deprenyl, Eldepryl™), in oral doses up to 10 mg/day, is a selective and irreversible inhibitor of monoamine oxidase type B (MAO-B). It is generally not associated with sympathomimetic crises ('cheese effect') caused by nonselective monoamine oxidase inhibitors and the concomitant ingestion of tyramine or other monoamines. MAO-B inhibition partially blocks dopamine metabolism, thereby increasing striatal dopamine. Selegiline may also stimulate dopamine synthesis and inhibit dopamine reuptake. Selegiline's plasma half life is approximately 40 hours, but loss of activity is dependent on the generation of new MAO-B enzyme in the brain. Selegiline may therefore provide clinical effects for several months after discontinuation, though rapid clinical deterioration in disease control has been seen when selegiline is rapidly withdrawn.

Selegiline is usually administered at a dose of 5 mg with breakfast and lunch. It is given early in the day to minimize the likelihood of insomnia, which could be caused by its amphetamine metabolites. As monotherapy in early disease, selegiline provides modest symptomatic benefit and delays the need for levodopa (Parkinson Study Group 1993). In patients with motor fluctuations on levodopa/PDI, selegiline reduces 'off' time and improves clinical response (Presthus and Hajbe 1983).

When used as an adjunct to levodopa/PDI, selegiline can exacerbate dopaminergic side effects including dyskinesia, thereby necessitating a reduction of the levodopa dose. Other possible side effects include gastrointestinal distress, insomnia, confusion or hallucinations, increased liver enzymes, and rarely, peptic ulcer disease (Golbe 1989).

Controversy exists as to whether selegiline confers a neuroprotective effect and whether in older patients selegiline is associated with increased mortality. In animal models selegiline promotes protein synthesis that inhibits apoptosis, a type of programmed cell death. However, a neuroprotective effect has yet to be clearly demonstrated in PD. An open label, prospective study from the PD Research Group of the United Kingdom found that selegiline, in combination with levodopa, was associated with more deaths than levodopa alone (Lees et al. 1995). However, the conclusions of this study are limited by a variety of methodological shortcomings and this finding has not been observed in other studies. Further analysis of mortality in this study has shown that the increase in mortality in the levodopa/selegiline arm is still increased, but was no longer significantly greater than in the levodopa monotherapy arm (Ben-Shlomo et al. 1998). Elderly patients in the combined treatment arm with a history of falls and dementia were more likely to die than similar patients on levodopa alone. Analysis of mortality in the DATATOP study did not show any increased mortality in patients assigned to selegiline combined with levodopa (Parkinson Study Group 1998). It would seem prudent to avoid the combination of levodopa with selegiline in frail elderly patients and to withdraw selegiline slowly in similar patients already taking this combination. Selective serotonin reuptake inhibitors (SSRIs), either alone or in combination with monoamine oxidase inhibitors such as selegiline, can theoretically cause a serotonin syndrome characterized by myoclonus, tremor, diaphoresis, incoordination, mental status changes and possibly death. However, the occurrence of the serotonin syndrome in patients receiving both selegiline and a SSRI has not been reported and does not appear to be a clinically relevant issue (Waters 1994, Richard et al. 1997).

Amantadine

Amantadine, or 1-amino-adamantine, is an antiviral medication found to provide antiparkinsonian benefit (Schwab et al. 1969). Its exact mechanism of action is unknown, but it may increase dopamine release, block dopamine reuptake, stimulate dopamine receptors, block n-methyl-d-aspartate receptors and have anticholinergic activity. Amantadine is excreted unchanged in the urine. It is well absorbed, and has a half-life of approximately 24 hours in young volunteers. The elimination half life correlates with creatinine clearance, and is approximately twice as long in the elderly.

Amantadine provides modest benefit for bradykinesia and rigidity (Butzer et al. 1975), and has less effect on tremor than anticholinergic drugs. Amantadine can be used as monotherapy in early PD or as an adjunct to levodopa/PDI in moderate and advanced disease.

Amantadine is administered at a maximum dose of 100 mg three times daily. Several case reports suggest that the withdrawal of amantadine may be associated with dramatic worsening of parkinsonian features. The side effects of amantadine, especially confusion and hallucinations, limit the usefulness of this drug in older patients (Schwab et al. 1969).

Anticholinergics

Anticholinergic (antimuscarinic) medications can be useful to treat tremor in young physiologically fit patients with PD, but their use requires very careful consideration. They have little or no place in the treatment of late stage or late onset PD and should be avoided in frail elderly patients. Those currently in use are structural analogues of atropine and are muscarinic antagonists. Anticholinergics were initially found to have beneficial effects in PD when they were used by Charcot to control sialorrhea. Today they are mostly used to treat isolated or treatment-resistant tremor. Trihexyphenidyl, cogentin, and benztropine are currently the most common anticholinergic medications used for the treatment of PD. They can delay gastric emptying, thereby slowing the delivery of levodopa to the small intestine. Anticholinergics have a greater incidence of side effects than levodopa. Elderly patients are especially susceptible to these side effects, which include confusion (Broe and Caird 1973), memory impairment, hallucinations and sedation. Cognitive impairment has been demonstrated in health young volunteers given this class of drugs. The risk of neuropsychiatric side effects increases with increasing dose, age, and coexistent dementia (Robertson and George 1990). Anticholinergics may also cause constipation, visual blurring, dry mouth and urinary difficulties (particularly in men with prostatism). They should be used with caution in patients with narrow angle glaucoma. The anticholinergics are best introduced at a low dose and slowly escalated. Trihexyphenidyl is started at a dose of 1 mg/day and increased gradually to as high as 2 mg four times daily. Benztropine is introduced at a dose of 0.5 mg/day and escalated to as high as 4–6 mg/day in divided doses. Anticholinergic treatment should never be withdrawn suddenly.

Theoretical considerations in the treatment of PD in elderly patients

Is selegiline neuroprotective?

That selegiline might slow the progression of PD was initially attributed to its ability to inhibit MAO-B. MPTP (1-methyl-4-phenyl-1,2,3,6-tetrahydropyridine) is a protoxin that causes dopamine cell death and induces parkinsonism in animals and man, because it is oxidized to the neurotoxin MPP^+ (1-methyl-4-phenylpyridinium ion) by MAO-B (see Fig. 9.3). When selegiline is administered prior to

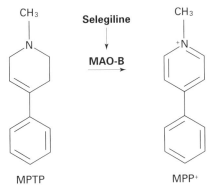

Fig. 9.3   Oxidation of MPTP (1-methyl-4-phenyl-1,2,3,6-tetrahydropyridine) to MPP+ (1-methyl-4-phenylpyridinium ion) is inhibited by selegiline, a selective inhibitor of MAO-B.

MPTP, MPTP is not converted to MPP^+ and parkinsonian symptoms are not elicited (Heikkila et al. 1984). If there is an environmental agent similar to MPTP that causes PD in man, selegiline might prevent its oxidation and protect against dopamine cell damage. Similarly, if free radical formation from the oxidative metabolism of dopamine by MAO-B contributes to disease progression, inhibition of MAO-B by selegiline may reduce free radical formation and slow dopamine cell degeneration. An early retrospective study found that patients taking selegiline lived longer than those not taking selegiline (Birkmeyer et al. 1985).

Based on these early observations, the Parkinson Study Group examined the ability of selegiline and tocopherol (vitamin E), alone or together, to slow the progression of PD (Parkinson Study Group 1993). The study conclusively demonstrated that selegiline in early PD delays the need for levodopa therapy and is consistent with the hypothesis that selegiline may slow disease progression. However, the study also found that selegiline alone provided a small symptomatic benefit and it cannot be excluded that the delay in need for levodopa was due entirely or in part to this small symptomatic effect. Another study designed to minimize symptomatic effects also suggested that selegiline slows progression of disability in PD (Olanow et al. 1995).

However, it is clear that selegiline does not stop disease progression and several studies have found that after several years of treatment, selegiline treated patients experience comparable disability to patients not treated with selegiline. Although several clinical studies have yielded results that are consistent with a neuroprotective action, this has yet to be conclusively demonstrated in PD patients. When selegiline monotherapy is used in early PD it is in the hope that dopamine neuronal degeneration may be slowed and that a delay in the introduction of levodopa may be associated with long-term benefit.

Medication strategies in the treatment of PD in elderly patients

General principles

The signs and symptoms of PD and their effect on function and handicap must be evaluated in each patient to determine the need for treatment changes at any point in time. For any treatment under consideration, the relative likelihood of benefit versus the risk of side effects must be considered. Symptoms of the disease will advance despite best medical management, and drug dosages will need to be adjusted as the disease progresses. Several guidelines for the drug treatment of PD have been developed (Koller et al. 1994, Bhatia et al. 1998).

We make only one medication change at a time so that the effects of that change are clear. Symptomatic medications are initiated at a low dose and escalated slowly so that most side effects that do occur will be mild and appropriate action can then be taken. The optimal medication dose is the lowest one that will maintain adequate function for the patient.

Treatment strategies in early PD

For older patients, we place less emphasis on long-term theoretical considerations and focus on providing adequate symptomatic benefit in the near term with the fewest possible side effects. If a medication provides neuroprotective effects in PD, it is likely to do so throughout the course of the disease and it should be administered from the time of diagnosis onward. We undertake a discussion with our patients to review current information regarding selegiline and interest in its potential neuroprotective effects. It is clear that selegiline administration in early disease will delay the need for symptomatic therapy. The younger the patient, the more critical is the need for therapy that will slow disease progression, and the more likely we are to initiate selegiline from the time of diagnosis.

Symptomatic therapy is introduced when a patient experiences functional disability. If disability is due to bradykinesia, rigidity, decreased fine coordinated movements, soft speech, or shuffling gait, a dopaminergic medication should be introduced. Most patients require symptomatic therapy within one to two years after diagnosis. Tremor is variably responsive to drug treatment (Koller et al. 1994). If bradykinesia or rigidity are present in addition to tremor, we introduce a dopaminergic medication and monitor the clinical response. If troublesome tremor occurs in isolation or does not respond to dopaminergic medication, an anticholinergic can be prescribed cautiously, though is best avoided in elderly patients. Disabling tremor not responsive to other medications warrants a trial of clozapine (Friedman and Lannon 1990, Friedman et al. 1997). A surgical procedure such as thalamotomy or thalamic stimulation may be considered for medically refractory disabling tremor.

In younger patients requiring more treatment to control akinesia and rigidity we prefer to initiate therapy with a dopamine agonist. For patients with dementia and older individuals who may be prone to side effects from dopamine agonists, we generally initiate symptomatic therapy with levodopa/PDI and rely more heavily on it throughout the disease. As a guideline we use early dopamine agonist mono-therapy and a levodopa sparing strategy in patients under 65 years of age and rely on levodopa in patients over 70 years of age. For patients between 65 and 70 we make a judgment based on their general health and cognitive status. The more robust and cognitively intact, the more likely we are to use dopamine agonist monotherapy followed by combination therapy (dopamine agonist plus levodopa/PDI) when necessary.

We usually introduce levodopa therapy using the controlled-release formulation. Fewer daily dosings may be required than with standard levodopa/PDI, thereby affording greater convenience. In addition, co-careldopa CR has been demonstrated to provide significantly better improvement in activities of daily living than standard formulation in a long-term study (Block et al. 1997).

Most patients with bradykinesia and rigidity will experience an obvious reduction in symptoms once levodopa/PDI therapy has been underway for several weeks. If no improvement is apparent, the reason why should be carefully considered. Focus may be placed on the wrong symptom, the diagnosis may be incorrect, or the levodopa dosage may be too low. Tremor may or may not respond to levodopa. If symptoms are minimal, improvement may be difficult to detect. For patients with moderate disability, the levodopa dose should be slowly escalated until symptoms are reduced or side effects are encountered. Failure to respond to levodopa raises serious doubts about the diagnosis of PD.

COMT inhibitors smooth levodopa serum fluctuations, and augment and extend the clinical response to levodopa/PDI. They are not known to provide efficacy except as adjuncts to levodopa/PDI therapy. We favour introducing a COMT inhibitor at the time levodopa/PDI therapy is begun. This may allow lower levodopa dosages and fewer levodopa administrations through the day. In addition, there is interest as to whether providing smoother levodopa-derived dopamine stimulation will afford a better long-term outcome and forestall motor fluctuations and dyskinesia. This strategy is usually well tolerated by both younger and older individuals.

Treatment strategies for motor fluctuations in PD

PD will continue to progress despite treatment with symptomatic medications. As clinical signs and symptoms increase, they may be controlled by increasing the levodopa/PDI dose, or by adding adjunctive medications including dopamine agonists, COMT inhibitors, selegiline, or amantadine. We attempt to maintain the

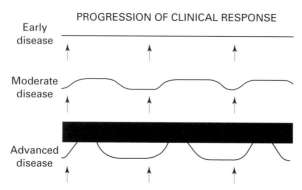

Fig. 9.4   Progression of clinical response. Despite the short half-life of levodopa/PDI, patients with
early disease experience a sustained response through the day. As the disease progresses,
patients begin to notice 'wearing off' fluctuations, with the benefit of levodopa/PDI
wearing off after a few hours. Ultimately, clinical response fluctuates more and more
closely in association with peripheral levodopa and patients develop choreiform
dyskinesias when dopamine peaks. Arrows indicate time of levodopa/PDI administration.
Reprinted with permission from Hauser and Zesiewicz (1997b).

levodopa/PDI dose at or below 600 mg per day for as long as reasonable function
can be maintained. If a patient experiences progression of symptoms on a low dose
of levodopa/PDI, we prefer to add adjunctive medication rather than increase the
levodopa dose.

End of dose / 'wearing off' motor fluctuations

Over time, nearly all patients regardless of age of onset of PD develop 'wearing
off / end of dose' motor fluctuations (see Fig. 9.4) in response to levodopa/PDI
(Chase et al. 1993). Patients will notice that levodopa provides benefit for a few
hours and then wears off as bradykinesia, rigidity and tremor return. Wearing off
motor fluctuations alone are relatively easy to treat. They can be alleviated by
increasing the levodopa/PDI dose, administering levodopa/PDI doses more frequently, switching from standard levodopa/PDI to a controlled-release formulation, or by adding a dopamine agonist, COMT inhibitor, or selegiline (see Fig. 9.5).
Adjustment of the antiparkinsonian medication regimen should eliminate 'off'
time unless increasing dopaminergic stimulation causes an intolerable side effect
such as peak dose dyskinesia, hallucinations, orthostatic hypotension or somnolence.

Patients with prominent motor fluctuations and those who find they turn 'off'
after a meal may benefit from a low protein or protein redistributed diet (Carter et
al. 1989). Minimizing serum protein fluctuations reduces the variability of levodopa transport and helps stabilize the clinical response.

Patients with both motor fluctuations and troublesome peak dose dyskinesia

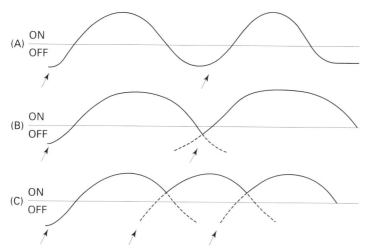

Fig. 9.5   Management of a patient with motor fluctuations and no dyskinesia (A). Off time can be
reduced by using a higher levodopa dose (B), switching to a long-acting preparation (B),
adding a dopamine agonist, COMT inhibitor or selegiline (B), or by shortening the
interdose interval (C). Arrows indicate time of levodopa administration. Reprinted with
permission from Hauser and Zesiewicz (1997b).

present a challenging management dilemma. Peak dose dyskinesias occur at the
peak of the dosing cycle, coincident with high levels of dopamine, and consist of
choreiform, twisting turning movements. They are exacerbated by increasing
dopaminergic stimulation and diminished by reducing dopaminergic stimulation.
Most patients prefer to be 'on' with mild peak dose dyskinesia than to be 'off'.
Dyskinesia that does not cause functional difficulty or distress may not require a
reduction of dopaminergic medication. However, dyskinesia can be severe in
amplitude and as disabling as 'off' time (Hauser et al. 1997b). Increasing dopaminergic medication in these patients will increase disability from dyskinesia and
decreasing dopaminergic medication will increase 'off' time. For patients with both
motor fluctuations and troublesome peak dose dyskinesia, it is important to
attempt to maximize good functional time (i.e. time 'on' without dyskinesia or with
nontroublesome dyskinesia). We find it very helpful to have patients complete a 24
hour home 'diary' (see Fig. 9.6) indicating their parkinsonian status at half hour
intervals to understand their response to medication and the proportion of the day
that they are under or over treated (Hauser et al.1997a). For patients with motor
fluctuations and dyskinesia we attempt to provide the most stable as possible
dopamingeric stimulation within the target zone (see Fig. 9.7).

Other motor fluctuations

Other types of dyskinesia in PD such as wearing off dystonia and diphasic dysto-
nia/dyskinesia are less commonly seen in elderly patients. Wearing off dystonia

PARKINSON'S DISEASE DIARY

NAME _____   DATE _____

Instructions: For each half-hour time period place one check mark to indicate your predominant status during most of that period.
ON = Time when medication is providing benefit with regard to mobility, slowness, and stiffness.
OFF = Time when medication has worn off and is no longer providing benefit with regard to mobility, slowness, and stiffness.
Dyskinesia = Involuntary twisting, turning movements. These movements are an effect of medication and occur during ON time.
Non-troublesome dyskinesia does not interfere with function or cause meaningful discomfort. Troublesome dyskinesia interferes with function or causes meaningful discomfort.
Tremor is shaking back and forth and is not considered dyskinesia.

Time	Asleep	OFF	ON without dyskinesia	ON with non-troublesome dyskinesia	ON with troublesome dyskinesia
6:00 AM					
:30					
7:00 AM					
:30					
8:00 AM					
:30					
9:00 AM					
:30					
10:00 AM					
:30					
11:00 AM					
:30					
12:00 PM					
:30					
1:00 PM					
:30					
2:00 PM					
:30					
3:00 PM					
:30					
4:00 PM					
:30					
5:00 PM					
:30					

Time	Asleep	OFF	ON without dyskinesia	ON with non-troublesome dyskinesia	ON with troublesome dyskinesia
6:00 PM					
:30					
7:00 PM					
:30					
8:00 PM					
:30					
9:00 PM					
:30					
10:00 PM					
:30					
11:00 PM					
:30					
12:00 AM					
:30					
1:00 AM					
:30					
2:00 AM					
:30					
3:00 AM					
:30					
4:00 AM					
:30					
5:00 AM					
:30					

Fig. 9.6   Parkinson's disease diary. Used with permission, copyright R. A. Hauser (1997).

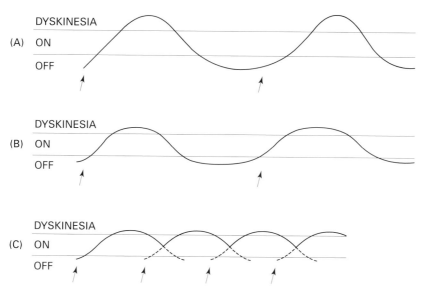

Fig. 9.7   Management of a patient with motor fluctuations and dyskinesia. The treatment of
patients with motor fluctuations and peak dose dyskinesia (A) generally involves providing
less levodopa more frequently. The levodopa dose should be lowered until it brings on
only mild dyskinesia (B). The time to wearing off then determines the interdose interval
(C). Arrows indicate times of levodopa administration. Reprinted with permission from
Hauser and Zesiewicz (1997b).

occurs in association with low or falling dopamine levels (McHale et al. 1990). It
can occur early in the course of the disease and consists of involuntary, sustained,
painful muscle contractions, often manifest as foot inversion or plantar flexion in
the early morning hours or at times when dopaminergic medication has worn off.
Wearing off dystonia may be improved by providing more sustained dopaminergic
stimulation. This can be accomplished with controlled-release levodopa/PDI preparations, adding a COMT inhibitor to levodopa/PDI therapy, or by introducing a
dopamine agonist.

Diphasic dystonia/dyskinesia (D-I-D dystonia) is uncommon, and occurs at the
beginning and end of the levodopa cycle. It may appear as a combination of dystonia and chorea, and commonly affects the lower extremities. D-I-D dystonia can be
difficult to treat, but attempts should be made to increase and smooth dopaminergic stimulation so as to avoid 'turning on' and 'wearing off' fluctuations.

Freezing is the momentary inability to walk. It can cause troublesome gait
difficulty and may affect up to one-third of patients with longstanding disease
(Giladi et al. 1992). Turning, walking through a doorway or anxiety often triggers
freezing. If freezing occurs during 'off' periods, it can be improved by eliminating
or minimizing 'off' time by increasing dopaminergic stimulation. However, the
management of 'on' period freezing is usually disappointing. Motor 'tricks' such as

marching in place or walking over masked tape placed across a hallway may be helpful.

Treatment of the secondary symptoms of PD

Sleep abnormalities

Sleeping problems are common in PD, affecting 75–98% of patients. Such problems usually take the form of fragmented sleep with frequent awakenings and result in excessive daytime sleepiness. Difficulty turning over in bed, leg cramps, nightmares, dystonia, dyskinesia and leg jerks are also frequently reported. Nocturia is a common cause of poor sleep maintenance, but motor problems, anxiety and depression may also play a role. Sleep abnormalities, if bothersome, should be evaluated with an overnight polysomnography (PSG).

In older patients, chronic use of sedative hypnotics is generally not recommended because of possible cognitive side effects, next day residual effects, physical dependence and tolerance. When a hypnotic is required, the short acting zolpidem, an imidazopyridine that acts at the benzodiazepine receptor, has the advantage of causing relatively little hangover effect. Patients are asked to try to sleep each night without hypnotic medication, but if they are unable to sleep to take the medication. Some patients require regular hypnotic medication.

If a patient complains of fragmented sleep due to nocturnal leg cramps or dystonia, a bedtime dose of a sustained release levodopa formulation or a long-acting dopamine agonist such as cabergoline may be useful. If vivid dreams and nightmares or dyskinesias are disturbing sleep, bedtime antiparkinsonian drugs may need to be stopped or reduced. It is important to recall that selegiline, which is metabolized to amphetamines, given too late in the day may lead to nightmares and insomnia. Depression, which is contributing to a sleep disorder, should be treated with an antidepressant, and tricyclics such as amitriptyline may reduce depression while promoting sleep.

Urinary incontinence

Symptoms of urinary dysfunction in PD include urgency, frequency and nocturia. Patients complaining of urinary symptoms should be evaluated by a urologist for prostatism and other structural problems, and undergo cystometric studies. The most common type of urinary dysfunction in PD is detrusor hyperreflexia (Andersen et al. 1976, Pavlakis et al. 1983). The extrapyramidal system generally exerts an inhibitory effect on micturition, and the basal ganglia abnormalities of PD may cause detrusor dysfunction.

Anticholinergic drugs are the mainstay of treatment for urge incontinence. Unfortunately, in elderly subjects these drugs often lead to significant side effects including cognitive impairment, constipation that can itself worsen bladder function, and postural hypotension. Anticholinergic drugs such as oxybutynin and propantheline may be used cautiously to improve incontinence. Newer drugs such as tolterodine and propiverin, both recently launched in the UK, may be associated with fewer central anticholinergic side effects. Patients with nocturia should be advised to maintain a good fluid intake of at least two litres per day, but should not take liquids late in the evening. Desmopressin, a synthetic analogue of vasopressin, in the form of a nasal spray is useful for troublesome, refractory nocturia (Suchowersky et al. 1995). Urea and electrolytes need to be monitored in these patients as hyponatraemia and fluid overload can develop.

Drooling

Drooling (sialorrhoea) is a late manifestation of PD that may occur in up to 70% of patients (Edwards et al. 1991). Drooling can potentially lead to serious problems including aspiration. In PD drooling results from saliva pooling in the mouth owing to swallowing difficulty, rather than increased production of saliva. Treatment is commonly undertaken with anticholinergic medications that can reduce saliva production. However, these medications should be used with caution in the elderly, as they cause cognitive impairment, constipation, and dry mouth. The peripheral anticholinergic glycopyrrolate is useful to reduce saliva production with minimal cognitive side effects. Alternatively, increased dopaminergic therapy can improve swallowing and if tolerated may improve drooling.

Seborrhoea

Excessive oiliness of the skin is a common problem in PD. Oiliness is most common in the forehead and central parts of the face (Flint 1977). Secretion of sebum, which is produced by sebaceous glands, is increased in patients with PD. Topical steroids and tar shampoo can be used daily for three days to treat seborrhea. Chronic use of topical steroids can lead to skin atrophy and should generally be avoided. A maintenance regimen consisting of frequent washing and the use of detergent shampoo will usually provide long-term benefit. Troublesome seborrhoea may warrant referral to a dermatologist.

Sexual dysfunction

Impotence is a common problem in the elderly. Kinsey et al. (1948) reported that by the age of 55 years, 7% of men are impotent, and by the age of 70 years, 27% are impotent. Verwoerdt et al. (1969) found that 35% of women aged 60–65 had no interest in sex. Difficulty with sexual function is particularly common in PD; roughly 60% of male patients may experience erectile dysfunction (Singer et al. 1992).

Sexual dysfunction usually has several causes, including decreased mobility, autonomic nervous system abnormalities, depression and side effects from drug treatment. Identification of the cause helps direct treatment. Antihypertensive medications including propranolol, clonidine, and methyldopa, as well as thiazide diuretics, digoxin and cimetidine, can cause sexual dysfunction. Antidepressants, especially the serotonin reuptake inhibitors, can also lead to impotence. If no cause is apparent, evaluation by a specialist should be undertaken. Vascular disease is a common cause of erectile dysfunction. The use of an externally applied device can help men achieve and maintain an erection.

Postural hypotension

Signs of postural (orthostatic) hypotension are commonly encountered in PD (Senard et al. 1997). One definition of orthostatic hypotension is a drop of 30 mmHg in systolic blood pressure or a drop of 20 mmHg in mean blood pressure (diastolic pressure plus one third of the pulse pressure) when going from the supine to standing position. Its mechanism in PD remains controversial. Recent data suggest that alpha-adrenergic supersensitivity may occur in response to low levels of plasma noradrenaline (Senard et al. 1990), but the pathophysiology may involve a decreased ability to secrete renin (Barbeau et al. 1970), and impairment of baro-receptor reflexes. Neuropathological evidence of involvement of the autonomic nervous system in PD has been described (Rajput and Rozdilsky 1976). Symptomatic postural hypotension usually causes feelings of dizziness or light headedness that occur during positional changes, but may cause unsteadiness, cognitive slowing, or other vague symptoms (Hillen et al. 1996). Postural hypotension can cause significant morbidity and mortality by contributing to falls, limiting mobility, and interfering with rehabilitation efforts.

Treatment of orthostatic hypotension includes discontinuing unnecessary medications, encouraging the patient to drink five or more glasses of fluid each day and adding salt liberally to the diet. Medical management includes the use of mineralocorticoids to increase intravascular volume (Hickler et al. 1959). Fludrocortisone is introduced at a dose of 0.1 mg once or twice a day, and can be increased to as high as 0.4 to 0.6 mg daily. Supine hypertension and dependent oedema are common side effects, and patients should be monitored for congestive heart failure. Midodrine is a peripherally acting alpha-1-agonist that causes vasoconstriction of both arterioles and venous capacitance vessels (McTavish and Goa 1989, Jankovic et al. 1993). The initial recommended dosage is 2.5 mg twice or three times daily. The maintenance dose is as high as 40 mg daily in divided doses. Side effects include scalp pruritus and tingling, pilomotor reactions, gastrointestinal complaints, headaches, and dizziness. It does not cross the blood–brain barrier, and is less likely to produce central side effects than ephedrine. Midodrine is a selective alpha-adrenergic agonist, and is relatively free of beta adrenergic side effects, including increased pulse rate. Several open label trials have found midodrine to control symptoms of orthostatic hypotension effectively in most patients (Kaufman et al. 1988).

Hallucinations

Drug-induced changes in mental state, including hallucinations (mostly visual), delusions, confusional states, and paranoid psychosis are common in elderly patients with PD (Goetz et al. 1982, Sage and Mark 1994, Sanchez-Ramos et al. 1996). The incidence of hallucinations is in the range of 20–33%. Elderly subjects may be particularly prone to hallucinations, especially in association with amantadine, anticholinergic, or dopamine agonist therapy. These medications appear to induce hallucinations and other psychiatric disturbances more readily than levodopa. Other possible risk factors for the development of hallucinations remain controversial, including disease duration, duration of levodopa exposure, and disease severity (Sanchez-Ramos et al. 1996).

Hallucinations should be treated if they are bothersome to the patient or interfere with function, by gradual withdrawal of drugs most likely to cause or worsen this problem, such as amantadine, selegiline, and anticholinergics. Following this, dopamine agonist drugs and lastly levodopa itself may need to be reduced in dose or withdrawn. If hallucinations occur at night, bedtime doses of antiparkinsonian medications may be reduced or discontinued. An atypical neuroleptic drug, such as clozapine, may be useful in controlling hallucinations when antiparkinsonian medication cannot be reduced. Clozapine predominantly antagonizes mesolimbic pathways rather than nigrostriatal pathways and causes fewer extrapyramidal side effects than traditional neuroleptics (Doraiswamy et al. 1995). Potential side effects include somnolence, orthostatic hypotension and hypersalivation. It also carries a risk for agranulocytosis, necessitating weekly complete blood counts. Patients with PD require much smaller doses of clozapine than that used to treat schizophrenia. We start patients on a small chip of a clozapine tablet (~ 3 mg, or one eighth of a 25 mg tablet) and slowly escalate. Most patients are controlled on 12.5–50 mg clozapine per day. For patients who cannot or will not comply with weekly blood monitoring, instead of clozapine we use the atypical neuroleptic risperidone, although it can worsen the motor signs of PD.

Depression

Depression (see Chapter 3) is the most common mood disturbance in PD, affecting 40–50% of patients (Cummings 1992). Tricyclic antidepressants, selective serotonin reuptake inhibitors (SSRIs), and atypical antidepressants have all been found to improve depression in PD (Laitenen 1969, Andersen et al. 1980, Goetz et al.

1984). Consistent with their popularity in the general population, SSRIs are probably the most commonly used antidepressants in PD in the US. However, several case reports have noted worsening of parkinsonian symptoms during treatment with some SSRIs (Jansen-Steur 1993, Jiminez-Jiminez et al. 1994). This has not been confirmed in population studies or open label studies of sertraline in depressed patients with PD (Hauser and Zesiewicz 1997a).

Constipation

Constipation is a common complaint in PD and transit time is prolonged in all segments of the colon (Jost and Schimrigk 1991). Both peripheral and central neurologic abnormalities may contribute to this problem. Lewy bodies have been found in the myenteric plexus of the colon and in the neurons of the dorsal group of the spinal cord (Oyanagi et al. 1990). Anismus, a dystonia causing paradoxical contraction of the striated sphincter muscles during defecation, may also contribute to constipation. As with other dystonias in PD, it may respond to dopamine agonist therapy (Jost and Schimrigk 1994). Treatment of constipation involves increasing stool bulk by adding fibre to the diet and by increasing daily liquid intake. Patients should be counselled to eat more fruit and vegetables, as well as bran products. Drugs that inhibit gastric motility, such as anticholinergics, should be discontinued. Cisapride enhances gastric motility, may improve colonic transit times (Jost and Schimrigk 1994) and can increase peak plasma levodopa levels by improving gastric emptying (Neira et al. 1995).

REFERENCES

Abrams WB, Coutinho CB, Leon AS, Spiegel HE (1971) Absorption and metabolism of levodopa. *Journal of the American Medical Association*, 218, 1912–14.

Adler CH, Sethi KD, Hauser RA, Davis TL, Hammerstad JP, Bertoni J, Taylor RL, Sanchez-Ramos J, O'Brien CF (1997) Ropinirole for the treatment of early Parkinson's disease. The Ropinirole Study Group. *Neurology*, 49, 393–9. Published erratum appears in *Neurology* 1997, 49, 1484.

Andersen J, Aabro E, Gulmann N, Hjelmsted A, Pedersen HE (1980) Anti depressive treatment in Parkinson's disease: a controlled trial of the effect of nortriptyline in patients with Parkinson's disease treated with L-dopa. *Acta Neurologica Scandinavica*, 52, 210–19.

Andersen JT, Hebjorn S, Frimodt-Moller C, Walter S, Worm-Petersen J (1976) Disturbances of micturition in Parkinson's disease. *Acta Neurologica Scandinavica*, 53, 161–70.

Avorn J (1990) Reporting drug side effects: signals and noise. *Journal of the American Medical Association*, 263,1823.

Barbeau A, Gillo-Joffroy L, Brossard Y (1970) Renin, dopamine and Parkinson's disease. In: L-*dopa and Parkinsonism*, eds. Barbeau A, McDowell FH, pp. 286–93. Philadelphia: Davis,

Ben-Shlomo Y, Churchyard A, Head J, Hurwitz B, Overstall P, Ockelford J, Lees AJ (1998)

Investigation by the PDRG of the United Kingdom into excess mortality seen with combined levodopa and selegiline treatment in patients with early, mild Parkinson's disease: further results of randomised trial and confidential inquiry. *British Medical Journal*, 316, 1191–6.

Bhatia K on behalf of Parkinson's Disease Consensus Working Group (1998) Guidelines for the management of Parkinson's disease. *Hospital Medicine*, 59, 469–80.

Birkmayer W, Knoll J, Riederer P (1985) Increased life expectancy resulting from the addition of L-deprenyl to Madopar treatment in Parkinson's disease; a long-term study. *Journal of Neural Transmission*, 64,113–27.

Block G, Liss C, Reines S, Irr J, Nibbelink D (1997) The CR First Study Group. Comparison of immediate-release and controlled-release carbidopa/levodopa in Parkinson's disease. A multi-centre 5 year study. *European Neurology*, 37, 23–7.

Broe GA, Caird FI (1973) Levodopa for parkinsonism in elderly and demented patients. *Medical Journal of Australia*, I, 630.

Bromocriptine Multicentre Trial Group (1990) Bromocriptine as initial therapy in elderly par-kinsonian patients. *Age and Ageing*, 19, 62–7.

Butzer JF, Silver DE, Sahs AL (1975) Amantadine in Parkinson's disease: a double-blind placebo-controlled cross-over study with long-term follow-up. *Neurology*, 25, 603–6.

Calne DB, Teychenne PF, Claveria LE, Eastman R, Greenacre JK, Petrie A (1974) Bromocriptine in parkinsonism. *British Medical Journal*, 4, 442–4.

Carlsson A, Lindqvist M, Magnusson R (1957) 3,4–Dihydroxyphenyl-alanine and 5-hydrox-ytryptophan as reserpine antagonists. *Nature*, 180, 1200.

Carter JH, Nutt JG, Woodward WR, Hatcher LF, Trotman TL (1989) Amount and distribution of dietary protein affects clinical response to levodopa in Parkinson's disease. *Neurology*, 39, 1036–9.

Cedarbaum JM (1987) Clinical pharmacokinetics of anti-parkinsonian drugs. *Clinical Pharmacokinetics*, 13, 141–78.

Chase TN, Mouradian MM, Engber TM (1993) Motor response complication and the function of striatal efferent systems. *Neurology*, 43, S23–S27.

Cotzias GC, Papavasiliou PS, Gellene R (1968) Experimental treatment of parkinsonism with L-dopa. *Neurology*, 18, 276–7.

Cummings JL (1992) Depression and Parkinson's disease: a review. *American Journal of Psychiatry*, 149, 443–54.

de Michele G, Mangano A, Filla A, Trombetta L, Campanella G (1989) A double-blind, cross-over trial with Madopar HBS in patients with Parkinson's disease. *Acta Neurologica*, 11, 408–14.

Doraiswamy M, Martin W, Metz A, Deveaugh-Geiss J (1995) Psychosis in Parkinson's disease: diagnosis and treatment. *Progress in Neuro-Psychopharmacology and Biological Psychiatry*, 19, 835–46.

Eden RJ, Costall B, Domeney AM, Gerrard PA, Harvey CA, Kelly ME, Naylor RJ, Owen DA, Wright A (1991) Preclinical pharmacology of ropinirole (SK and F 101468–A) a novel dopa-mine D2 agonist. *Pharmacology, Biochemistry and Behavior*, 38, 147–54.

Edwards LL, Pfeiffer RF, Quigley EM, Hofman R, Balluff M (1991) Gastrointestinal symptoms in Parkinson's disease. *Movement Disorders*, 6, 151–6.

Ehringer H, Hornykiewicz O (1960) Verteilung von Noradrenalin und Dopamine (3-hydroxy-tyramin) im Gehirn des Menschen und ihr Verhalten bei Erkrankungen des exrapyraminalen Systems. *Klinische Wochenschrift*, 38, 1236–9.

Evans MA, Triggs EJ, Broe GA, Saines N (1980) Systemic activity of orally administered L-dopa in the elderly Parkinson patient. *European Journal of Clinical Pharmacology*, 17, 215–21.

Feldman RG, Mosbach PA, Kelly MR, Thomas CA, Saint-Hilaire MH (1989) Double-blind comparison of standard Sinemet and Sinemet CR in patients with mild to moderate Parkinson's disease. *Neurology*, 39, Suppl. 2, S96–S101.

Flint A (1977) The skin in Parkinson's disease. *Primary Care*, 4, 475–80.

Friedman JH, Koller WC, Lannon MC, Busenbark K, Swanson-Hyland E. Smith D (1997) Benztropine versus clozapine for the treatment of tremor in Parkinson's disease. *Neurology*, 48, 4, 1077–81.

Friedman JH, Lannon MC (1990) Clozapine treatment of tremor in Parkinson's disease. *Movement Disorders*, 5, 225–9.

Giladi N, McMahon D, Przedborski S, Flaster E, Guillory S, Kostic V, Fahn S (1992) Motor blocks in Parkinson's disease. *Neurology*, 42, 333–9.

Goetz CG, Stebbins GT (1995) Mortality and hallucinations in nursing home patients with advanced Parkinson's disease. *Neurology*, 45, 669–71.

Goetz CG, Tanner CM, Klawans HL (1982) Pharmacology of hallucinations induced by long-term drug therapy. *American Journal of Psychiatry*, 139, 494–7.

Goetz CG, Tanner CM, Klawans HL (1984) Bupropion in Parkinson's disease. *Neurology*, 34, 1092–4.

Goetz CG, Tanner CM, Klawans HL, Shannon KM, Carroll VS (1987) Parkinson's disease and motor fluctuations: long-acting carbidopa/levodopa (CR4–Sinemet). *Neurology*, 37, 875–8.

Golbe LI (1989) Long-term efficacy and safety of deprenyl in advanced Parkinson's disease. *Neurology*, 39, 1109–11.

Goldstein M, Leiberman A, Lew JS, Asano T, Rosenfeld MR, Makman MH (1980) Interaction of pergolide with central dopamine receptors. *Proceedings of the National Academy of Sciences*, 77, 3725–8.

Hauser RA, Friedlander J, Zesiewicz TA, Adler CH, Seeburger LC, O'Brien CF, Molho ES, Factor SA (1997a) Evaluation of a new home diary to assess functional status in Parkinson's disease patients with fluctuations and dyskinesia (abstract). *Movement Disorders*, 12, 843.

Hauser RA, Molho E, Shale H, Pedder S, Dorflinger EE, and Tolcapone De Novo Study Group (1998) A pilot evaluation of the tolerability, safety, and efficacy of tolcapone alone and in combination with oral selegiline in untreated Parkinson's disease patients. *Movement Disorders*, 13, 643–7.

Hauser RA, Zesiewicz TA (1997a) Sertraline for the treatment of depression in Parkinson's disease. *Movement Disorders*, 12, 756–9.

Hauser RA, Zesiewicz TA (1997b) *Parkinson's Disease: Questions and Answers*, Second Edition. London: Merit Publishing.

Hauser RA, Zesiewicz TA, Friedlander J, Seeburger LC , O'Brien CF, Adler CH, Molho ES, Factor SA (1997b) Impact of different severities of dyskinesia on patient-defined functional status in Parkinson's disease (abstract). *Movement Disorders*, 12, 843.

Heikkila RE, Manzino L, Cabbat FS, Duvoisin RC (1984) Protection against the dopaminergic neurotoxicity of 1-methyl-4-phenyl-1,2,5,6-tetrahydropyridine by monoamine oxidase inhibitors. *Nature*, 311, 467–9.

Hickler RB, Thompson GR, Fox LM, Hamlin JT (1959) Successful treatment of orthostatic hypotension with 9-alpha-fludrohydrocortisone. *New England Journal of Medicine*, 261, 788–91.

Hillen ME, Wagner ML, Sage JI (1996) 'Subclinical' orthostatic hypotension is associated with dizziness in elderly patients with Parkinson's disease. *Archives of Physical Medicine and Rehabilitation*, 77, 710–12.

Hindle JV, Meara RJ, Sharma JC, Medcalf P, Forsyth DR, Huggett IM, Cassidy TP, Morris J, Dunn A, Hobson JP (1998) Prescribing pergolide in the elderly – an open label study of pergolide in elderly patients with Parkinson's disease. *International Journal of Geriatric Psychopharmacology*, 1, 78–81.

Hutton JT, Morris JL, Brewer MA (1993) Controlled study of the antiparkinsonian activity and tolerability of cabergoline. *Neurology*, 43, 613–6.

Jankovic J, Gilden JL, Hiner BC, Kaufman H, Brown DC (1993) Neurogenic orthostatic hypotension: a double-blind placebo-controlled study with midodrine. *American Journal of Medicine*, 95, 38–48.

Jansen-Steur EN (1993) Increase of Parkinson disability after fluoxetine medication. *Neurology*, 43, 211–13.

Jimenez-Jimenez FJ, Tejeiro J, Martinez-Junquera G, Cabrera-Valdivia F, Alarcon J, Garcia-Albea E (1994) Parkinsonism exacerbated by paroxetine. *Neurology*, 44, 2406.

Jost WH, Schimrigk K (1991) Constipation in Parkinson's disease. *Klinische Wochenschrift*, 69, 906–9.

Jost WH, Schimrigk K (1994) The effect of cisapride on delayed colonic transit time in patients with idiopathic Parkinson's disease. *Wiener Klinische Wochenschrift*, 106, 673–6.

Kaakkola S, Rinne UK, Gordin A (1996) *COMT Inhibition with Entacapone: a New Principle of Levodopa Extension*, p. 27. Finland: Koteva Oy.

Kaufman H, Brannan T, Krakoff L, Yahr MD, Mandeli J (1988) Treatment of orthostatic hypotension due to autonomic failure with a peripheral alpha-adrenergic agonist (midodrine). *Neurology*, 38, 951–6.

Kieburtz K for the Parkinson Study Group (1996) The COMT inhibitor entacapone improves parkinsonian features in fluctuating patients. *Movement Disorders*, 11, Suppl. 1, 268.

Kinsey AC, Pomeroy WB, Martin CE (1948) *Sexual Behaviour in the Human Male*. Philadelphia: W.B. Saunders Company.

Koller WC, Pahwa R (1994) Treating motor fluctuations with controlled-release preparations. *Neurology*, 44, S23–S28.

Koller WC, Silver DE, Lieberman A (1994) An algorithm for the management of Parkinson's disease. *Neurology*, 44, Suppl. 10, S1–S51.

Kreider M, Know S, Gardiner D, Wheadon D (1996) A multicentre double-blind study of ropinirole as an adjunct to L-dopa in Parkinson's disease. *Neurology*, 46, Suppl. A475.

Kurth MC, Adler CH, St. Hilaire M (1997) Tolcapone improves motor function and reduces levodopa requirement in patients with Parkinson's disease experiencing motor fluctuations: A multicentre, double-blind, randomised placebo-controlled trial. *Neurology*, 48, 81–7.

Laitenen L (1969) Desipramine in treatment of Parkinson's disease. *Acta Neurologica Scandinavica*, 45, 109–13.

Larsen JP and the Norwegian Study Group of Parkinson's disease in the Elderly (1991) Parkinson's disease as community health problem: study in Norwegian nursing homes. *British Medical Journal*, 303, 741–3.

Lees AJ on behalf of the Parkinson's disease Research Group of the United Kingdom (1995) Comparison of the effects and mortality data of levodopa and levodopa combined with selegiline in patients with early, mild Parkinson's disease. *British Medical Journal*, 311, 1602–7.

LeWitt PA, Calne DB (1982) Pleuropulmonary changes during long-term bromocriptine treatment for Parkinson's disease. *Lancet*, I, 44.

Lieberman A, Ranhosky A, Korts D (1997) Clinical evaluation of pramipexole in advanced Parkinson's disease: results of a double-blind, placebo-controlled, parallel-group study. *Neurology*, 49, 162–8.

Mannisto PT, Kaakkola S (1990) Rationale for selective COMT inhibitors as adjuncts in drug treatment of Parkinson's disease. *Pharmacology and Toxicology*, 66, 317–23.

Mannisto PT, Tuomainen P, Tuominen RK (1992) Different in vivo properties of three new inhibitors of catechol O-methyltransferase in the rat. *British Journal of Pharmacology*, 105, 569–74.

McHale DM, Sage JI, Sonsalla PK, Vitagliano D (1990) Complex dystonia of Parkinson's disease: clinical features and relation to plasma levodopa profile. *Clinical Neuropharmacology*, 13, 164–70.

McNeely W, Davis R (1997) Entacapone. *CNS Drugs*, 8, 79–90.

McTavish D, Goa KL (1989) Midodrine: a review of its pharmacological properties and therapeutic use in orthostatic hypotension and secondary hypotensive disorders. *Drugs*, 38, 757–77.

Mear JY, Barroche G, de Smet Y, Weber M, Lhermitte F, Agid Y (1984) Pergolide in the treatment of Parkinson's disease. *Neurology*, 34, 983–6.

Mearrick PT, Wade DN, Birkett DJ, Morris J (1974) Metoclopramide, gastric emptying and L-dopa absorption. *Australian and New Zealand Journal of Medicine*, 4, 144–8.

Mieraau J, Schingnitz G (1992) Biochemical and pharmacological studies on pramipexole, a potent and selective dopamine D2 receptor agonist. *European Journal of Pharmacology*, 215, 161–70.

Montastruc JL, Rascol O, Senard JM (1993) Current status of dopamine agonists in Parkinson's disease management. *Drugs*, 46, 384–93.

Myllyla VV, Sotaniemi KA, Illi A, Keranen T (1992) Effects of entacapone, a novel COMT inhibitor, on levodopa pharmacokinetics and cardiovascular responses (CVRs) in Parkinson's disease patients. *Neurology*, 42, Suppl. 3, 442.

Neira WD, Sanchea V, Mena MA, Yebenes JG (1995) The effects of cisapride on plasma – dopa levels and clinical response in Parkinson's disease. *Movement Disorders*, 10, 66–70

Nissinen E, Linden I-B, Schultz E, Pohto P (1992) Biochemical and pharmacological properties of a peripherally acting catechol-O-methyltransferase inhibitor Entacapone. *Naunyn-Schmiedebergs Archives of Pharmacology*, 346, 262–6.

Nutt JG, Fellman JH (1984) Pharmacokinetics of levodopa. *Clinical Neuropharmacology*, 7, 35–49.

Nutt JG, Woodward WR, Anderson JL (1985) The effect of carbidopa on the pharmacokinetics of intravenously administered levodopa: the mechanism of action in the treatment of parkinsonism. *Annals of Neurology*, 18, 537–45.

Nutt JG, Woodward, WR, Gancher ST, Merrick D (1987) 3–O-methyldopa and the response to levodopa in Parkinson's disease. *Annals of Neurology*, 21, 584–8.

Olanow C (1988) Dopamine agonists in early Parkinson's disease. In: *The Comprehensive Management of Parkinson's Disease*, eds. Stern B, Hurtig I, pp. 89–100. New York: PMA Publications.

Olanow CW, Fahn S, Muenter M (1994) A multicentre double-blind placebo-controlled trial of pergolide as an adjunct to Sinemet in Parkinson's disease. *Movement Disorders*, 9, 40–7.

Olanow CW, Hauser RA, Gauger L, Malapira T, Koller W, Hubble J, Bushenbark K, Lilienfeld D, Esterlitz J (1995) The effect of deprenyl and levodopa on the progression of Parkinson's disease. *Annals of Neurology*, 38, 771–7.

Oyanagi K, Wakabayahi K, Ohama E, Takeda S, Horikawa Y, Morita T, Ikutai F (1990) Lewy bodies in the lower sacral parasympathetic neurons of a patient with Parkinson's disease. *Acta Neuropathologica*, 80, 558–9.

Parkinson Study Group (1993) Effects of tocopherol and deprenyl on the progression of disability in early Parkinson's disease. *New England Journal of Medicine*, 328,176–83.

Parkinson Study Group (1998) Mortality in DATATOP: a multicentre trial in early Parkinson's disease. *Annals of Neurology*, 43, 318–25.

Pavlakis AJ, Siroky MB, Goldstein I, Krane RJ (1983) Neurologic findings in Parkinson's disease. *Journal of Urology*, 129, 80–3.

Pezzoli G, Martignoni E, Pacchetti C, Angeleri VA, Lamberti P, Muratorio A, Bonuccelli U, De Mari M, Foschi N, Cossutta E, Nicoletti F, Giammona F, Canesi M, Scarlato G, Caraceni T, Moscarelli E (1994) Pergolide compared with bromocriptine in Parkinson's disease: a multicentre crossover, controlled study. *Movement Disorders*, 9, 431–6.

Presthus J, Hajbe A (1983) Deprenyl (selegiline) combined with levodopa and a decarboxylase inhibitor in the treatment of Parkinson's disease. *Acta Neurologica Scandinavica*, 95, 127–33.

Rajput AH, Martin W, Saint-Hilaire MH, Dorflinger E, Pedder S (1997) Tolcapone improves motor function in parkinsonian patients with the 'wearing off' phenomenon: A double-blind, placebo-controlled, multicentre trial. *Neurology*, 49, 1066–71.

Rajput AH, Rozdilsky B (1976) Dysautonomia in parkinsonism: a clinicopathological study. *Journal of Neurology, Neurosurgery, and Psychiatry*, 39, 1092–100.

Rascol O (1996) A double-blind L-dopa-controlled study of ropinirole in patients with early Parkinson's disease. *Neurology*, 46, A160.

Richard IH, Kurlan R, Tanner C, Factor S, Hubble J, Suchowersky O, Waters C, Parkinson Study Group (1997) Serotonin syndrome and the combined use of deprenyl and an antidepressant in Parkinson's disease. *Neurology*, 48, 1070–7.

Rinne UK (1987) Early combination of bromocriptine and levodopa in the treatment of Parkinson's disease: a 5 year follow-up. *Neurology*, 37, 826–8.

Rinne UK, Bracco F, Chouza C, Dupont E, Gershanik O, Marti Masso JF, Montastruc JL, Marsden CD, Dubini A, Orlando N, Grimaldi R (1997) Cabergoline in the treatment of early Parkinson's disease: results of the first year of treatment in a double-blind comparison of cabergoline and levodopa. The PKDS009 Collaborative Study Group. *Neurology*, 48, 363–8.

Rinne UK, Sonninen V, Siirtola T (1973) Plasma concentration of levodopa in patients with Parkinson's disease. *European Neurology*, 10, 301–10.

Robertson DR, George CF (1990) Drug therapy for Parkinson's disease in the elderly. *British Medical Bulletin*, 46, 124–46.

Rodnitzky R (1992) The use of Sinemet CR in the management of mild to moderate Parkinson's disease. *Neurology*, 42, Suppl. 1, 44–50.

Ropinirole Study Group (1996) To compare the efficacy at six months of ropinirole vs bromo-criptine as early therapy in Parkinsonian patients. *Movement Disorders*, 11, Suppl. 1, 188.

Sage JI, Mark MH (1994) Diagnosis and treatment of Parkinson's disease in elderly. *Journal of Geriatric and Internal Medicine*, 9, 583–9.

Sanchez-Ramos JR, Ortoll R, Paulson GW (1996) Visual hallucinations associated with Parkinson's disease. *Archives of Neurology*, 53, 1265–8.

Schwab RS, England AC, Poskanzer DC, Young RR (1969) Amantadine in the treatment of Parkinson's disease. *Journal of the American Medical Association*, 208, 1168–70.

Senard JM, Rai S, Lapeyre-Mestre M, Brefel C, Rascol O, Rascol A, Montastruc JL (1997) Prevalence of orthostatic hypotension in Parkinson's disease. *Journal of Neurology, Neurosurgery, and Psychiatry*, 63, 584–9.

Senard JM, Valet P, Durrieu G, Berlan M, Tran MA, Montastruc JL, Rascol A, Montastruc P (1990) Adrenergic supersensitivity in parkinsonians with orthostatic hypotension. *European Journal of Clinical Investigation*, 20, 613–19.

Shannon KM (1996) New alternatives for the management of early Parkinson's disease (Parkinson's disease). *Movement Disorders*, 11, Suppl. 1, 266.

Shannon KM, Bennett JP Jr, Friedman JH, for the Pramipexole Study Group (1997) Efficacy of pramipexole, a novel dopamine agonist, as monotherapy in mild to moderate Parkinson's disease. *Neurology*, 49, 724–8.

Singer C, Weiner WJ, Sanchez-Ramos JR (1992) Autonomic dysfunction in men with Parkinson's disease. *European Neurology*, 32, 134–40.

Spencer CM, Benfield P (1996) Tolcapone. *CNS Drugs*, 5, 6, 475–81.

Suchowersky O, Furtado S, Rohs G (1995) Beneficial effect of intranasal desmopressin for nocturnal polyuria in Parkinson's disease. *Movement Disorders*, 10, 337–40.

Tison F, Dartigues JF, Dubes L, Suber M, Alperovitch A, Henry P (1994) Prevalence of Parkinson's disease in the elderly: a population study in Gironde, France. *Acta Neurologica Scandinavica*, 90, 111–15.

Verwoerdt A, Pfeiffer E, Wang HS (1969) Sexual behaviour in senescence. *Geriatrics*, 2, 137–54.

Waters CH (1994) Fluoxetine and selegiline – lack of significant interaction. *Canadian Journal of Neurology*, 21, 259–61.

Waters CH, Kurth M, Bailey P, Shulman LM, LeWitt P, Dorflinger E, Deptula D, Pedder S (1997) Tolcapone in stable Parkinson's disease: efficacy and safety of long-term treatment. The Tolcapone Stable Study Group. *Neurology*, 49, 665–71.

Wilding IR, Davis SS, Melia CD, Hardy JG, Evans DF, Short AH, Sparrow RA (1989) Gastrointestinal transit of Sinemet CR in healthy volunteers. *Neurology*, 39, Suppl. 2, 5333–58.

Williamson J (1978) Prescribing problems in the elderly. *Practitioner*, 220, 749–55.

Zurcher G, Keller HH, Kettler R, Borgulya J, Bonetti EP, Eigenmann R, Da Prada M (1990) Tolcapone a novel, very potent, and orally active inhibitor of catechol-*O*-methyl-transferase: a pharmacological study in rats. *Advances in Neurology*, 53, 497–503.

10

Rehabilitation in Parkinson's disease and parkinsonism

Christopher D Ward

Introduction

This chapter presents an overview of rehabilitation in Parkinson's disease (PD) and in parkinsonism not due to PD, prior to a series of chapters reviewing specific types of nonmedical intervention. The first part of the chapter discusses conceptual issues relevant to progressive neurological conditions such as PD and parkinsonism. What counts as rehabilitation? How (if at all) can rehabilitation be distinguished from care and support? Is rehabilitation effective and cost effective? What are the general service requirements for people with PD and parkinsonism? The second part of the chapter considers how services can be designed to meet the needs of people with these syndromes. How specific are the needs? What resources are required? The chapter ends with an outline of rehabilitation interventions relevant to different stages of PD and to other syndromes resembling PD.

Rehabilitation concepts in PD/parkinsonism

What counts as rehabilitation?

If people with PD/parkinsonism (the two terms are used interchangeably in this section) are to benefit from health and social services their individual needs must always occupy centre stage: each medical and each nonmedical intervention must be relevant, in one way or another, to everyday life. All too often physicians forget this truism, for example in prescribing a drug to suppress a tremor that is unimportant to the patient or in mechanically continuing six-monthly outpatient appointments when neither the doctor nor the patient has clear objectives in mind. Unfocused, essentially aimless activities of this sort maintain a distinction that need hardly exist between medical management and rehabilitation. Rehabilitation in its broadest sense is a pragmatic approach common to all worthwhile interventions; the desired outcomes are relevant in the daily lives of patients and families.

Our broad definition of rehabilitation rules out any distinction between 'treatment' and rehabilitation: all treatments (including cures) are potentially rehabilitative. Rehabilitation is sometimes contrasted with 'active' or 'medical' treatment (one junior doctor wrote in the hospital notes that 'nothing further could be done so the patient was referred for physiotherapy'), but the distinction is spurious. Medical and surgical interventions are rarely curative – all interventions in PD, for example, are essentially palliative. Moreover, nonmedical modalities such as physiotherapy can in some circumstances be used as direct alternatives to interventions such as drugs or surgery (see Chapter 12). Rehabilitation includes all technologies that can reduce handicap.

How should rehabilitation be distinguished from care? The crucial point is that rehabilitation is active and goal directed. Designing a care package to meet the need for continuing care or support is a rehabilitation activity; routine delivery of care is not rehabilitation. However, care staff can and should participate in rehabilitation goals, for example by detecting changing needs and by collaborating in routine activities designed to prevent complications such as contractures and skin sores.

Finally, is there a boundary between rehabilitation and palliation? Does there come a point where rehabilitation has outlived its usefulness in the course of progressive illness, and where symptomatic treatment (palliation) must take its place? In PD and similar disorders a balance must often be struck between symptom control and achieving functional goals that risk exacerbating symptoms such as pain or anxiety. Rehabilitation assessment in progressive disease is a constant process of discovering what is (and what is not) an appropriate intervention. Even in terminal illness there are ways in which a person's functional abilities can be facilitated or impeded. Rehabilitation concepts are therefore just as relevant to a good death as to a good life.

Implementing rehabilitation

Rehabilitation can be more precisely understood within the framework endorsed by the World Health Organization International Classification of Impairments, Disabilities and Handicaps (WHO 1980). Interventions are directed in various combinations towards pathologies (disease processes), impairments (deficits in anatomy or physiology), and disabilities (failure to perform specific tasks to an agreed standard). However, in each case all interventions must finally be evaluated in terms of their separate or combined impact on handicaps (disadvantages). A current revision of the ICIDH framework (WHO 1997) is likely to redesignate disabilities as 'activities' and handicap as 'participation', but with no fundamental change in concepts. A further proposed level will include the person's environment – social and physical factors that often largely determine the extent of disadvantage.

When the scope for reducing impairment or disability is limited, rehabilitation can often be directed towards modifying the environment.

Disadvantage should be understood to include subjective as well as objective states. For example, the mere fact of carrying the diagnosis of PD, irrespective of any disabilities, could weigh a person down with a sense of doom or worthlessness. Another reason for not equating handicaps with physical disabilities is that handicaps include *potential* as well as *actual* states. Thus, in comparison with others of the same age a person with PD is severely disadvantaged by an increased risk of falls and fractures and will be still further disadvantaged by not being made aware of how such risks could be reduced.

Disadvantage provides a philosophical focus for the rehabilitation approach but is a difficult concept to handle in routine practice because disadvantages are subjective and variable and notoriously difficult to evaluate objectively. Moreover, in progressively disabling disorders such as parkinsonism we need to accommodate potential as well as actual disadvantages. We have been experimenting with a scheme called PILS, which breaks down handicap or disadvantage into four broad areas that are targets for rehabilitation: Prevention, Independence, Lifestyle and Social Resources (the PILS scheme resulted from discussions with Professor Paul Dieppe, Dr Ted Cantrell and Dr John Burn).

In the PILS scheme, *Prevention* encompasses assessment and reduction of risks of physical, psychological and social complications. Prevention receives little emphasis in conventional models of rehabilitation since these, along with the ICIDH, have largely been designed to accommodate acquired, nonprogressive disabilities such as stroke. In PD, by contrast, rehabilitation must be a process extended across time and orientated towards future problems as well as to those which have already occurred. The anticipatory stance, so fundamental to the practice of geriatric medicine, is crucial in PD. Physicians have an important role in anticipating disease behaviour and future disability, in contributing to the planning of future patterns of care and rehabilitation and in helping patients and families to take avoiding action. Rehabilitation in this context can therefore be seen as a specialized form of health promotion, empowering individuals to promote future autonomy and well-being (Anderson 1996).

Independence, the second target domain in the PILS scheme, includes activities of daily living and mobility. Note that we place independence in a broader context than is customary. As implied earlier, dependency is not always the crucial determinant of handicap. Whilst dependency can be a major disadvantage the person with full independence may still be severely disadvantaged. However, individuals with similar levels of dependency vary in their degree of disadvantage. Note also that dependency and physical disability are by no means synonymous.

Impairments in communication and in cognition often require others to take over practical tasks (for example control of personal finances). Similarly, depression, and especially anxiety, often adds to dependency in parkinsonism. Studies of carers of people with severe head injuries have demonstrated that behavioural problems outweigh physical disabilities as sources of carer stress (Florian et al. 1989) and the testimony of PD carers suggests that for them, too, physical difficulties are easier to cope with than psychological impairments (McCarthy and Brown 1989).

Lifestyle refers to the person's roles and aspirations and for reasons already given must not be identified with independence. Thus, for someone whose life revolves around grandchildren the role of grandparent can be conserved despite severe physical disabilities. Physicians are not in a good position to understand what is meaningful to their patients and what they most value in their lives. The artificial environment of a clinic, day hospital or inpatient unit produces a limited and unrepresentative picture of the individual. More can be gleaned from a home visit, although even there the doctor–patient relationship often inhibits communication. Information from other sources, for example professional colleagues, is essential if 'lifestyle' is to be understood and valid rehabilitation goals negotiated.

The fourth PILS target area, *Social resources*, includes the environmental level identified in the revised ICIDH. An important goal in rehabilitation is to review a person's assets and to narrow the gap (the disadvantage) caused by lack of resources. Money, housing and transport are three important resource categories. Under the category of prevention we need to consider how physical assets can be conserved in the future. For example, exploring the insurance and financial implications of PD at the time of diagnosis can be considered a rehabilitation activity. However, a person's key assets (so to speak) are people such as family members, other informal carers and professional carers. Catering for their current needs and anticipating future difficulties is always a central goal in rehabilitation. Two important issues arise. Firstly, the needs of spouses and others extend beyond any role they may have in physical care and the designation 'carer' must be used carefully. Secondly, no one is required to care *for* people with PD when they are fully independent but one or more relatives or friends are likely to care *about* them and therefore may require information, education and psychological support. A third general issue regarding carers is that when their needs diverge radically from those of the patient the focus of rehabilitation must be carefully reviewed. This dilemma is often encountered when cognitive or behavioural factors prevent someone with PD from fully acknowledging the needs of a spouse. This justifies regarding the two individuals as separate 'clients' (Ward and McIntosh 1993).

Rehabilitation in PD generates a complex pattern of linkages between personal and professional perspectives, between pathologies, impairment, disabilities, and disadvantages, and between intervention targets such as prevention, independence, lifestyle and social resources. Such complexity has two implications, which are the cornerstones for rehabilitation. Firstly, complexity often requires a *multi professional* approach. One reason for this is that the pre-eminence of personal values calls for a subtle and multifaceted approach to assessment, rather than one that is dominated by doctors or by other professional groups. Not all rehabilitation is team based, but a single individual can rarely meet any but the simplest functional needs without the advice and support of others. A very wide range of health and social technologies and interventions has to be considered. Secondly, complexity calls for a *structured* response: feasible goals must be identified and agreed.

In summary, progressive disorders such as PD require the term rehabilitation to be extended beyond its conventional usage to describe a process that is continuous (even though punctuated by time limited goals). Rehabilitation describes the full range of activities which are directed towards reducing disadvantages, including not only actual handicaps, but also risks of future complications. Rehabilitation also includes interventions to increase a person's ability to 'participate' in their chosen activities (to use the terminology of the revision of the ICIDH), or to sustain their chosen 'lifestyle' (in PILS terminology) both now and in the future. Rehabilitation is a person centred, active, structured and usually multidisciplinary process.

The effectiveness of rehabilitation

Does rehabilitation work? This question makes little sense when addressed to the totality of potential rehabilitation approaches and technologies (Soderback 1995). Rehabilitation as a whole cannot be evaluated comprehensively because it is inseparably bound to a multiplicity of medical and nonmedical processes. Individual rehabilitation 'technologies', especially physiotherapy, have been the subject of formal evaluation (Ward 1992) as described in more detail in the next chapters. Many such studies, however, demonstrate effects of therapies on impairments (Comella et al. 1994, Johnson and Pring 1990) and can therefore scarcely be counted as evidence of the effectiveness of rehabilitation in reducing disability and disadvantage. Evaluations of rehabilitation should assess the benefits of the two key processes identified earlier, notably multidisciplinary working and effective goal setting. There is some evidence, for example on the effectiveness of stroke units (Kalra 1996), that can be interpreted to suggest that structured specialist teams have a positive effect on outcomes of people with neurological disabilities. Evidence is beginning to emerge on the effectiveness of structured rehabilitation processes in multiple sclerosis, a progressive neurological disorder with some similarity to PD (Freeman et al. 1997). There is still, however, a severe paucity of published evidence on the benefits of multidisciplinary interventions for people with PD or other progressive disabling neurological disorders.

The PILS framework provides a starting point for evaluating evidence on PD and for extrapolating, where possible, from studies on other disabling conditions. Regarding the first PILS dimension, *prevention*, there is a remarkable lack of evidence on the effectiveness of interventions in PD. It is likely that some at least of the multifactorial interventions shown to reduce falling in at-risk elderly people (Tinetti et al. 1994, Campbell et al. 1997) should be applicable to people with PD. Demonstration of reduction in rates of other adverse events (for example episodes of aspiration pneumonia or unwanted nursing home admissions), or even of reduced level of risks of such events, has not yet been attempted in PD.

Demonstrating improvements in *independence*, the second PILS domain, is difficult in a progressive disorder such as PD. No studies have demonstrated a sustained improvement in independence as a result of rehabilitation interventions although mobility has benefited from impairment focused physiotherapy. The most important and yet the most elusive outcomes concern the effect of rehabilitation interventions on the third PILS domain, *lifestyle*. A controlled evaluation of a specialist PD community team based in a small Hampshire town showed, by comparison with controls, a significant improvement in mood as measured by the General Health Questionnaire (Goldberg and Hillier 1979) in people with PD and in their carers. This suggested that the team had an overall effect on improving quality of life (C. D. Ward et al. unpublished observations). Anecdotes abound, although without quantitative confirmation, to suggest that providing specialized multidisciplinary support to people with PD facilitates the achievement of individual goals such as resuming a social activity, or undertaking a short trip independently. In the realm of *social resources*, specialist advice undoubtedly increases the uptake of entitlements to benefits although, again, formal evidence is lacking.

Rehabilitation in PD and parkinsonism: matching services to needs

The aim of this and subsequent chapters is to develop an overall description of rehabilitation services for PD and parkinsonism not due to PD, taking into account firstly the epidemiology and clinical characteristics of PD and parkinsonism, and secondly the concepts of rehabilitation proposed in this chapter.

Must services be diagnosis specific?

The needs of people with PD/parkinsonism, and therefore the services and resources they require, can be divided into those common to all people with disabilities, those shared by people with progressive neurological disorders and those unique to individual syndromes. By grouping needs in this way we should be able to determine the extent to which services must be specialized and the extent to which they can be delivered in populations of different sizes.

Generic social and healthcare needs

The fascination of parkinsonism as a specialist field may sometimes tempt us to lose sight of an obvious fact. Many needs of people with PD/ parkinsonism are common to other causes of long-term disabilities whether neurological or otherwise. Disabled people rightly insist that most of their needs are better described in social than in medical terms. Although the clinical profile of each parkinsonian syndrome is highly distinctive the experience of disability is dominated, for many, by nonspecific burdens such as reduced independence, impaired mobility, increased reliance on informal carers and associated psychological stresses. Professional service providers sometimes over value their own specialist contributions whilst underestimating the importance of, for example, daily home care.

Even from the medical point of view there is a generic aspect to PD/parkinsonism, which gives rise to a range of problems experienced by older people in general. Thus people with PD/parkinsonism are liable to *multiple pathologies,* which tend to interact with the parkinsonism or to be masked by it. Symptoms such as pain, dyspnoea, constipation, weight loss and incontinence can sometimes be linked to the neurological disorder but may, alternatively, have independent causes that the rehabilitation team is likely to overlook unless expert medical surveillance is available.

Needs common to progressive neurological disorders

A somewhat more specific group of needs are shared by those with progressive neurological disorders (excluding Alzheimer's disease/dementia), with a total prevalence of perhaps 400 per 100000. PD and parkinsonism together constitute the largest proportion of these conditions in the community (Mutch et al. 1986). Multiple sclerosis (prevalence around 100–200 per 100000) accounts for most of the remainder (Rodriguez et al. 1994). Motor neurone disease and Huntington's disease affect a much smaller number of people although with a disproportionately high impact on services.

The most obvious feature shared by these conditions is progressiveness, so that rehabilitative management must be forward looking and preventive in approach. The progression of PD gives rise to phases in which different needs predominate, from the time of diagnosis, when information and support are especially important, through the phases of increasing disability to the late stage when palliation and family support are emphasized, although the rehabilitation approach remains relevant. The British Multiple Sclerosis Society has suggested that needs can be divided into those associated with (1) the time of diagnosis, (2) mild disability (3) severe disability and (4) terminal disease (Multiple Sclerosis Society 1997). A very similar division could apply to PD and parkinsonism although age related issues would be different. Thus, the need for information and support at the time of diagnosis is strongly expressed by individuals and by organizations representative of all the progressive neurological disorders (The Neurological Alliance 1996). Nonparkinsonian syndromes share many of the opportunities for health promotion, for example prevention of falling. Similarly, there is a shared need for forward planning on issues such as finances. However, in a recent community survey of people with progressive neurological disorders in Derbyshire, we found that few had been provided with information to enable them to plan ahead in view of their progressive disabilities, or knew where to obtain such information.

Striking parallels have been reported between consecutive service users with PD and with MS (McKinney et al. 1998). The range and frequency of symptoms reported by the two groups were surprisingly similar, as were the profile of restrictions in activities of daily living and the degree of psychological stress in patients and carers, as measured by the General Health Questionnaire – 28. In conclusion, it appears likely that there are large overlaps in the service requirements for people with progressive neurological disorders and that the specificity of needs associated with PD and with parkinsonism could be overstated.

Needs specific to PD/parkinsonism

Whilst it is important to appreciate the generic context of disability, rehabilitation cannot be fully effective unless there is full recognition of the pattern of needs associated with PD and specific parkinsonian syndromes. One dominant need in PD/parkinsonism is for medical and nursing support to institute an appropriate drug regime and especially to monitor it *in relation to functional objectives*. The importance of linking the drug regime with pragmatic goals can hardly be overstated. As the next chapter describes, a specialist nurse is likely to improve the relevance of medical treatment to everyday life. Provision of information and training to patients has been shown to improve the quality of medical management, with gains in mobility, independence and subjective sense of self-efficacy (Montgomery et al. 1994).

A woman reported that the burden of caring for her husband was nearly intolerable. He requested her help several times nightly to get him to the toilet. The use of controlled-release levodopa at night helped the situation.

A woman with inadequate response to levodopa was receiving three different formulations of levodopa with inter-dose intervals as short as 30 minutes. The sheer complexity of the drug regime inhibited her from going out and was a source of distress for her somewhat obsessional husband. A simpler regime had no adverse effects on mobility but considerably reduced the requirement for care.

A man with severe 'on-off' fluctuations was taught to administer subcutaneous apomorphine, initially to enable him to give a speech at his wedding without fear of unpredictable akinesia.

A second important distinguishing characteristic of PD/parkinsonism has already been mentioned; in these syndromes physical and psychological deficits are characteristically combined. Psychiatric disorders are sometimes the critical determinants of overall disability and handicap in PD. These include not only anxiety and depression (Gotham et al. 1986, Routh et al. 1987), but also hallucinations and drug related psychotic symptoms (Saint Cyr et al. 1993). Dementia, that is progressive multimodality cognitive failure, affects 10–30% of patients with PD (Brown and Marsden 1984). Even at the level of physical disability one might describe PD as a behavioural as much as a physical disorder. The everyday observation that environmental stimuli such as obstacles or thresholds cause akinetic freezing provides evidence that even motor tasks such as walking have a cognitive aspect. The communicative impairments in PD are a complex blend of motor and cognitive deficits, including not only reduced expressive fluency, impaired articulation and phonation (Critchley 1981), but also deficits in perception of prosodic cues from other speakers (Pell 1996). Psychometric evidence of deficits in selective attention (Cooper et al. 1991, Brown and Marsden 1991) help to explain the familiar observation that distraction, for example through anxiety, impedes motor performance and increases disability. Dramatic changes in a mood state termed 'affect-arousal' occur in parallel with fluctuations in mobility as a result of response to levodopa treatment (Brown et al. 1984). There is thus at least one potential link between motor disability, cognitive impairment and disturbances in mood in PD.

A man with recently diagnosed, relatively mild PD had become incapacitated by an anxiety state that had compounded his physical disability. A series of therapy sessions with a clinical psychologist helped him and his wife to resume some of their previous social activities. One root cause of the anxiety was that he had been traumatized by the abrupt way in which the diagnosis had been communicated and by the lack of subsequent information about his future outlook.

An important distinguishing characteristic of PD (as opposed to parkinsonism) is the variability of disability. Health and social care professionals, as well as the general public, have difficulty in acknowledging that motor disabilities in PD are highly variable. Variability is most dramatic in people with erratic response to levodopa but was observable before the levodopa era (Granger 1961). Predictable diurnal fluctuations place additional restrictions on people's lives whilst unpredictable fluctuations cause intense psychological distress as well as practical inconvenience. Rehabilitation must take account of both the minimum and maximum abilities experienced from day to day and from hour to hour.

A woman aged 65 was reluctant to use her disabled parking sticker in the local supermarket. Other shoppers often made critical comments when they saw her able to walk apparently normally from the car – despite the fact that an hour later she was barely able to walk 10 metres unaided.

A woman with severe motor fluctuations was described by nursing home staff as 'wilful' and 'malingering' because she asked for assistance in dressing, having been observed to be able to knit skilfully at other times.

Rehabilitation resources in PD/parkinsonism

The three groups of needs, those associated with disability in general, with progressive neurological disorders, and specifically with PD and parkinsonism, provide some indications of the range of services required for the rehabilitation and ongoing support of people with these diseases. Existing resources, whether adequate or underprovided, must be coordinated, preferably by a nominated key worker, and some degree of teamwork is essential between health and social services. Rehabilitation in PD/parkinsonism is a continuous process and must therefore be largely community based. A general framework (see Table 10.1) can be adapted to local conditions, which will largely determine the possible form taken by such a team. The team can be based in a specialist movement disorder clinic, in a day hospital, or within a service developed for people with progressive neurological disorders.

Sensitivity to the specific characteristics of PD/parkinsonism requires all health and social service providers to have access to the advice of at least one clinician with experience of the full range of impairments and disabilities which can be encountered. Because of the rarity of PD/parkinsonism such experience cannot be gained within a social services area or primary care group, which typically serve a population of around 100 000. A hospital-based specialist is essential to enable the team to take full account of key principles such as medical management, variability of disability and psychological factors. The medical roles can be fulfilled in various ways (see Table 10.1). A neurologist is appropriate for some roles such as assessment of diagnosis and review of complex treatment regimes. However, as a recent survey of British neurologists and trainees demonstrated (C. D. Ward and C. Young, unpublished observations), neurologists are likely to be relatively inexperienced in assessing disability in the context of home or family, and nor are they well positioned to handle emergent medical complications or to liaise with community services. A geriatrician is often better placed to acquire the necessary specialist experience and to work effectively within a multidisciplinary team. Old age psychiatry has an important role (Wilkinson 1992), as has clinical psychology.

The roles of other health professionals are described more fully in succeeding chapters. The contribution of a specialist PD nurse (see Chapter 11) can often be to provide professionals less experienced in PD (including doctors) with advice and support, as well as contributing directly to the management of individuals with

Table 10.1 Key functions of a rehabilitation service for PD/parkinsonism

The multiprofessional team (health and social services)	– jointly assess and negotiate goals with the patient/client and family – identify key worker (health or social services professional as appropriate) – inform and educate patient/client and family – establish strategies to prevent future complications – jointly monitor progress – joint training programme
Medicine	– establish diagnosis and interpret and control emerging symptoms – assess prognosis – monitor treatment in liaison with nursing colleagues – provide psychiatric assessment
Nursing	– liaise with medical colleagues (consultant and GP) – inform and advise on symptoms – negotiate and monitor drug regimes and associated functional goals
Therapy	– assess functional abilities and provide therapy programmes
Social services	– provide and coordinate information on available resources – assess social needs – provide or organize resources for care and support
Voluntary organizations (local and national)	– provide information – give support
Specialist information and advisory services	– allow access to local and national information databases on statutory and voluntary services – provide coordination of information and education strategy for local service users

complex medical or nursing needs. With expert advice a community nurse can develop some of the roles of the specialist nurse at a local level. This can include supervision of interventions such as apomorphine. The community nurse is often in a better position than the specialist nurse to act as a key worker who is locally accessible and in touch with the activities of other members of the rehabilitation team. Depending on individual needs a therapist may prove to be appropriate as the key worker, through being the team member currently most actively involved. Such a fluid approach to team working and key working is only possible when a group of professionals have established a pattern of trust and collaboration, usually facilitated by effective leadership. Quality of service then depends not so much on the particular professional qualifications of individuals as on the competence of the team as a whole. Some degree of management and leadership is required to control case loads, to prevent over dependency of patients/clients on professionals and to ensure continuing follow-up and support as needs change over time. There are opportunities to rationalize the roles of health and social services so as to ensure that people with PD and their families have continuous access to available information and services. In the UK, voluntary organizations such as the Parkinson's Disease Society (PDS) and the private sector can play a complementary role, especially if they employ voluntary or paid welfare workers. People with PD will also benefit from organizations providing general information for disabled people, such as details of locally available specialized transport facilities and from organizations such as the Citizens Advice Bureau (see Table 10.1).

Is there a role for intensive inpatient rehabilitation?

Faced with complex disabilities and distressed relatives, physicians have often been tempted to offer hospital admission for 'a good sort out' and 'to give the family a break'. There is a need, firstly, to disentangle rehabilitation from respite care, and secondly, to recognize the limitations of hospital as a context for assessment. Hospital admission can precipitate mental confusion, with disastrous results. A further argument against hospital admission and other forms of intensive rehabilitation is that most if not all problems in PD are long standing, and permanent solutions require behavioural changes that take weeks or months rather than days to bring about. Short term functional gains have often not been sustained for long periods after intensive therapy courses for PD.

Rehabilitation strategies in PD

Rehabilitation is relevant at all stages in PD but different strategies are required at different stages. People with PD typically experience two or three obvious lifetime milestones. The first of these, always, is the time of diagnosis. A second milestone may be perceived at the time when disabilities begin to impact significantly on daily life, leading perhaps to early retirement or to the need for home adaptations. A third stage is initiated by recognition of dependency, often an insidious process marked by a progressive shift in family relationships and responsibilities, such that a wife or husband is acknowledged as a carer. Finally there is a terminal stage calling for intensified support and palliative care.

Each milestone marks a shift in a person's subjective experiences and perceived needs and there is a parallel shift in requirements for information. Accessible and appropriate information has a large part to play in ensuring that high quality rehabilitation services are available at critical junctures. We are experimenting with a signpost leaflet designed to enable people to select topics of interest to them at different phases of their disease, from diagnosis onwards. Piloting the leaflet in an outpatient clinic has shown that people are selective in their requests for information, although the majority request more information about their disease.

PD – from diagnosis to disability

The rehabilitation priorities in this phase are for prevention. The best outcomes are likely to result from setting up productive long-term relationships (partnerships) between patients and professionals so as to allow access to timely advice while avoiding excessive dependency. Professional support can probably help to reduce the likelihood of depression, anxiety, and social dysfunction; expert advice prevents impulsive and inappropriate life decisions, for example premature retirement or premature discontinuance of driving.

One determinant of the quality of such relationships, beyond the control of professionals, is the approach initially adopted by the individual and the family to the fact of chronic disease. For some, maintaining some distance from professional help facilitates adjustment (Bury 1991). Opportunities for setting up preventive strategies are then limited. The likeliest source of useful practical advice for this group will be through voluntary organizations such as the PDS. All patients should be made aware of the PDS at the time of diagnosis so that they can make their own choices about involvement at local or national level.

For many people, resistance to professional help can be traced partly to the way in which they were informed about the diagnosis and prognosis. Lack of communication, lack of information and lack of family support at the time of diagnosis are common experiences that contribute subsequently to resistance to professional help, and to dysfunctional responses to illness. Inaccurate or misconstrued information can also be damaging:

A man was excessively preoccupied with quite mild symptoms of PD, which persisted despite partial response to levodopa. He claimed that a junior doctor had assured him that drugs would 'cure' him.

Another elderly man, whose significant disabilities eventually responded well to levodopa, delayed accepting treatment because he had been told that the drug produced distressing involuntary movements and other adverse effects.

Such pitfalls can be avoided or minimized by ensuring that the person communicating the diagnosis is adequately trained. A hospital specialist who has no contact with patients with late stage PD is likely to communicate a misleadingly positive prognosis while those with little experience of PD may be correspondingly over pessimistic. At the time of diagnosis there should be *multiple* opportunities to receive and absorb information. Ideally, as in the system pioneered in Romford (Oxtoby 1988), the physician charged with communicating the diagnosis is

Table 10.2 Preventive advice in early PD

	Advice	Rationale
Psychological issues	Be well informed about PD	Dispel unjustified anxieties
		Realistic expectations
	Promote communication	Discourage social isolation
	Maintain social roles	Discourage social withdrawal
Social issues	Financial advice	Optimize resources for future
	Employment advice	Prevent premature (unwanted) retirement
	Housing advice	Discourage move to unsuitable house
	Review of transport needs	Anticipate eventually being unable to drive
Physical fitness	Promote general health	Reduce risks (cardiovascular etc)
	Monitor body weight	Useful long-term index of well-being in PD
	Dental care	Reduce future speech/swallowing problems
	Anti-osteoporosis strategy	High risk of falls, reduced bone density and fractures in late PD (Taggart and Crawford 1995)
	Specific exercises	Reduce future dystonic postural deformity

supported by a professional colleague such as a social worker or nurse who can continue to answer questions and to provide support both at the initial appointment and subsequently. A follow-up phone call by a nurse or doctor from the clinic, the day after an initial appointment, is an option when resources are limited.

In contrast to those who keep professionals at arm's length, some people will wish to be actively engaged in 'fighting' the disease – they will ask 'What can I do?'. Whilst there is little scientific evidence to support preventive strategies early in PD, it is reasonable to offer a menu of rational advice, which could include the issues listed in Table 10.2. Physiotherapists routinely recommend programmes of exercises to discourage postural deformity and to maintain the quality of gait. This advice can be supported, although as yet there is only weak evidence for the efficacy of physiotherapy in reducing the severity of long-term disability in PD (Doshay 1962).

A subjective sense of self-efficacy – the feeling that one's actions can influence at least some aspects of the present and future – contributes positively to well-being and in other contexts appears to influence physical health (Mendes de Leon et al. 1996). Some activities without solid scientific foundation can nevertheless be health promoting if they enhance self-efficacy. A range of so called complementary therapies can be justified on these grounds and also because they are a means of reducing anxiety and increasing social confidence.

PD – early disability

Even when drug treatment is effective most people will begin to experience significant disabilities within a few years of diagnosis and treatment. Acknowledgement of disabilities – or even of the word disability – is psychologically challenging for many people and may trigger a radical reappraisal of their situation, requiring psychological support. Those who were previously reluctant to accept advice may now do so, and rehearsal of the educational process begun at diagnosis may be more productive at this stage. People should be given the opportunity to be better informed across a range of topics that previously seemed irrelevant to them. Many will be unaware of their full entitlement to benefits and may be interested in information on other social topics such as housing and transport as well as on medical aspects of PD. Those with several years' experience of PD cannot be assumed to be well informed and a signpost leaflet, as described above, provides an opportunity to meet the individual's perceived needs for information as disability progresses.

Many interventions can be helpful in response to the onset of specific impairments or disabilities (Caird 1991), as shown in Table 10.3.

PD – late stage PD

Whilst the division of disease progression into phases is artificial, there is a qualitative distinction between the stage when disabilities are moderate and compatible with full independence, and a stage when dependency is unavoidable. There is then open acknowledgement of a spouse as a carer – with momentous effects on relationships. Disability and dependency result from increasing physical deficits, declining communicative ability and cognitive impairment. Response to drugs is less satisfactory and less predictable. There are escalating risks of physical complications such as falls, fractures, pressure sores and dysphagia and nutritional problems. There are also increasing risks of adverse psychological and social events: for example psychiatric symptoms including drug related psychosis; and physical or psychological ill health of carers.

The rehabilitation agenda remains relevant in late stage PD, although the goals of the multidisciplinary team take account of a sharper decline in physical (and sometimes cognitive) function (see Table 10.4).

Table 10.3 Interventions in early PD

Problem	Interventions
Disturbed sleep	Physiotherapy advice and equipment to facilitate turning in bed Drug treatment, including changes to antiparkinsonism drugs
Dysarthria/dysphonia	Speech therapy advice to maintain communication Dental care
Dysphagia	Speech and language therapy advice to reduce risks Dental care
Impaired dexterity	Occupational therapy (OT) advice and provision of small items of equipment (crockery, adapted pen, etc)
Self-care difficulties	OT advice, adapted clothing (eg Velcro fastenings), equipment (e.g. electric toothbrush)
Reduced mobility, Truncal instability	OT home assessment (reduce risks, improve function) Physiotherapy advice : remedial treatment programme and maintenance exercises OT advice on car transfers, car adaptations (Dubinsky et al. 1991) Assessment of driving competence (mobility centre)
Sexual dysfunction (Brown et al. 1990, Koller et al. 1990)	Skilled assessment of physical, pharmacological and psychological factors Counselling Alteration in drug regimes to reduce adverse factors such as impaired mobility

Rehabilitation strategies in parkinsonism not due to PD

Rehabilitation strategies in degenerative parkinsonian syndromes are qualitatively similar to those for PD. One important difference is that drug treatment is less likely to play a critical role in controlling disability (although significant response to dopaminomimetic agents may sometimes be seen in multiple system atrophy). Another point of contrast is the more rapid rates of progression typically seen in both multiple system atrophy (MSA) and in progressive supranuclear palsy (PSP). Rehabilitation of many people with these syndromes is complicated by delayed recognition of the true nature of the disorder (initially, PD may be mimicked). There is often a consequent failure to keep pace with disabilities as they develop. The rehabilitation programme may fail to take full account of disabilities not commonly observed in PD. For example, visual deficits resulting from reduced range of conjugate gaze occur in PSP and incontinence is an early feature in MSA. For the most

Table 10.4 Interventions in late stage PD

Problem	Interventions
Erratic response to drugs	Intensive monitoring and revision of drug regime, with specific functional aims
Prolonged akinetic freezing	Use of 'tricks', including inverted walking stick (Dietz et al. 1990) Apomorphine therapy
Impaired mobility	Walking aids; e.g. wheeled walking frame Wheelchair (with good postural support to discourage scoliosis) Equipment to assist transfers Home adaptations or rehousing to reduce carer burden and to reduce risk of falling
Pain (Quinn et al. 1984)	Improved postural support (seating and sleeping) to control musculoskeletal pain. Use of apomorphine to treat 'off' period pain
Feeding and nutrition (Kempster and Wahlqvist 1994)	Monitor nutritional status (dietician); equipment for feeding (e.g. Neater eater); monitor dysphagia, remedial treatment (speech and language therapist); use of thickeners for fluids and modified diet; rarely alternative feeding route (e.g. PEG tube or night time fine bore nasogastric feeding)
Bladder symptoms (Gray et al. 1995)	Review medication (anticholinergics) Urinary urgency: OT advice for improved mobility and undressing Nocturnal frequency: optimize sleeping and night-time mobility (see below); night-time antidiuretic treatment (desmopressin spray); use of pergolide; apomorphine for 'off' period voiding difficulty Consider unrelated urological problem
Constipation (Jost 1997)	Review medication (anticholinergics)
Disturbed nights	Optimize mobility in bed Optimize antiparkinsonism medication at night Review home environment for safety Review needs of carer Hypnotic or antidepressant drugs if appropriate
Skin care (risk of sores)	Monitor and manage pressure areas, transfers, continence, nutrition
Psychiatric drug reactions	Review of drug regime Antipsychotic medication Counselling and support for patient and family
Dementia	Monitor cognitive function; acknowledge implications for family; appropriate support services (including Alzheimer's Disease Society for severe dementia)

part, however, impairments and disabilities encountered in parkinsonism are qualitatively similar to those seen in PD, even though often of greater severity. In MSA the severity of dysphagia frequently requires percutaneous endoscopic gastrostomy (PEG) feeding and the early use of a wheelchair may be necessary due to severe postural hypotension. The ethics of life sustaining measures in degenerative parkinsonism, particularly in PSP, which is often rapidly progressive, need to be carefully considered before embarking on procedures such as PEG feeding.

Conclusion

The quality of life of people with PD and parkinsonism, and of their families, can be improved through rehabilitation. Multidisciplinary, goal directed interventions should be focused on handicaps – the disadvantages incurred by disease and disability. Many of these are generic but some can only be understood in terms of the pattern of neurological impairments characteristic of specific parkinsonian syndromes. One point repeatedly stressed in this chapter is the importance of adopting a preventive approach. One of the dimensions of handicap/disadvantage is risk: progressive disorders bring about physical, psychological and social complications that can be avoided if they are anticipated. A second recurring theme has been information: people with PD and parkinsonism need continuing access to sources of information and education throughout the course of their disease to enable them to promote their own independence and well-being.

REFERENCES

Anderson JM (1996) Empowering patients: issues and strategies. *Social Science and Medicine*, 43, 697–705.

Brown RG, Jahanshahi M, Quinn NP, Marsden CD (1990) Sexual function in patients with Parkinson's disease and their partners. *Journal of Neurology, Neurosurgery, and Psychiatry*, 53, 480–6.

Brown RG, Marsden CD (1984) How common is dementia in Parkinson's disease? *Lancet*, 2, 1262–5.

Brown RG, Marsden CD (1991) Dual task performance and processing resources in normal subjects and in patients with Parkinson's disease. *Brain*, 114, 215–31.

Brown RG, Marsden CD, Quinn NP, Wyke MA (1984) Alterations in cognitive performance and affect-arousal state during fluctuations in motor function in Parkinson's disease. *Journal of Neurology, Neurosurgery, and Psychiatry*, 47, 454–65.

Bury M (1991) The sociology of chronic illness: a review of research and prospects. *Sociology of Health and Illness*, 13, 451–68.

Caird FI ed. (1991) *Rehabilitation in Parkinson's disease*. London: Chapman & Hall.

Campbell AJ, Robertson MC, Gardner MM, Norton RN, Tilyard MW, Buchner DM (1997)

Randomised controlled trial of a general practice programme of home based exercise to prevent falls in elderly women. *British Medical Journal*, **315**, 1065–9.

Comella CL, Stebbins GT, Brown-Toms N, Goetz CG (1994) Physical therapy and Parkinson's disease: a controlled clinical trial. *Neurology*, **44**, 376–8.

Cooper JA, Sagar HJ, Jordan N, Harvey NS, Sullivan EV (1991) Cognitive impairment in early, untreated Parkinson's disease and its relationship to motor disability. *Brain*, **114**, 2095–122.

Critchley EMR (1981) Speech disorders in parkinsonism: a review. *Journal of Neurology, Neurosurgery, and Psychiatry*, **46**, 140–4.

Dietz MA, Goetz CG, Stebbins GT (1990) Evaluation of a modified inverted walking stick as a treatment for parkinsonian freezing episodes. *Movement Disorders*, **5**, 243–7.

Doshay LJ (1962) Method and value of physiotherapy in Parkinson's disease. *New England Journal of Medicine*, **266**, 878–80.

Dubinsky RM, Gray C, Husted D, Busenback K, Vetere-Overfield B, Wiltfong D (1991) Driving in Parkinson's disease. *Neurology*, **41**, 517–20.

Florian V, Katz S, Laman V (1989) Impact of traumatic brain damage on family dynamics and functioning: a review. *Brain Injury*, **3**, 219–33.

Freeman JA, Langdon DW, Hobart JC, Thompson AJ (1997) The impact of inpatient rehabilitation on progressive multiple sclerosis. *Annals of Neurology*, **42**, 236–44.

Goldberg DP, Hillier VF (1979) A scaled version of the General Health Questionnaire. *Psychological Medicine*, **9**, 139–45

Gotham A-M, Brown RG, Marsden CD (1986) Depression in Parkinson's disease: a quantitative and qualitative analysis. *Journal of Neurology, Neurosurgery, and Psychiatry*, **49**, 381–9.

Granger ME (1961) Exacerbations in parkinsonism. *Neurology*, **11**, 538–43.

Gray R, Stern G, Malone-Lee J (1995) Lower urinary tract dysfunction in Parkinson's disease: changes relate to age and not disease. *Age and Ageing*, **24**, 499–504.

Johnson JA, Pring TR (1990) Speech therapy in Parkinson's disease: a review and further data. *British Journal of Disorders of Communication*, **25**, 183–94.

Jost WH (1997) Gastrointestinal motility problems in patients with Parkinson's disease. Effects of antiparkinsonian treatment and guidelines for management. *Drugs and Aging*, **10**, 249–58

Kalra L (1996) Organization of stroke services: The role of stroke units. *Cerebrovascular Diseases*, **6**, 7–12.

Kempster PA, Wahlqvist ML (1994) Dietary factors in the management of Parkinson's disease. *Nutrition Reviews*, **52**, 51–8.

Koller WC, Vetere-Overfield B, Williamson A, Busenbark K, Nash J, Parrish D (1990) Sexual dysfunction in Parkinson's disease. *Clinical Neuropharmacology*, **13**, 461–3.

McCarthy B, Brown R (1989) Psychosocial factors in Parkinson's disease. *British Journal of Clinical Psychology*, **28**, 41–52.

McKinney M, Douglas S, Ward CD (1998) The needs of people with progressive neurological disorders: how different are Parkinson's disease and multiple sclerosis? *Clinical Rehabilitation*, **12**, 169–70.

Mendes de Leon CF, Seeman TE, Baker DI, Richardson ED, Tinetti ME (1996) Self-efficacy, physical decline, and change in functioning in community-living elders: A prospective study. *Journals of Gerontology, Series B, Psychological Sciences and Social Sciences*, **51**, S183–90.

Montgomery EB, Lieberman A, Singh G, Fries JF, Calne D, Koller W, Muenter M, Olanow CW,

Stern M, Tanner C, Tintner R (1994) Patient education and health promotion can be effective in Parkinson's disease: A randomised controlled trial. *American Journal of Medicine,* **97,** 429–35.

Multiple Sclerosis Society (1997) *Standards of Healthcare for People with MS.* London.

Mutch WJ, Strudwick A, Roy SK, Downie AW (1986) Parkinson's disease: disability, review and management. *British Medical Journal,* **293,** 675–7.

Oxtoby M (1988) *A Strategy for the Management of Parkinson's Disease and for the Long-term Support of Patients and their Carers.* London: Parkinson's Disease Society.

Pell MD (1996) On the receptive prosodic loss in Parkinson's disease. *Cortex,* **32,** 693–704.

Quinn NP, Koller WC, Lang AE, Marsden CD (1984) Painful Parkinson's disease. *Lancet,* 2, 1366–9.

Rodriguez M, Siva A, Ward J, Stolp-Smith K, O'Brien P, Kurland L (1994) Impairment, disability and handicap in multiple sclerosis: A population-based study in Olmsted County, Minnesota. *Neurology,* **44,** 28–33.

Routh LC, Black JL, Ahlskog JE (1987) Parkinson's disease complicated by anxiety. *Mayo Clinic Proceedings,* **62,** 733–5.

Saint Cyr JA, Taylor AE, Lang AE (1993) Neuropsychological and psychiatric side effects in the treatment of Parkinson's disease. *Neurology,* **43,** S47–S52

Soderback I (1995) Effectiveness of rehabilitation. *Critical Reviews in Physical and Rehabilitation Medicine,* **7,** 275–86.

Taggart H, Crawford V (1995) Reduced bone density of the hip in elderly patients with Parkinson's disease. *Age and Ageing,* **24,** 326–8.

The Neurological Alliance (1996) *Living with a Neurological Condition: Standards of Care.* London.

Tinetti ME, Baker DI, McAvay G, Claus EB, Garrett P, Gottschalk M, Koch ML, Trainor K, Horwitz RI (1994) A multifactorial intervention to reduce the risk of falling among elderly people living in the community. *New England Journal of Medicine,* **331,** 821–7.

Ward CD (1992) Rehabilitation in Parkinson's disease. *Reviews in Clinical Gerontology,* **2,** 254–68.

Ward CD, McIntosh S (1993) The rehabilitation process: a neurological perspective. In: *Neurological Rehabilitation,* eds. Greenwood R, Barnes MP, McMillan TM, Ward CD, pp.13–27. Edinburgh: Churchill Livingstone.

Wilkinson D (1992) The psychogeriatrician's view: management of chronic neurological disability in the community. *Journal of Neurology, Neurosurgery, and Psychiatry,* **55,** Suppl. 41–4.

World Health Organization (1980) *The International Classification of Impairments, Disabilities, and Handicaps – a Manual of Classification Relating to the Consequences of Disease.* Geneva: WHO.

World Health Organization (1997) *The International Classification of Impairments, Disabilities, and Handicaps.* Draft Revision, 1-beta, Geneva: WHO.

11

Rehabilitation, nursing and elderly patients with Parkinson's disease

Sally Roberts

Introduction

The successful nursing assessment and management of Parkinson's disease (PD) in elderly patients requires a sound knowledge not only of the natural history of PD in older people, but also the important principles that underpin geriatric medicine and social aspects of aging. The role of the nurse will be considered specifically in relation to PD though much of the discussion is equally applicable to other causes of parkinsonism. Parkinsonism due to multisystem degenerative disease is usually more rapidly disabling than PD and also has a shorter natural history. Rehabilitation is at the core of successful management in PD and involves a joint effort between the patient, carer and multidisciplinary team.

Nursing care provision in PD

Best nursing care depends upon an understanding of the impairments, disabilities and handicaps that result from PD. This is not always easy to achieve as PD is, except in extreme old age, a relatively rare disorder. Many nurses in primary health care and in hospital service may have little experience or knowledge of this disease. However, the principles underlying the planning of nursing care in PD are common to chronic progressive neurological disease in general. This is an important area for nurse education, as the prevalence of Alzheimer's disease, PD and motor neurone disease will substantially increase in the twenty-first century. The continuity of care for the elderly patient with PD (and other coexisting illness) is also a nursing priority – whether the care provision setting is the person's own home, a residential or nursing home, the GP surgery, the hospital outpatient department or during a period of inpatient care. Continuity of nursing care is increasingly difficult to achieve in all of these care settings and 'team' nursing is often a poor substitute.

The nature of PD and the special aspects of this condition must always be taken into account in planning nursing activity, even if the episode may not be directly related to PD (e.g. an acute or planned surgical admission to hospital). An example of this is seen with 'routine' drug administration when the availability of antiparkinsonian medication is restricted only to the times of formal drug rounds on the ward.

Role of nursing assessment in PD care

A balanced and holistic nursing assessment will assist the rehabilitation team members in making appropriate choices in care and treatment regimes. The nurse is often ideally placed to recognize the links between medication change and altered behaviour (or symptoms) and can 'alert the prescriber' to such changes (Smith 1998). Re-assessment will provide measurable outcomes of intervention and allow the evaluation of the patient's current health status before further nursing diagnosis and care planning takes place. Demographic detail, functional abilities and drug history are all a part of the general nursing assessment. Vital signs (lying and standing blood pressure and weight) are important in the baseline assessment of the elderly patient with PD. Standardized assessment tools, covering the domains of importance in the nursing assessment, can be used to measure impairments, disabilities and handicap related to PD and any existing comorbidities. Such tools can be generic measures (such as the Barthel measure of ADL) or specific to aspects of PD (such as the Unified Parkinson's Disease Rating Scale). A more detailed account of assessment tools is given in Chapter 3. Comprehensive assessment by the whole rehabilitation team should avoid overlap and duplication in the assessment process. Economy of effort can be achieved by prior agreement between health professionals about the assessment tools to be used and who should assess what and when. The nurse is ideally placed to coordinate the comprehensive assessment process at baseline and at times of reassessment after drug and non-drug therapeutic interventions. Of all health professionals the nurse is most likely to spend the longest period of time with an elderly person with PD and their family. This contact is likely to take place over an extended period of time. The psychological support and encouragement of patient and carer together during care planning improves communication and gains mutual confidences. The nurse can actively promote the direct involvement of the patient in the process of care planning. This will assist in identifying, prioritizing and focusing on the *real* problems faced at that time by that patient, rather than those perceived by health professionals.

The goals of nursing care for a person with PD will include improvement and maintenance of the individual's optimum levels of quality of life for as long as possible by preventing or reducing unwanted or negative influences. A conceptual model of nursing can be used as a guide for the nurse towards action, producing positive health gains for the patient with PD, as discussed by Kelly (1995) in a case study using Orem's Model of nursing care (Orem 1980). The nurse acts as a contact and resource, able to recognize needs then initiate appropriate referral in order to optimize care provision.

Core nursing components in PD care

The key components to the nursing care plan and management for PD are shown in Fig. 11.1.

Medication

Treatment regimes become more complicated with disease progression. Elderly patients are also likely to be on concurrent medication for other diseases. Timing of oral medication becomes more crucial in maintaining optimum 'on' time in the patient's life, as does the relationship of oral medication to food intake. The nurse can provide a careful explanation of drug actions to help improve and maintain compliance and can also explain the potential side effects of antiparkinsonian drugs. In order to assist the patient with tablet administration the nurse may suggest the introduction of a suitable portable container with labelled partitions (often called a 'dosette'), which the patient or carer can fill with the scheduled tablets for the day. This method allows the patient to see at a glance when tablets are due and helps maintain a complex drug regime. This approach can be particularly useful when significant cognitive impairment is present.

The nurse can also provide a written list of medication that may have an adverse effect on PD (such as neuroleptic drugs and cinnarazine). The nurse may play a particularly vital role in the assessment of elderly patients for apomorphine treatment, organizing and performing an apomorphine challenge test, assessing treatment response, monitoring side effects, and initiating and maintaining patients on continuous apomorphine pump treatment (see Chapter 3).

Communication

Communication is directly impaired by PD and this is a major source of handicap for patients with PD. Difficulties with communication between patient and carer, patient and therapist, and patient and doctor can lead to misunderstanding and increased anxiety and handicap in the patient. The nurse can make an early referral to a speech and language therapist for assessment and advice on how best to maintain functional communication. A physiotherapist will be able to give advice on exercise to make the person more aware of breathing control to improve speech. The nurse can motivate and encourage the patient to maintain the programme of therapy interventions. Family and carers can be made aware that as communication becomes more difficult it is important for patients to be allowed time to talk,

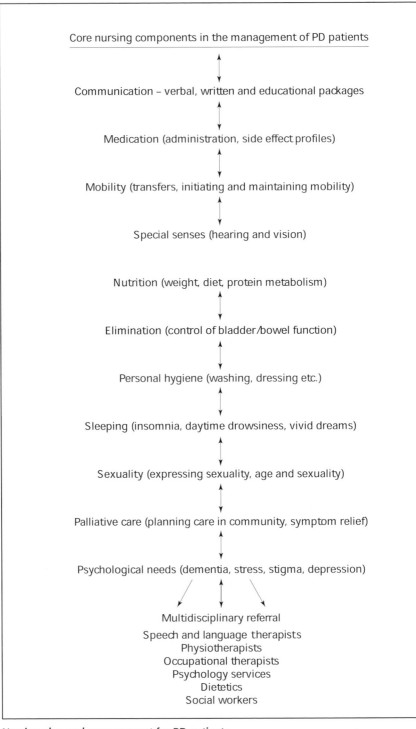

Core nursing components in the management of PD patients

Communication – verbal, written and educational packages

Medication (administration, side effect profiles)

Mobility (transfers, initiating and maintaining mobility)

Special senses (hearing and vision)

Nutrition (weight, diet, protein metabolism)

Elimination (control of bladder/bowel function)

Personal hygiene (washing, dressing etc.)

Sleeping (insomnia, daytime drowsiness, vivid dreams)

Sexuality (expressing sexuality, age and sexuality)

Palliative care (planning care in community, symptom relief)

Psychological needs (dementia, stress, stigma, depression)

Multidisciplinary referral
Speech and language therapists
Physiotherapists
Occupational therapists
Psychology services
Dietetics
Social workers

Fig. 11.1   Nursing plan and management for PD patients.

not to have sentences finished for them, and to speak for themselves. Recognition that, despite communication difficulties, the person retains the same personality, humour and feelings, needs to be tactfully reinforced by the nurse, especially when the burden of caring brings about family frustrations.

Handwriting also deteriorates in PD though usually not to the extent of losing financial control by being unable to sign a document or cheque. If this does occur, the patient should seek legal advice so that a new signature or the signature of a designated person can be accepted as financial authority.

A second problem is that in PD there is a large amount of often complex and confusing information that may need to be discussed with patients and families. Critical communication needs to take place on at least three stages in the disease: at diagnosis, when dependency due to PD first develops, and at the palliative stage of PD.

Most individuals fail to retain much of even the most basic information given to them at the time the diagnosis of PD is first given. It is a shattering diagnosis to many people fuelled by fears of a progressive neurological disease and knowledge of other people, or elderly relatives with PD recollected from childhood. It is also a time of considerable fear and anxiety about the future. Feelings of anger, frustration, denial and despair may be very evident at this time. The nurse can provide timely and accurate information concerning PD and the likely impact this will have on the patient's future. Such information can be reinforced in writing and also by the provision of appropriate leaflets and videotapes from the Parkinson's Disease Society. The knowledge of an individual and their family and lifestyle gained over the time of the nurse's involvement with the patient can help determine the timing, the amount and the detail of information that needs to be given about PD.

Mobility

The nurse, who often has more frequent contact with the patient and their family, can motivate and encourage the patient to maintain the programme of exercises recommended by the physiotherapist. One of the most useful exercises can be walking with good stride length, putting the heel down first, toes upwards and feet well apart (to assist balance). However, sitting or standing exercises may be also useful, depending on the patient's abilities.

When rising from a chair, the nurse can instruct the person to put their feet together, lean forwards and using the arms of the chair for stability push upwards with the legs. The nurse can encourage the use of the arms of the chair to help the patient sit down safely. The patient may need reminding of these strategies regularly, encouraged by family and carers. Independent foot care may become difficult; the nurse will be in a position to monitor the need for referral to a chiropodist (podiatrist). Neglected foot care may result in pain and mobility problems.

Mobility can fluctuate widely in PD and this needs to be explained to carers and family and also other health care professionals, particularly if the patient is admitted to hospital. Motor fluctuations have provided the basis for the erroneous conclusion that the patient 'isn't trying' on occasions throughout the day and night. When in hospital (and other care settings) the knowledge of fluctuations in mobility can influence not only possible bed positioning in relation to toilets and other facilities on the ward, but also the expectations of staff placed on the patient. Assessments for state disability allowances, such as Attendance Allowance in the UK, usually have set eligibility criteria that need to be met in terms of disability. Patients assessed in the 'on' state, when maximally mobile, may fail to reach eligibility criteria even though most of the day mobility would be very much worse.

Mobility is often closely linked with impaired balance and falls. Falls cause a dramatic loss of confidence in elderly patients with PD, which in turn leads to reduced mobility and increased risk of falls. The nurse can help overcome this spiral of immobility that develops after such a life threatening event by promoting safe exercise and confidence boosting activities.

The elderly person with PD needs to be regularly assessed for risk of developing pressure sores due to possible periods of immobility, weight loss, incontinence and general decline associated with the aging process. Appropriate aids to pressure relief can be discussed with the patient and family as a preventative rather than curative intervention.

The issue of safe driving in PD may need to be discussed with patients and families by the nurse. It is important that a full assessment of driving ability is made, otherwise the elderly person with PD may prematurely stop driving, possibly as a result of family pressure. In the absence of sensory loss and cognitive problems a practical test of driving skills is often the best way to assess fitness to drive.

Special senses – hearing and vision

Although hearing and visual impairment do not arise directly as a result of PD, impairment of special senses is very common in elderly people and magnifies the impairments due to PD. The nurse should assess vision and hearing ability so that remediable impairment in these areas can be treated appropriately. Visual problems due to ocular causes can increase the mobility and balance problems of PD and can increase difficulties with communication. Hallucinosis is also more common in the presence of impaired vision and hearing from whatever cause. Impaired hearing is extremely common in older adults and is often helped by the removal of wax in the external auditory meatus and/or the provision of a hearing aid.

Nutrition

Oral hygiene can be a problem due to the patient having difficulty clearing their mouth of food properly. The stale food residue can lead to infection and ulceration. The nurse can remind the patient to check oral cleaning, promote oral hygiene and also ensure dentures are well fitting. The altered saliva in PD and the tendency to a dry mouth despite drooling can result in poorly fitting dentures.

Eating is, for most people, a pleasurable and often social event. The nurse needs to support the patient in maintaining their confidence and ability in independent feeding. The family may already be aware of difficulties the patient is experiencing and can be encouraged to participate in levels of social function at meal times with which the patient can cope. Presentation and the preference of patients for taste need to be taken into account when preparing meals. A person with PD may have impaired sense of smell and taste, so the appearance of food is very important in appetite stimulation and meal enjoyment. It may take great ingenuity to offer a liquidized meal that looks interesting, appealing and tasty. Smaller, more frequent meals and snacks may be more acceptable, as large meals can be exhausting and time consuming with food getting cold long before being finished.

Excessive and uncontrollable drooling will cause embarrassment and discomfort if clothing is penetrated. Many patients eventually resort to the use of padding under the clothes. The nurse needs to be aware of this and advise on skin care to prevent soreness developing under the pad.

Maintenance of body weight is important. Calorie intake normally needs to match energy expenditure. The person with PD may require many more calories to compensate for increased muscle tone and dyskinesia (Davies et al. 1994). Regular weight monitoring needs to be a part of the ongoing nursing assessment in conjunction with expert advice from the dietician.

Elimination

Problems with urinary continence are common in elderly people and are also frequent in PD. The extent to which incontinence in elderly patients with PD is due to aging or directly to PD is still unclear. Incontinence is rarely a part of day to day discussion or debate with family and friends and as a result may be accepted as inevitable by elderly subjects. This is coped with by whatever means available to the patient, sometimes for a long period until containment becomes impossible, causing social embarrassment and distress, before medical help is sought.

Following careful assessment the nurse will be able to establish the nature of any problem with bowel and bladder function and refer the patient on to specialist medical or nursing advice. Urinary difficulties are rarely simply urge incontinence due to detrusor hyperactivity or pure stress incontinence due to pelvic floor muscle weakness. Bladder dysfunction in elderly patients with PD is usually multifactorial in nature and not all causes are likely to be responsive to treatment.

Constipation is a common problem encountered by elderly subjects and patients with PD. In elderly patients with PD constipation can result from a reduced intake of oral fluids or dietary bulk, immobility, autonomic dysfunction, drug side effects, or focal dystonia of the pubococcygeus causing 'anisnus' – a failure of muscular relaxation when attempting to defecate. The nurse can provide relevant and appropriate nutritional advice and encouragement in participating in regular exercise, which will promote bowel function. Many elderly patients need to take stimulant laxatives regularly to avoid constipation.

Sexuality

Nurses, along with other health care professionals, tend to skirt around the impact of disability on sexual function. In relation to aging Catesby Ware (1998) found that 25% of the 80 years plus group reported normal sexual relations. The feeling of insufficient skill in dealing with needs of the chronically disabled in terms of sexuality, as described by Conine and Evans (1982), suggests a more proactive nursing approach than is often provided. Burgener and Logan (1989) consider that the nurse, before embarking on the role of sexual counsellor, needs to be comfortable with their own sexuality. Other considerations should include knowledge of normal sexual response in older adults and the possible limitations set by physical impairment. A nurse can more easily inquire about the effect of PD on the patient's sexual relations, and this will provide a starting point for more sensitive concerns. This will give the patient 'permission to ask' (Burgener and Logan 1989), as it is unlikely that the elderly patient will broach the subject – possibly feeling it to be inappropriate. Patient ownership of the problem may pose certain barriers to the nurse in her assessment. Encouragement to the patient to see the problem as not just theirs, but shared with their partner, will assist in providing a more complete and mutually beneficial picture.

Sexual problems may not be directly associated with PD. Gillie (1990) suggests that one in ten men suffer from impotence and reports that 50–80% of impotence is due to a physical cause. In a study of very elderly subjects Catesby Ware (1989) reports that loss of erectile capability seems to be due to multiple causes. In women, reduced lubrication and vaginismus may play a role in decreased sexual desire. Through discussion, the nurse may establish whether the problem is of a physical nature or due to other influences.

Conine and Evans (1982) endorse the feeling that sexual intimacy is dependent on effective communications between a couple, especially if there is limited movement or spontaneity – as occurs in PD. The decline in verbal and nonverbal sexual responsiveness can be mutual. Reduced frequency of touch and caressing may become evident (with or without the intention of having sex).

Timetabling of sexual activity around best medication responses, continence problems and privacy will require open discussion by the couple. The nurse's role will be to facilitate and encourage such enhanced communication.

Practical advice can be offered regarding alternative positioning, devices available, and minimizing the risk of incontinence during sex. Literature sources can be provided, and many helpful leaflets are available in the UK from The Association to Aid the Sexual and Personal Relationships of People with a Disability (SPOD) and the Parkinson's Disease Society (PDS).

Admission to hospital

Individuals with PD are sometimes placed in considerable difficulty when admitted to hospital either for elective procedures, a period of planned respite admission, or as an emergency admission to medical, surgical or orthopaedic wards. Busy ward staff do not always appreciate the critical nature and timing of medication in PD. The spontaneous motor fluctuations of PD and the sometimes unpredictable response to medication are often poorly appreciated. Standard procedure on admission to hospital is often the removal of medication from patients, with medication only being dispensed at the fixed times of drug rounds. This situation is clearly undesirable for patients with PD on complex drug regimes. After admission to hospital patients with PD should be allowed to self-medicate whenever practical, given the circumstances of their admission.

There has been very little scientific study of the impact of PD on common medical and surgical emergencies. Considerably more work needs to be done in this area to inform clinical practice. Clinical anecdote suggests that patients with PD have less good outcome after both elective and emergency orthopaedic surgery. This impression is supported by some (Coughlin and Templeton 1980, Eventov et al. 1983, Gialanella et al. 1991), but not all studies of femur fracture in patients with PD (Turcotte et al. 1988). These were all retrospective case note studies.

Anaesthesia presents particular problems for patients with PD (Severn 1988). Intubation can be difficult due to axial deformity and laryngospasm (Backus 1991). Swallowing problems in PD increase the risk of perioperative aspiration and may lead to increased risk of postoperative chest infections (Vincken et al. 1984). Muscular rigidity can make adequate ventilation throughout the operative period difficult to achieve (Stoelting et al. 1988). Tremor can be mistaken on the heart monitor for ventricular fibrillation (Reed and Han 1992). Several anaesthetic agents may worsen PD (halothane, neuroleptics, opioids), cause electrolyte imbalance (succinylcholine), or result in unstable blood pressure control due to the additional underlying autonomic dysfunction of PD.

Table 11.1 Guidelines for the management of the patient with PD over a surgical admission

On admission	• Accurately determine existing drug treatment for PD (family physician may need to be contacted to confirm this) and the usual timing of drug treatment
	• Carefully note the descriptions of disease pattern and fluctuation reported by the patient and/or carer. The timing of fluctuations are important for optimal patient care
	• Inform team normally looking after the patient's PD of their admission
Pre-operative care	• Continue antiparkinsonian drug treatment as closely to the point of anaesthesia as possible (in consultation with senior anaesthetist)
	• Restart medication if surgery cancelled
	• Subcutaneous apomorphine or parenteral anticholinergic drug treatment should be considered
	• Maintain adequate hydration
Operative care	• The surgical and anaesthetic team need to be aware of potential problems and hazards of anaesthesia in PD
Post-operative care	• Recommence antiparkinsonian medication as soon as possible after recovery
	• Avoid anti-emetics, sedatives and analgesics that worsen parkinsonism

There is still uncertainty about how best to handle the drug treatment for PD in the patient undergoing surgery. Generally, it is advised that levodopa should be given right up to the operative period to minimise complications and improve the speed of postoperative recovery (Hyman et al. 1988, Katz et al. 1990, Reed and Han 1992). However, it has also been claimed that levodopa can be discontinued up to one day preoperatively without adversely effecting outcome (Pollard and Harrison 1989). It would seem prudent to maintain antiparkinsonian drug treatment for as long preoperatively as possible and to restart medication as soon as possible after surgery. Apomorphine by subcutaneous infusion can control parkinsonian symptoms before, during and after surgery. Domperidone can be given rectally to control nausea and vomiting. Apomorphine needs to be seriously considered to control symptoms in patients with moderate to severe PD undergoing elective surgical procedures.

Guidelines can be developed for managing PD on general medical, surgical and orthopaedic wards (see Table 11.1) to reflect local procedures and needs. The PD specialist nurse can play an important role in developing good practice by involving relevant stakeholders in developing guidelines for managing PD on medical, surgical and orthopaedic wards.

Palliative care

Towards the end of life many people express wishes to be in familiar surroundings, and with the people closest to them. It is the nurse's role to facilitate these requests and then coordinate the best care in this setting.

Lindop et al. (1997) suggest that current trends for palliative care are now moving from hospital to community – again requiring multidisciplinary and interagency working, but to a much greater degree than has been previously been thought. Responsibility lies with the nurse to liaise with relatives about all aspects of nursing care in these final stages.

The PD specialist nurse – the future of nursing care in PD

Due to the rarity of PD it is unlikely that primary health care teams can independently develop the necessary expertise to optimally manage PD. In the UK, where primary health care groups are becoming increasingly responsible for purchasing health care, a new trend is emerging with commissioners 'buying in' specialist nursing services from established specialist sites for PD care.

In the UK the PDS, supported by the pharmaceutical industry, has actively promoted the development of the PD specialist nurse/nurse advisor. The PD specialist nurse can fulfil the entire major nursing roles in the care of patients with PD and their families. The success of the initial PDS funded pilot study (Oxtoby et al. 1988) has led to a significant expansion of these posts around the UK. Specialist nurses have been based in primary care and have been linked to established movement disorder clinics run by geriatricians and neurologists. Publication of a detailed study currently in progress in the UK evaluating the effectiveness and cost effectiveness of the PD specialist nurse is eagerly awaited.

The qualification requirements for employment as a specialist nurse are constantly being reviewed in order to improve academic and clinical standards of nursing care. The necessary clinical supervision may be difficult for specialist nurses to find, and guidance relating to clinical practice can be difficult to achieve due to the autonomy of many PD nurses. Guidelines referring to clinical and professional practice for PD specialist nurses are presently being widely debated by professional nursing groups in the UK, including the Royal College of Nursing. In the future the specialist nurse may be responsible for direct prescribing in PD and already nurse specialists are competent in the accurate diagnosis of parkinsonism in primary care. The specialist nurse can increase the awareness of the possibility of parkinsonism in elderly people by involving primary health teams and nursing home staff in screening procedures to detect early signs of this condition.

Summary

The nurse has a central role in the long-term management of PD and parkinsonism in elderly subjects. The successful and effective management of these conditions is dependent upon the skill, knowledge and organizational abilities of nursing staff. The nurse's role covers not only traditional nursing care, but also an extended medical role supporting the drug treatment of PD. Other important aspects of the specific nursing role in PD include education, promotion of rehabilitation interventions, support and counselling of patient, and enhancing communication between the patient, carer and other health professionals. The nurse can provide a pivotal role in the integration and planning of care in the traditional multidisciplinary team.

REFERENCES

Backus WW, Ward RR, Vitkun SA, Fitzgerald D, Askanazi J (1991) Postextubation laryngeal spasm in an unanesthetized patient with Parkinson's disease. *Journal of Clinical Anesthesia*, 3, 314–16.

Burgener S, Logan G (1989) Sexuality: Concerns of the post-stroke patient. *Rehabilitation Nursing*, 14, 4, 178–81.

Catesby Ware J (1989) Impotence and ageing. *Clinics in Geriatric Medicine*, 5, 2, 301–14.

Conine TA, Evans JH (1982) Sexuality reactivation of chronically and disabled adults. *Journal of Allied Health*, 11, 261–70.

Coughlin L, Templeton J (1980) Hip fractures in patients with Parkinson's disease. *Clinical Orthopaedics and Related Research*, 148, 192–5.

Davies KN, King D, Davies H (1994) A study of the nutritional status of elderly patients with Parkinson's disease. *Age and Ageing*, 23, 142–5.

Eventov I, Moreno M, Geller E, Tardiman R, Salama R (1983) Hip fractures in patients with Parkinson's syndrome. *Journal of Trauma*, 23, 2, 98–101.

Gialanella B, Mattioli F, D'Alessandro G, Bonomelli M, Zancan A, Luisa A (1991) Prognosis of femur fractures in parkinsonian patients. In: *Parkinson's Disease and Extrapyramidal Disorders. Pathophysiology and Treatment*, eds. Agnoli A, Fabbrini G, Stocchi F, pp. 591–4, London: John Libbey.

Gillie O (1990) *Impotence: One in Ten Men*. Channel 4 Television Publication. London: Calvert's Press.

Hyman SA, Rogers WD, Maciunas RJ, Allen GS, Berman ML (1988) Perioperative management for transplant of autologous adrenal medulla to the brain for parkinsonism. *Anesthesiology*, 69, 618–22.

Katz J, Benumof JL, Kadis LB (1990) *Anesthesia and Uncommon Diseases*. Philadelphia: WB Saunders Company.

Kelly G (1995) A Self-care approach. *Nursing Times*, 91, 2, 40–1.

Lindop E, Beach R, Read S (1997) A composite model of palliative care for the UK. *International Journal of Palliative Nursing*, 3, 5, 287–92.

Martz DG, Schreibman DL, Matjasko MJ (1990) Neurological diseases. In: *Anesthesia and Uncommon Diseases*, eds. Katz J, Benumof JL, Kadis LB, pp. 560–89. Philadelphia: W B Saunders Company.

Orem DE (1980) *Nursing: Concepts of Practice*. New York: McGraw-Hill.

Oxtoby M, Findley L, Kelson N, Pearce P, Porteous A, Thurood S, Wood A (1988) *A Strategy for the Management of Parkinson's Disease and for the Long-term Support of Patients and their Carers*. London: Parkinson's Disease Society.

Pollard BJ, Harrison MJ eds (1989) Parkinson's disease. In: *Anaesthesia for Uncommon Diseases*, p. 194. Oxford: Blackwell Scientific Publications.

Reed AP, Han DG (1992) Intraoperative exacerbation of Parkinson's disease. *Anesthesia and Analgesia*, 75, 850–3.

Severn AM (1988) Parkinsonism and the anaesthetist. *British Journal of Anaesthesia*, 61, 761–70.

Smith S (1998) A new look at elderly care. *Nursing Times*, 94, 14, 42–3.

Stoelting RK, Dierdorf SF, McCammon MD eds (1988) Diseases of the nervous system. In: *Anesthesia and Co-existing Disorders*, 2nd edition, pp. 263–354. New York: Churchill Livingstone.

Turcotte R, Godin C, Duchesne R, Jodoin A (1988) Hip fractures and Parkinson's disease. *Clinical Orthopaedics and Related Research*, 256, 132–6.

Vincken WG, Gauthier SB, Dollfuss RE, Hanson RE, Darauay CM, Cosio MG (1984) Involvement of upper airway muscles in extrapyramidal disorders. A cause of airflow limitation. *New England Journal of Medicine*, 311, 438–42.

12

Rehabilitation, physiotherapy and elderly patients with Parkinson's disease

Hilary Chatterton and Brenda Lövgreen

Introduction

A primary motor disorder, such as Parkinson's disease (PD), appears to be an ideal target for physiotherapy intervention. Referral to physiotherapy is recommended in the early stages of the disease (Dobbs et al. 1992) and there is evidence of the clinical effectiveness of physiotherapy at this time (Comella et al. 1994). Unfortunately it is still more common for referral to be delayed until the disease is advanced (Oxtoby 1982), when the opportunity to initiate a preventative treatment strategy has passed.

Physiotherapy has a significant role to play in the short and long-term management of PD. Physiotherapy must be integrated with other therapies. This will maximize the benefits of therapy for the patient and carer by ensuring consistency of approach, reinforcement of treatment aims, and by developing appropriate compensatory strategies (Kauser and Powell 1996).

The pathophysiology of the motor disorder in PD

Due to a deficiency of dopamine in the basal ganglia motor control is impaired in PD. Patients experience this in terms of difficulties with initiating, maintaining, and changing from one sequence of voluntary movement to another. Excess abnormal involuntary movement, such as tremor, may also be present. Balance is often impaired in elderly patients with PD. Clinical examination defines these difficulties in terms of akinesia, bradykinesia, tremor, rigidity and impaired postural reflexes. Impaired integration of normal control may contribute to these problems and a sense of increased effort of movement may result (Lövgreen and Cody 1997). During active voluntary movements sensory feedback is utilized by the central nervous system to interpret the ongoing action in terms of forces that are being generated and trajectories of movements produced. Impulses, known as corollary discharges, are generated in the higher levels of the nervous system and are integrated with afferent feedback to give an internal sense of the movement. In PD there

Table 12.1 Aims of physiotherapy treatment in PD

- Ensure each patient is functioning to maximum potential
- Maintain the patient at the highest level of functional independence for as long as possible
- Slow the rate of decline and onset of movement problems within the constraints imposed by the disease process
- Prevent the secondary complications of immobility
- Educate both the patient and carers to enable them to take the lead role in the physical management of this disease

appears to be some failure in this model with kinaesthetic information generated during a movement being incorrectly compared to original motor commands (Moore 1987, Sanes and Shadmer 1995, Dietz et al. 1993).

Movement problems may not only be of a physical origin, but may also result from deficits of communication and/or cognition. Cognitive problems may present in many forms and may be initially recognized when advice is not followed due to lack of understanding.

Clinical guidelines

In the United Kingdom (UK), guidelines for clinical practice in the management of neurological and elderly patients have been published by the Association of Chartered Physiotherapists Interested in Neurology (ACPIN 1995) and the Association of Chartered Physiotherapists with a Special Interest in Elderly People (ACSIEP 1991). Physiotherapy in PD should be assessment based, taking a holistic and individualized approach to meet the needs of patients, and should involve joint goal setting between therapist, patient and carer (Baker et al. 1997, Greenfield et al. 1995).

The overall aims of physiotherapy treatment in PD are shown in Table 12.1. To achieve the aims of treatment it is necessary for patients with PD to be referred to the physiotherapist at or even before diagnosis is confirmed. An open referral system is advocated, where initial referral should be for a lifetime, not just a course of treatment.

Assessment

Frequent reassessment is necessary to evaluate efficacy of treatment, to identify the need for modification, and to ensure pertinent issues are addressed. There is a tendency within the profession for physiotherapists to use assessment procedures that are individual to their own practice or institution (Lövgreen et al. 1996). One small survey reported that 74% of therapists do not use existing standardized assessments (Robb and Lennon 1997). A standardized assessment is available from the Parkinson's Disease Society in the UK (Franklyn 1986). Other scales commonly used by physiotherapists include the internationally recognized Webster Rating scale and the Hoehn and Yahr scale (Lövgreen et al. 1996).

Assessment procedures should give an overview of the general status of the patient, as well as addressing all relevant physical aspects. This should include functional ability with reference to initiation, sequencing, timing and quality of movement, posture, balance, and underlying muscle tone. Soft tissue length and extensibility is also an important area to assess (Williams 1990), as is respiratory function and exercise tolerance (Hovestadt et al. 1989, Sabate et al. 1996). The relevance of autonomic disturbances affecting activity should also be considered (e.g. dizziness on standing due to postural hypotension). Assessment should take place at a defined time in relation to antiparkinsonian drug-induced motor improvement (Morris et al. 1996).

A model for assessment has been developed that acknowledges the composite effects of physical, psychological and social problems (Schenkman and Butler 1989). Standardized scales such as the Webster scale, Parkinson's Disease Society Scale and the Functional Limitations Profile may also be utilized (Wade 1992).

Communication, which is necessary for the patient's understanding, education and compliance with the management programme, can initially be assessed in a subjective way followed, when indicated, by more detailed assessment in collaboration with a speech and language therapist. Mood disorders, such as depression and anxiety, can also influence a patient's performance. Disease specific health related quality of life measures such as the PDQ-39 (Jenkinson et al. 1995) and PDQL (DeBoer et al. 1996) have also recently been developed. A further area of therapeutic liaison between disciplines is in assessing cognitive function. Assessment of cognitive function is essential in treatment planning and in the interpretation of outcome measures of treatment. The Mini-Mental State Examination (MMSE) is an easily applied screening test for cognitive impairment (Folstein et al. 1975), though allowance needs to be made for age and prior education achievement, before the score can be correctly interpreted.

A problem solving approach to treatment is preferred, which should facilitate the clinical reasoning process (Higgs 1992). Assessment needs to address not only the functional problems experienced by the patients, but also their underlying causes. For example, difficulty experienced in getting up from sitting could be due to soft tissue shortening, weakness in the extensors of the hip and knee, inability to transfer weight over the new base of support, difficulty initiating the movement, or problems in timing and sequencing the movement. Therapists must be able to differentiate between possible causes so that treatment can be directed appropri-

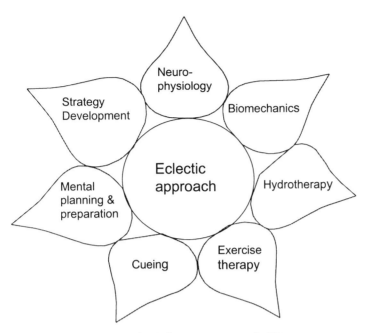

Fig. 12.1   The eclectic approach to physiotherapy treatment in PD.

ately to resolve underlying problems, prior to patient re-education within a functional movement context. Assessment should lead to joint goal setting and an individualized treatment plan.

Treatment approaches

There are a variety of approaches to the physical treatment of patients with PD (see Fig. 12.1). The development of the physiotherapy management of PD lends itself to a problem solving approach, which is mirrored in the evolution of approaches to the physical management of other neurological conditions, e.g. stroke. Approaches identified as being in current use, singly or in combination, include Bobath, Conductive Education and Flewitt–Handford (Lövgreen et al. 1996). The traditional approach in the UK is the Flewitt–Handford. This is an exercise based approach aiming to correct gait. It places a particular emphasis on the rotatory components of movement (Handford 1986). Patients are instructed in a series of exercises, which they are expected to continue at home. These exercises appear to be standard to all patients. The literature suggests that the treatment aims of various approaches are similar to those listed in Table 12.1 (Schenkman et al. 1989, Cutson et al. 1995, Brown and Read 1996). There are also other recognized approaches, such as the Motor Relearning Programme, which could be used in the treatment of PD (Carr and Shepherd 1987).

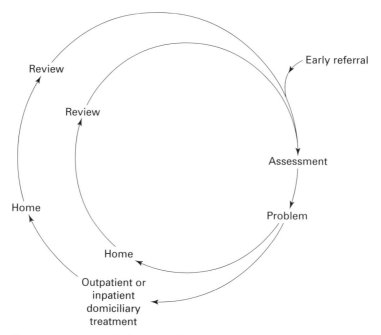

Fig. 12.2   The management cycle for physiotherapy interventions in PD.

Ideally regular contact with the patient should be maintained and once initial referral has been received the patient should have open access to the physiotherapist. This will ensure that if the patient deteriorates an urgent review can take place. The physiotherapist should also initiate regular reviews with the patient so that the patient's condition can be monitored and management programmes adapted accordingly. This may take the form of alterations to the patient's home maintenance programme and/or a course of physiotherapy on either an inpatient or domiciliary basis, as appropriate (see Fig. 12.2). It is the authors' experience that patients with PD, unlike other patients with degenerative neurological conditions such as multiple sclerosis, are poor at initiating contact with the therapist, and therefore the responsibility should be on the therapist to maintain contact with the patient.

Physiotherapy in early PD

In the early stage of PD key goals are: coping with the impact of diagnosis, patient education, the promotion of a healthy lifestyle, and good habits relating to posture and regular activity. The main emphasis at this stage is attempting to slow down the rate of deterioration and maintain normal function. Early referral is necessary so that these aspects of management can be established prior to the onset of significant movement deficits. Patients may be reassured that they may exercise safely, as it has

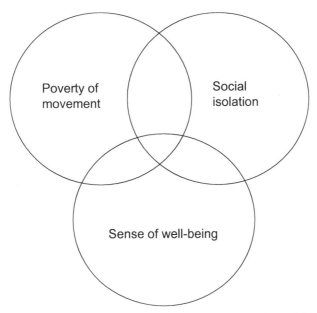

Fig. 12.3   The relationship between social, physical and psychological factors and mobility in PD.

been established that cardiovascular and metabolic responses to exercise do not differ between early stage PD and age matched subjects without PD (Protas et al. 1996). Where available, patients and carers can contact societies specific to the disease and gain access to the regional and local support groups. Information in the form of advice, literature and videos relating to many aspects of the disease are currently available from specific societies. Physiotherapy departments often produce their own information and advice sheets.

Physiotherapy and disease progression

With disease progression motor impairments become more pronounced. At this stage it is necessary to begin correcting the movement disorders. The secondary problems that arise from these disorders (e.g. soft tissue shortening, loss of confidence, weakness through disuse, etc.) must also be addressed. Functional re-education of movement should include all aspects of the patient's lifestyle. Social isolation leading to fears of not being socially accepted has a large impact on patients with movement disorders (see Fig.12.3). As the disease progresses there is a reduction in the proportion of patients participating in activities outside the home in comparison to activities that are home based (Oxtoby 1982). This was most apparent where group activities were concerned.

Ongoing education of patient and carers is important to deal with the impact of this gradual decline. It is necessary to maintain their involvement with a management programme to minimize or delay the effects of the disease process, whilst not raising unrealistic expectations of treatment outcomes (Nolan and Grant 1989).

Physiotherapy in late stage PD

With further disease progression the emphasis towards a corrective and compensatory approach increases. The patient will require more assistance to perform exercise programmes at home or in the physiotherapy department. Compensatory strategies may need to be taught to overcome irreversible or severe movement deficits. Close liaison must exist with other members of the multidisciplinary team to ensure appropriate prescription of aids and adaptations to promote independent function. This may involve home visits by the community therapists. Inappropriate timing of the introduction of aids may increase the rate of decline as patients rely on the aid, rather than using the movement still available to them. The introduction of walking aids is a particularly difficult area to deal with as common aids, such as sticks and frames, are designed to cope with instability in anterior and lateral directions, not posteriorly. Assessment for walking aids must include the reason for their prescription, such as a balance tool. As the patient moves into the palliative stage of the disease a more compensatory approach is required. Treatment moves from active assisted activities towards more passive treatment as the patient becomes less able to participate and goals become more limited. The management of the impact of the emotional and psychological effects of severe disability requires careful handling by the therapist. Over time an extension from the treatment of a pure movement disorder to a more holistic approach is required (Kauser and Powell 1996). The carer's subjective burden also has important implications for the therapist (Zarit and Zarit 1982).

Hospital, community and domiciliary physiotherapy

The environment for treatment is important. If the main aim of treatment is for the patient to function effectively in their own home, then it may be most appropriate to treat them there. Treatment at home can be adapted to specific conditions, such as selection of a chair from which to practice sit to stand movement in order to strengthen the quadriceps. Domestic stairs are often narrower and steeper than those in hospital settings and therefore practice at home is likely to be of more benefit. However, space may be insufficient for certain activities and specialized equipment lacking, in which case hospital-based therapy may be more appropriate. The difference in effectiveness between hospital-based and domiciliary physiotherapy has been the subject of attention in the literature on stroke (Gladman and Lincoln 1994, Gladman et al. 1994). Similar research data needs to be available to inform purchasers of care for PD. Banks and Caird (1989) in a small study, found domiciliary physiotherapy to have more effect than hospital-based therapy.

Hospital physiotherapy may occur on an individual or group basis, or as a combination of both. To some extent the selection of individual or group treatment is reliant on the philosophy underlying the treatment approach. A group allows patients to recognize common problems and share solutions, giving mutual support and encouragement. An example of this format was a six week interdisciplinary group intervention that one of the authors has been involved with. This featured speech therapy, occupational therapy and physiotherapy sessions. During each of the half day sessions a variety of therapeutic assessment and treatment was offered. Educational input from a pharmacist, social worker, PD Society local branch officer, dietician and medical staff was also included. A significant improvement in patients' psychological well-being has been suggested after participation in a group programme (Gauthier et al. 1987).

Hydrotherapy

Hydrotherapy may have a role in the management of PD. The warmth of the water can assist in the reduction of rigidity prior to undertaking a stretching programme in the water. Buoyancy can be used to assist movement to increase range and may also be used as a resistance to movement when strengthening muscles. Patients with poor balance on land often find walking in the water easier, as the hydrostatic pressure of the water increases stability. The warmth of the water also promotes general relaxation and eases the pain associated with stiff muscles. Hydrotherapy has known psychological benefits and is often a treatment that patients enjoy and may increase patients' confidence. Hydrotherapy can also be used as a recreational activity increasing social contacts.

Patients fearful of the water, with unstable cardiac or pulmonary conditions, or with continence problems, are unsuitable for this therapy. Patients with autonomic dysfunction may be at risk from syncope due to vasodilatation induced by warm water.

Treating specific movement components/deficits

Rotational components of movement

All normal movements possess rotatory components. These are essential for normal function. Axial mobility in particular has been shown to correlate positively with overall physical performance (Schenkman et al. 1996). In PD rotation is one of the first movements to be lost and is reflected in the difficulties patients experience in turning over in bed, turning in an enclosed space and during gait. Loss of trunk and pelvic rotation results in a 'legs only gait' with inability to turn (Yekutiel et al. 1991). Whole body rotation using a swivel chair in which the patient is rotated to stimulate the vestibular system has also been suggested as a way of improving posture, increasing stride length, and facilitating movement initiation (McNiven 1986).

Range of movement

Stretching exercises to maintain soft tissue length and range of movement frequently form part of the physiotherapy session and the patient's home maintenance programme. Muscle that is immobilized in a shortened position has been demonstrated to undergo structural changes. These changes include: reduction in number of sarcomeres, an increase in the proportion of connective tissue, muscle fibre atrophy, changes in fibre type, and abnormal cross-bridge formation (Williams 1990, Carey and Burghardt 1993). Working in a shortened range has been shown to increase the speed at which these changes occur (Williams 1990). In PD an increase in percentage of Type I muscle fibres with decreased percentage and atrophy of Type II fibres has been reported (Edstrom 1970).

Placing muscle on a stretch, and advice regarding posture at rest and during specific daily activities, has been shown to be beneficial in preventing length associated changes. A stretch of 30 minutes every two days is recommended to prevent changes in immobilized muscle (Williams 1990). Exercises should encourage movement through full range. The use of sensory targets to give feedback as to whether full range has been achieved may be beneficial, as there is a tendency for patients to lose amplitude, as well as speed of movement, during repeated movements. For example, knee rolling from side to side in crook lying is a suitable exercise, but the patient should be aware of touching the bed with the outer surface of the knees as the lower limbs are lowered.

Flexor musculature is at particular risk of shortening due to the flexed posture adopted by the patient, particularly when more time is spent in the sitting position. Therefore these muscles need to be the focus of treatment, even in the early stages, in order to maintain length. Flexor muscle shortening causes extensor muscle lengthening with resulting muscle imbalance. Lengthening also puts muscle at a mechanical disadvantage. Correcting the flexed posture of the trunk and limbs will have a beneficial effect on the re-education and strengthening of the extensors, allowing them to work in their physiological range of movement.

Gait disturbances

Physiotherapy may be targeted towards one or more aspects of gait re-education and to improving confidence in walking. Achilles tendon stretches, re-education of active dorsiflexion, and of dorsiflexion in the ankle strategy of balance, with its incorporation into gait pattern, are used for decreased heel strike and retropulsion. Muscle strengthening may be required. Visual and auditory cues have been used to aid initiation of movement and to increase step size (McIntosh et al. 1997). Counting and singing may aid dysrhythmia. Distraction techniques, rocking, getting heels to floor, and the use of external cues may be ways of coping with freezing episodes. Trunk mobilization techniques may improve the rotational component of gait and therefore arm swing. Objective evaluation of gait may include simple measures such as 360° turn, six minute or ten minute walk tests. These have been shown to be reliable measures of gait in early and moderate PD (Schenkman et al. 1997).

The patient should practise manoeuvring in small spaces, negotiating doorways and obstacles. It is important that re-education should include walking on different surfaces, such as wooden floors, carpets, grass, and rough ground including slopes, kerbs and steps and should include functional activities as well as distance walking (Schenkman et al. 1989). Stairs need to be practised with and without a rail, and with differing size of step rise.

Compensatory strategies

A characteristic of PD is the difficulty a patient experiences in initiating movement and changing the direction of movements. This involves the complex integration of sensory and motor functions (Schneider et al. 1987). The physiotherapist can have a valuable role in teaching strategies to overcome this deficit (Ype et al. 1995). Simple strategies such as visual cues, for example upturned walking sticks, walking through ladder rungs or over sticks, and the use of 'flip flap' frames, have commonly been used in gait re-education (Dunne et al. 1987). Significant improvements in some temporal aspects of gait have been demonstrated using visual cues (Bagley et al. 1991), though there was no carry over when cues were removed. There is a need to investigate how long training needs to continue before the long-term effects suggested by Worm (1988) may occur. Visual cues, in the form of tapes used as markers to form patterns on the floor, were investigated by Martin (1967) in the laboratory setting to facilitate ongoing movement for patients with freezing problems. However, using floor or low level visual cues may increase the patient's tendency towards a flexed posture, further impairing balance (Weissenborn 1993). The chosen stationary objects used by Bagley et al. (1991) may have implications for others in the patient's environment, such as carers. Mobile cues such as those used by Dunne et al. (1987) and Worm (1988) may be more acceptable. The successful use of visual targets above eye level demonstrates how visual targets can be carried over into normal environmental conditions, both in and out of doors

(Weissenborn 1993). In this single case report it is difficult to determine if the gait improvements noted were due to use of visual targets, or to postural improvement caused by use of targets above eye level.

Falls and balance problems

Patients with PD frequently fall, particularly backwards, although falls are rarely reported. One study suggests that over a third of patients with PD give a history of falls with around a tenth of patients falling at least once a week (Koller et al. 1989). Falling has been shown to correlate positively with postural instability, bradykinesia and rigidity (Koller et al. 1989). The cause of the fall may be related to the changes in posture altering the centre of gravity in relation to the base of support. Plantar flexion and trunk flexion move the centre of gravity backwards so that the line of gravity is displaced towards the back of the base of support. Decreased hip and ankle movements and an inability to extend the trunk have been shown to be associated with falls (Gehlsen and Whaley 1990). The increase in onset latency of the ankle dorsiflexor stretch reflex contributes to the difficulties in coping with posterior perturbation (Woolacott and Shumway-Cook 1990). Primary and/or secondary muscle weakness, in particular the ankle dorsiflexors, may also be associated with falls (Gehlsen and Whaley 1990). Foot and nail deformities, increasingly common in older subjects, have also been identified as independent risk factors for falls (Speechley and Tinetti 1990). It is important that foot problems are identified and early referral made to a podiatrist (chiropodist). Falls lead to loss of confidence and fear of further falling. Patients tend to reduce activity to lessen the risk of falling, though this leads to secondary muscle weakness, further deterioration of balance mechanisms, and increased risk of further falls.

The therapeutic management of the fall should address all components of normal movement and should include soft tissue length, range of movement, muscle tone and strength, and the initiation of appropriate levels of activity. Environmental factors that may contribute to the fall should be identified and adaptations made as required. Balance must be re-educated in static and dynamic functional activities in a variety of settings. Patient confidence will improve as the patient learns to function safely again. The patient and carer must also be taught how to get up from the floor in the event of a fall occurring. The provision of personal alarm systems that can be activated by the patient in the event of a fall and rapidly summon help will also increase the confidence of both patient and carer.

Evaluation of balance

A number of methods of clinical evaluation of balance in the elderly exist, such as the Berg Scale (Berg et al. 1989) and the 'Get up and Go' test (Mathias et al. 1986). Although these may test balance in relation to function, they do not predict those at risk of falling. Tinetti et al. (1986) describe a balance and gait assessment that fulfils both of these roles or, alternatively, the 'Falls' questionnaire (Isaacs 1986) could be used. A new clinical measure of dynamic balance, the functional reach measure, has been found in elderly subjects to correlate significantly with physical frailty (Duncan et al. 1990). The Balance Performance Monitor is of frequent use in the physiotherapy departments as a means of objectively measuring postural sway (Sackley et al. 1992).

Walking aids

A walking aid is rarely a solution to falls, and the patient, having been told an aid will be supplied, arrives in the Physiotherapy Department with false expectations. It does not take a great deal of imagination to work out that, in a patient at risk of falling backwards, conventional aids such as sticks and frames serve no purpose other than to land on top of the patient when they fall. A more appropriate referral would be for the *management* of falls.

In PD walking frames may only serve to increase trunk flexion by further compensating for the inability to dorsiflex the ankle, and inhibit a reciprocal gait pattern. It is often useful to supply an aid that is higher than would normally be the case. Most frames supplied to patients with PD are 'correctly' sized and tend to worsen trunk flexion. A reciprocal gait pattern is easier to achieve using a rollator, though these can 'run away' with patients who have a festinant gait, and braking systems are not easy to operate. The 'Arrow Walker' overcomes the problem of backwards instability but, due to size, is only practical for use in rehabilitation and institutional settings (Farley et al. 1996). Sticks may serve more as a useful warning to others that a person is unsteady on their feet than as a way of improving balance. When to give an aid is a complicated issue. The unnecessary provision of aids may render the patient unnecessarily dependent, with secondary weakness and increasingly impaired balance. If an aid is given and secondary complications are anticipated, these may be minimized by including in the rehabilitation or home exercise programme activities to counteract this effect. For example, if a frame increases trunk flexion additional exercises to encourage trunk extension and strengthen back and neck extensors would be prescribed.

Dystonia

Dystonia in PD can significantly impair functional ability. Several types of dystonia occur in PD (Kidron and Melamed 1987). Therapists need to be aware that even though the patient does not present in the physiotherapy department with dystonia, it may be present at other times. Physiotherapists can assist the patient with dystonia to develop strategies to enhance function. For example, compensatory fixing of the trunk and lower limbs can allow upper limb function and weight bearing to reduce dystonia prior to functional activities. In all aspects of the treatment programme therapists can learn from listening to how patients already deal with their disabilities. Dystonia may be painful (Kidron and Melamed 1987) and physiotherapeutic modalities for pain relief can be helpful in this situation. Dystonia may also cause changes in the mechanical properties of muscle, which in turn may lead to contracture. Clinically decreased range of movement has been observed in the affected muscle groups (Edwards 1996). Massage and specific soft tissue mobilization techniques may be beneficial in preventing these changes.

Exercise tolerance

As PD progresses some patients report an increasing sense of fatigue and reduction in exercise tolerance that can undermine home based exercise programmes. This can result from many causes including an increase in the perception of the sense of effort of moving due to abnormal central motor control. A further cause may be increased force generation during the production of a movement. This phenomenon has been studied in newly diagnosed patients with unilateral PD. The affected limb was found to produce more force during weight matching experiments than the unaffected limb, which could lead to earlier fatiguability (Lövgreen and Cody 1997).

Respiratory function

Restrictive respiratory deficits have been shown to have an impact on activities of daily living in PD (Sabate et al. 1996). Restrictive deficits may be caused by rigidity, contracture or tremor in trunk muscles (Estenne et al. 1984). Alternating abduction and adduction of the vocal chords and tremor of the glottal and supra-glottal areas has been noted during laryngoscopy in patients with PD. Flow volume loop abnormalities show regular acceleration and deceleration with a frequency similar to that of tremor recorded in the extremities (Vincken et al. 1984). The above changes may be superimposed on a pre-existing obstructive deficit in elderly patients, coupled with age related changes in lung function (Renwick and Connolly 1996). This may explain the obstructive deficits noted in some patients by Sabate et al. (1996).

In the early stages of the disease it is important to encourage the patient to undertake regular aerobic activity, which will assist in maintaining respiratory muscle strength and thoracic mobility. Raising postural awareness and postural correction are an essential part of management, emphasizing strengthening of the extensor musculature. Patients may also receive instructions in specific exercises to maintain trunk mobility. In the middle stages of the disease the patient may need to be instructed in breathing exercises. Respiratory muscle training devices to increase respiratory strength and endurance may be useful, but have not been evaluated in

PD (Chatham et al. 1996). In the later stages, attention to posture, seating advice, and breathing exercises to maintain a clear airway are the aspects of treatment on which to focus. In the middle and late stages of PD it may be necessary for the physiotherapist to work in conjunction with the speech and language therapist to enable the patient to achieve adequate respiratory support for speech. This may involve assistance with positioning and improvement of thoracic mobility prior to speech therapy.

Other considerations

Therapists need to consider all aspects of the patient's problems. Orthostatic hypotension has been associated with subjective reports of dizziness, possibly due to increased blood supply to muscles on exercise (Hillen et al. 1996). Pain and limb oedema have also been reported in PD (Hillen and Sage 1996). These are areas to which physiotherapy can contribute. Transcutaneous nerve stimulation (TENS) and acupuncture may be used in the management of pain in neurological conditions. Limb oedema may be improved by advice and exercises, prescription of anti-embolic stockings, and the use of massage or the Flowtron.

Sensory dyspnoea, anxiety and panic attacks are frequent in PD and require sensitive and careful handling (Hillen and Sage 1996). Relaxation techniques may be appropriate for some of these patients.

Evidence base for physiotherapy treatment

Physiotherapy has often been criticized for the lack of formal justification of its efficacy. Evaluation has been hampered by a lack of sensitive and reliable measures that reflect treatment aims in conditions where the signal may be small compared to the large volume of noise. Therapy interventions rely on the interaction and relationship between patient and therapist, as well as the treatment administered. In this context the medical model of the randomized controlled trial is rarely a suitable methodology. Medication effects can also confound assessments of physical therapy interventions around the time of acute admissions when drug therapy is commonly altered.

There is little published evidence concerning the effectiveness of physiotherapy in PD. Most published studies display the problems that are frequent in rehabilitation research: poor descriptions of treatment schedules, small numbers of subjects, poor classification of subjects, flawed or incomparable methodologies, bias, and insufficient power to detect clinically meaningful improvements even if present. Comella et al. (1994) in a small, single blind, randomized, crossover trial of moderately disabled patients found a significant improvement in the total United Parkinson's Disease Rating Scale (UPDRS) score and in the motor and ADL subsections. The trial consisted of a four week intensive programme of exercise therapy with timed motor tasks measured before and after intervention. Chan et al. (1993) in a multiphase single case study demonstrated improvement in gait parameters (step and stride length, cadence), during the treatment phase. A significant improvement in a 10 metre walking test was found in a group receiving a combination of physiotherapy and drug therapy as opposed to the group receiving drug therapy alone (Formisano et al. 1992). Yekutiel et al. (1991) identified after a treatment programme improvements in posture and gait and a reduction in the number of falls. Palmer et al. (1986) reported improvements in grip strength, gait, fine motor co-ordination, and reduction in tremor after a 12 week treatment period. Hurwitz (1989) found beneficial effects after a domiciliary exercise programme. Worringham and Stelmach (1990) studied the effects of practice on reaction time and suggested that patients with PD can use advanced information to programme activities reducing reaction time. However, in a small uncontrolled study Pedersen et al. (1990) found no long-term effect from a physical therapy programme. Weiner and Singer (1989), while reviewing evaluative studies of physiotherapy intervention for Parkinson's disease, suggest that the psychological effects of exercise may be important. They suggest that physiotherapy is the primary motivating factor. Kuroda et al. (1992) found that physical exercise reduced mortality in PD. Participation in a group occupational therapy programme has been found to significantly improve Barthel Index scores (Gauthier et al. 1987).

The way forward

A conference organized by the European Parkinson's Disease Society in 1996 confirmed the poor co-ordination, funding and prescription of physiotherapy across Europe. Arising from this a research group of physiotherapists from the UK, working in close contact with the UK Parkinson's Disease Society, have formulated proposals for seeking European agreement on the most effective methods of physiotherapy (service models and treatment modalities) to facilitate evaluation of best practice. The last phase of this project is now underway. Additionally, the Open Learning Project (Baker et al. 1997) has identified an educational need to improve the communication skills of health and social care professionals to better deal with the complex situations faced by severely handicapped and chronically ill patients.

REFERENCES

ACPIN: Association of Chartered Physiotherapists Interested in Neurology (1995) *Standards of Physiotherapy Practice in Neurology.* London: Chartered Society of Physiotherapy.

ACSIEP: Association of Chartered Physiotherapists with a Special Interest in Elderly People (1991) *Physiotherapy and Older People. Standards of Clinical Practice.* London: Chartered Society of Physiotherapy.

Bagley S, Kelly B, Tunnicliffe N, Turnbull GI, Walker JM (1991) The effect of visual cues on the gait of independently mobile Parkinson's disease patients. *Physiotherapy*, 77, 6.

Baker M, Fardell J, Jones B (1997) *Disability and Rehabilitation, Open Learning Project. Survey of Educational Needs of Health and Social Service Professionals.* London: Prince of Wales Trust.

Banks MA, Caird FI (1989) Physiotherapy benefits patients with Parkinson's disease. *Clinical Rehabilitation*, 3, 11–16.

Berg KO, Wood-Dauphinee S, Williams JI, Gayton D (1989) Measuring balance in the elderly. *Physiotherapy Canada*, 41, 304–11.

Brown M, Read J (1996) Conductive education for people with Parkinson's disease. *British Journal of Therapy and Rehabilitation*, 3, 11, 617–20.

Carey JR, Burghardt TP (1993) Movement dysfunction following central nervous system lesion: A problem of neurologic or muscular impairment. *Physical Therapy*, 73, 8, 538–47.

Carr JH, Shepherd RB, (1987) *A Motor Relearning Programme for Stroke.* London: Heinemann Physiotherapy.

Chan C, Lee J, Neubert C (1993) Physiotherapy intervention in Parkinsonian gait. *New Zealand Journal of Physiotherapy*, 4, 23–8.

Chatham K, Summers L, Baldwin J, Griffiths H, Oliver W (1996) Fixed load incremental respiratory muscle training: A pilot study. *Physiotherapy*, 82, 7, 422–6.

Comella CL, Stebbins GT, Brown-Toms N, Goetz CG (1994) Physical therapy and Parkinson's disease: a controlled clinical trial. *Neurology*, 44, 376–8.

Cutson T, Laub KC, Schenkman M (1995) Pharmacological and nonpharmacological interventions in the treatment of Parkinson's disease. *Physical Therapy*, 75, 5, 363–73.

DeBoer AGEM, Wijker W, Speelman JD, de Haes JCJM (1996) Quality of life in patients with Parkinson's disease: development of a questionnaire. *Journal of Neurology, Neurosurgery, and Psychiatry*, 61, 70–4.

Dietz V, Zijlstra W, Assiante C, Trippel M, Berger W (1993) Balance control in Parkinson's disease. *Gait Posture*, 6, 2, 77–84

Dobbs RJ, Dobbs SM, Bowes SG, O'Neill CJA (1992) Parkinsonism: Myths, dogma and the hope of prophylaxis. *Age and Ageing*, 21, 389–92.

Duncan PW, Weiner DK, Chandler J, Studenski S (1990) Functional reach: A new measure of balance. *Journal of Gerontology*, 43, 6, 192–7

Dunne JW, Hankey GJ, Edis HE (1987) Parkinsonism: upturned walking stick as an aid to locomotion. *Archives of Physical Medicine and Rehabilitation*, 68, 380–1.

Edstrom L (1970) Selective changes in sizes of red and white muscle fibres in upper motor neurone lesions and parkinsonism. *Journal of the Neurological Sciences*, 11, 537–50.

Edwards S (1996) Abnormal tone and movement as a result of neurological impairment: considerations for treatment. In: *Neurological Physiotherapy. A Problem Solving Approach*, ed. S Edwards, pp. 63–86. London: Churchill Livingstone.

Estenne M, Hubert M, De Troyer A (1984) Respiratory muscle involvement in Parkinson's disease. *New England Journal of Medicine*, 311, 23, 1516.

Farley R, Douglas W, Szadurski M, Hood M, Findlay A (1996) The arrow walker for adults: design, evaluation and commercial development. *Physiotherapy*, 82, 3, 176–83.

Folstein MF, Folstein SE, McHugh PR (1975) 'Mini-Mental State': a practical method for grading the cognitive state of patients for the clinician. *Journal of Psychiatric Research*, 12, 189–98.

Formisano R, Pratesi L, Modrelli FT, Bonifati V, Meco G (1992) Rehabilitation and Parkinson's disease. *Scandinavian Journal of Rehabilitation Medicine*, 24, 157–60.

Franklyn S (1986) User's guide to the physiotherapy assessment form for Parkinson's disease. *Physiotherapy*, 72, 7, 359–61.

Gauthier L, Dalziel S, Gauthier S (1987) The benefits of group occupational therapy for patients with Parkinson's disease. *American Journal of Occupational Therapy*, 41, 6, 360–5.

Gehlsen GM, Whaley MH (1990) Falls in the elderly: Part II: Balance, strength and flexibility. *Archives of Physical Medicine and Rehabilitation*, 71, 739–41.

Gladman JRF, Lincoln NB (1994) Follow-up of a controlled trial of domiciliary stroke rehabilitation (DOMINO study). *Age and Ageing*, 23, 9–13.

Gladman JRF, Whynes D, Lincoln NB (1994) Cost based comparison of domiciliary and hospital-based stroke rehabilitation. *Age and Ageing*, 23, 241–5.

Greenfield S, Kaplan S, Ware JE (1995) Expanding patient involvement in care. *Annals of Internal Medicine*, 102, 520–8.

Handford F (1986) The Flewitt–Handford exercises for parkinsonian gait. *Physiotherapy*, 72, 7, 382.

Higgs J (1992) Developing clinical reasoning competencies. *Physiotherapy*, 78, 8, 575–81.

Hillen ME, Sage JI (1996) Non motor fluctuations with Parkinson's disease. *Neurology*, 47, 1180–3.

Hillen ME, Wagner ML, Sage JI (1996) 'Subclinical' orthostatic hypotension is associated with dizziness in elderly patients with Parkinson's disease. *Archives of Physical Medicine and Rehabilitation*, 77, 7, 710–12.

Hovestadt A, Bogaard JM, Meerwaldt JD, Van der Meche FGA, Stigt J (1989) Pulmonary function in Parkinson's disease. *Journal of Neurology, Neurosurgery, and Psychiatry*, 52, 329–33.

Hurwitz A (1989) The benefit of a home exercise regimen for ambulatory Parkinson's disease patients. *Journal of Neuroscience Nursing*, 21, 180–4.

Isaacs B (1986) Question the patient; answers explain the fall. *Geriatric Medicine*, 2, 19–20.

Jenkinson C, Peto V, Fitzpatrick R, Greenall R, Hyman N (1995) Self-reported functioning and well-being in patients with Parkinson's disease: comparison of the short form health survey (SF-36) and the Parkinson's disease questionnaire (PDQ-39). *Age and Ageing*, 24, 505–9.

Kauser R, Powell GE (1996) Subjective burden on carers of patients with neurological problems. *Clinical Rehabilitation*, 10, 159–65.

Kidron D, Melamed E (1987) Forms of dystonia in patients with Parkinson's disease. *Neurology*, 37, 6, 1009–11.

Koller WC, Glatt S, Vetere-Overfiled B, Hassanein R (1989) Falls and Parkinson's disease. *Clinical Neuropharmacology*, 12, 2, 98–105.

Kuroda K, Tatara K, Takatorige T, Shinso F (1992) Effect of physical exercise on mortality in patients with Parkinson's disease. *Acta Neurologica Scandinavica*, 86, 55–9.

Lövgreen B, Cody FJW (1997) Bilateral matching of human isometric contractile force in health and Parkinson's disease. Published abstract *XXXIII International Congress of Physiological Sciences*, IUPS, St Petersburg.

Lövgreen B, Howe TE, Cody FWJ (1996) Physiotherapy provision for patients with Parkinson's disease: Results of a pilot questionnaire. Published abstract as conference proceedings. *1st World Congress for Research into Neurological Rehabilitation.*

McIntosh GC, Brown SH, Rice RR, Thaut HH (1997) Rhythmic auditory motor facilitation of gait patterns in patients with Parkinson's disease. *Journal of Neurology, Neurosurgery, and Psychiatry*, 62, 423–8.

McNiven DR (1986) Rotational impairment of movement in the Parkinsonian patient. *Physiotherapy*, 72, 8, 381.

Martin JP (1967) *The Basal Ganglia and Posture.* Philadelphia: J.B. Lippincott Co.

Mathias S, Nayak USL, Isaacs B (1986) Balance in elderly patients: The 'Get up and go' test. *Archives of Physical Medicine and Rehabilitation*, 67, 387–9.

Moore AP (1987) Impaired sensorimotor integration in Parkinsonism and dyskinesia: a role for corollary discharges. *Journal of Neurology, Neurosurgery, and Psychiatry*, 50, 544–52.

Morris ME, Matyas TA, Lansek R, Summers JJ (1996) Temporal stability of gait in Parkinson's disease. *Physical Therapy*, 76, 7, 763–77.

Nolan N, Grant G (1989) Addressing the needs of informal carers: a neglected area of nursing practice. *Journal of Nursing, Midwifery and Health Visiting*, 14, 950–61.

Oxtoby M (1982) *Parkinson's Disease Patients and Their Social Needs.* London: Parkinson's Disease Society.

Palmer SS, Mortimer JA, Webster DD, Dickinson GL (1986) Exercise therapy for Parkinson's disease. *Archives of Physical Medicine and Rehabilitation*, 6, 7, 741–5.

Pederson SW, Oberg B, Insulander A, Vretman M (1990) Group training in Parkinsonism: Quantitative measurements of treatment. *Scandinavian Journal of Rehabilitation Medicine*, 22, 207–11.

Protas EJ, Stanley RK, Jankovic J, Macneill B (1996) Cardiovascular and metabolic responses to upper and lower extremity exercise in men with idiopathic Parkinson's disease. *Physical Therapy*, 76, 1, 34–40.

Renwick D, Connolly M (1996) Prevalence and treatment of chronic airways obstruction in adults over the age of forty five. *Thorax*, 51, 164–8.

Robb C, Lennon SM (1997) A survey of current physiotherapy practice in Parkinson's disease patients in Northern Ireland. *Synapse.* Spring issue, 23.

Sabate M, Rodriguez M, Mendez E, Enriquez E, Gonzalez I (1996) Obstructive and restrictive pulmonary dysfunction increases disability in Parkinson's disease. *Archives of Physical Medicine and Rehabilitation*, 77, 1, 29–34.

Sackley CM, Baguley BI, Gent S, Hodgson P (1992) The use of a balance performance monitor in the treatment of weight bearing and weight transference problems after stroke. *Physiotherapy*, 78, 12, 907–13.

Sanes JN, Shadmer R (1995) Sense of muscular effort and somaesthetic afferent information in humans. *Canadian Journal of Physiology and Pharmacology*, 73, 223–33.

Schenkman M, Butler RB (1989) A model for multisystem evaluation treatment of individuals with Parkinson's disease. *Physical Therapy*, 69, 11, 932–3.

Schenkman M, Cutson TM, Kuchibhatla M, Chandler J, Pieper C (1997) Reliability of impairment and physical performance measures for persons with Parkinson's disease. *Physical Therapy*, 77, 1, 19–27

Schenkman M, Donovan J, Tsubota J, Kluss M, Stebbins P, Butler RB (1989) Management of individuals with Parkinson's disease: Rationale and case studies. *Physical Therapy*, 69, 11, 944–55.

Schenkman M, Shipp KM, Chandler J, Studenski SA, Kuchibhatla M (1996) Relationships between mobility of axial structures and physical performance. *Physical Therapy*, 76, 3, 276–85.

Schneider JS, Diamond SG, Markham CH (1987) Parkinson's disease; sensory and motor problems in arms and hands. *Neurology*, 37, 951–6.

Speechley M, Tinetti M (1990) Assessment of risk and prevention of falls among elderly persons: role of the physiotherapist. *Physiotherapy Canada*, 42, 4, 75–9.

Tinetti ME, Williams TF, Mayewski R (1986) Fall risk index for elderly patients based on number of chronic disabilities. *American Journal of Medicine*, 80, 429–34.

Vincken WG, Gauthier SG, Dollfuss RE, Hanson RE, Darauay CM, Cosio MG (1984) Involvement of upper airway muscles in extrapyramidal disorders. *New England Journal of Medicine*, 311, 438–42.

Wade DT (1992) *Measurement in Neurological Rehabilitation*. Oxford: Oxford University Press.

Weiner S, Singer C (1989) Parkinson's disease and non pharmacological treatment programmes. *Journal of the American Geriatrics Society*, 37, 359–63.

Weissenborn S (1993) The effect of using a two step verbal cue to a visual target above eye level on the Parkinsonian gait: A case study. *Physiotherapy*, 79, 1, 26–31.

Williams PE (1990) Use of intermittent stretch in the prevention of serial sarcomere loss in immobilized muscle. *Annals of the Rheumatic Diseases*, 49, 316.

Woolacott MH, Shumway-Cook A (1990) Changes in postural control across the life span – A systems approach. *Physical Therapy*, 70, 12, 799–807.

Worm GM (1988) Recovery of motion in Parkinson's disease. *Archives of Physical Medicine and Rehabilitation*, 69, 463–4.

Worringham CJ, Stelmach GE (1990) Practice effects on the programming of discrete movement in Parkinson's disease. *Journal of Neurology, Neurosurgery, and Psychiatry*, 53, 702–4.

Yekutiel MP, Pinasov A, Shahar G, Sroka H (1991) A clinical trial of the re-education of movement in patients with Parkinson's disease. *Clinical Rehabilitation*, 5, 207–14.

Ype PT, Wiebo H, Bruwoer H, Johannes PWFL (1995) Training of compensational strategies for impaired gross motor skills in Parkinson's disease. *Physiotherapy Theory and Practice*, 11, 209–29.

Zarit SH, Zarit JM (1982) Families under stress: Interventions for caregivers of senile dementia patients. *Psychological Therapy and Research Practice*, 19, 461–71.

13

Rehabilitation, occupational therapy and elderly patients with Parkinson's disease

Jackie Hughes

Introduction

Occupational therapy (OT) has been defined as the prescription of occupations, interactions and environmental adaptations to enable the individual to regain, develop or retain occupational skills and roles required to promote personal well-being. OT should also be concerned with helping an individual to achieve meaningful, purposeful goals and relationships appropriate to the relevant social and cultural setting (Hagedorn 1992). This definition emphasizes the uniqueness of each individual and the importance of establishing goals in rehabilitation that are relevant to the patient. OT intervention in PD is likely to take place over the whole of the natural history of the disease, which may last for many years. This chapter describes some of the areas in rehabilitation in PD that are the particular concern of the occupational therapist. A model and frame of reference for OT is suggested. The value of multidisciplinary team working is emphasized, as is the need for assessment in OT and greater commitment to evidence based practice.

Aims of intervention of OT in PD

For people with PD daily life can become consumed with coping with social isolation, estranged relationships, loss of roles, changing roles and changes in physical appearance. Not surprisingly, PD is associated with significant levels of stress, anxiety and depression in both patients and carer. Older patients with PD will also be limited in daily roles by other concurrent disease states that will summate with the effects of PD. The therapist needs to be aware of the potential for problems in elderly patients and to anticipate these whenever possible by emphasizing active prevention of complications and general health promotion.

The therapist is concerned with maximizing abilities and compensating appropriately for limitations that PD will produce. The aims of intervention are to prevent disability and maintain maximum physical, emotional, spiritual, social, vocational and psychological function for as long as possible (see Table 13.1).

Table 13.1 Aims of intervention of OT in PD

- To provide an understanding of the disease
- To provide education and support
- To assist the individual and carer to achieve a positive attitude towards keeping independent
- To prevent or delay disability
- To restore function, roles and relationships
- To plan interventions that are appropriate to the needs of the patient, carer and family
- To maintain quality of life near to the end of life in palliative care settings

A frame of reference and a model of practice for OT

A humane frame of reference emphasizes holistic practice and is flexible enough to allow a rehabilitative approach to those with deteriorating conditions. A frame of reference provides an organization for the knowledge, principles and research findings that underpin practice. A model is the system or process in which theories or ideas are presented in an organized format, and provides a framework for practice. One such model, the Reed and Sanderson Model, works well in practice in PD (see Fig.13.1). Occupation is seen as being fundamental to human health and this model emphasizes autonomy, functional independence, actualization and self-actualization.

Assessment in OT

Standardized methods of assessment are required to objectively measure the complex disabilities and handicaps that result from PD. The domains of importance in assessment by the OT consist of activities of daily living, handicap, quality of life and cognitive function (see Table 13.2). Unfortunately, the most popular and simple indexing systems are not standardized due to a long standing reluctance of therapists to adopt such schemes. Standardized and validated assessment tools are needed to establish the clinical effectiveness of OT in chronic diseases such as PD. Assessment tools can be generic or disease specific and a combination of these two types of assessments is often the most practical way forward (Wade 1992 and see Chapter 3).

Specific assessments in OT

The Canadian Occupational Performance Measures (COPM) measures performance that is both important and specific to the individual (Law et al. 1994). It includes self-care assessment, domestic activity, work and leisure. The emphasis on occupational work makes parts of this assessment less relevant to elderly people.

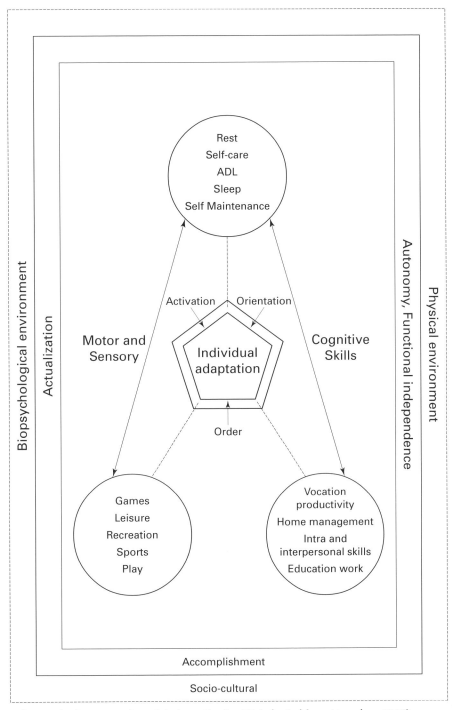

Fig. 13.1   A frame of reference and model of practice for OT (adapted from Hagedorn 1992).

Table 13.2 Assessment areas for the therapist in PD

- Range of movement – grip and pinch strength
- Fine motor control – coordination, handwriting
- Gross motor control – rolling, turning, positioning, balance and transfers
- Tolerance and endurance
- Sensory loss
- Cognitive function
- Self-concept
- Mood
- Coping skills
- Social situation and support network
- Role performance
- Daily living skills – kitchen work, aids
- Personal care
- Productivity – work skills
- Leisure interests and hobbies
- Home environment – risk assessment
- Environmental barriers – adaptations

The Barthel Index (Collin et al. 1988) has been widely used in occupational therapy and is the 'gold standard' assessment of physical ADL. The Functional Independence Measure (FIM 1993), and the Assessment of Motor Processing and Skills (Fisher 1995) can also be used to determine dependency in PD.

Several factors need to be considered before interpreting the results of functional assessment in PD. These include the natural variability and fluctuating nature of PD, the presence of comorbidity, the influence of depression and anxiety, the interaction of medication and communication problems. Assessment should lead to focused and planned interventions that deal with problems relevant to the patient, carer and family. Motivation on the part of the patient and carer is crucial to the success of any intervention and will depend upon the intervention being linked to meaningful goals.

Specific areas for OT intervention in PD

Dressing and grooming

The importance of an individual's style must be recognized when giving advice on clothing. Whereas some individuals will be happy to change lifelong habits to increase independence, others may not. The main points of dressing advice is to promote clothes that are easily taken off, with fastenings that are easy to use and accessible. Most clothing can be adapted easily. Dressing encompasses cognitive skills such as thought processing, planning and sequencing and is also a treatment activity that can be used to promote balance and coordination (Turner 1992).

Washing and bathing

Bathing and washing may need to be more frequent in PD due to the oiliness of the skin. The bathroom is a common site for accidents in elderly patients with balance and mobility problems and as a priority the therapist must ensure the safety of the individual whilst carrying out these activities. Good lighting, non-slip bath mats and the provision of shower units can help reduce accidents. Toilet and bathroom doors should be hung to open outwards with a locking mechanism accessible from both sides. It may be necessary to introduce some equipment such as a perching stool to reduce the fatigue of standing and when balance is impaired. In later stages it may be necessary to suggest hoists or strip washes in the home involving personal home carers or family members.

Toileting

In PD constipation is common as is frequency and urgency of micturition due to an unstable bladder. Physical disability compounds these problems by making getting to and using the toilet more difficult. Grab rails and a seat raise can help with getting on and off the toilet. Clothing needs to be manageable and all requirements for hygiene should be close to hand and easy to use.

Eating and drinking

Due to problems with tremor, akinesia and swallowing difficulties, meal times can be a nightmare for patients and their families. The OT needs to work closely with the physiotherapist to establish appropriate positioning at meal times and with the speech therapist and dietician to ensure adequate and safely administered nutrition. General advice can be given such as taking smaller more frequent meals and on occasions adapted cutlery and non-slip table mats can be usefully supplied. Eating meals when the response to medication is maximal may also be worth trying.

Promoting a safe environment

Helping to maintain home safety, particularly in the kitchen when preparing meals and on outside paths leading around the house, is a very important aspect to the work of the therapist. The risk of falling increases with disease progression in PD and patients need to be advised on what best to do after having fallen. The provision of personal alarms can help to maintain confidence. Advice can be given on the positioning of kitchen appliances and how to safely move and handle items (e.g. by sliding a kettle rather than lifting it).

Table 13.3 Provision of equipment in PD

Timing	Is it appropriate; is there still scope for further treatment?
Appropriateness	Is it practical; does it improve quality of life or encourage dependency?
Environment	Is the home physically suitable and practical (e.g. space, floor surfaces)?
Safety	Is it safe for the individual in his/her environment?
Choice	Is it what the patient wants and will the carer support its use?

Providing equipment

The use of equipment needs careful consideration (see Table 13.3). If introduced too soon it can promote an environment of dependency, rather than maintain independence. Inappropriate provision of equipment can worsen impairment in PD. For example, the use of a wheeled trolley may exacerbate spinal flexion because it is pushed too far ahead and increases the risk of falls. Walking equipment that works well in the clinic or Day Hospital, such as a wheeled zimmer frame, may be inappropriate at home due to thick pile carpet or other environmental hazards! In late stage PD, particularly if falls are a major problem, it may be necessary to consider a wheelchair for outside use and then even perhaps in the home if internal distances are long. A powered wheelchair, either self or attendant operated, may also significantly improve quality of life in late stage disease. Equipment must be seen to be useful to the patient and carer and also as a result be actually used. A considerable number of inappropriately prescribed aids and appliances remain unused and often further clutter up the home.

Transfers and mobility

The patient should be encouraged to assist in transfers for as long as possible. Carers may need back care education. The OT should work closely with the physiotherapist and carer. Specialist programmes of dance and movement run in conjunction with the physiotherapist may help to maintain mobility and balance. Conductive education programmes may benefit some patients. The most effective elements of this group therapy approach can be incorporated in generic rehabilitation programmes by therapists.

Driving

The ability to drive is a major factor determining the quality of life of many elderly people. Although in the UK, for example, there is a legal responsibility for the driver to inform the Driver and Vehicle Licensing Agency of the onset of PD, this diagnosis alone does not necessarily preclude safe driving (Anthony 1997). Problems with akinesia, tremor and dyskinesia may make driving less safe in PD. In PD reaction times and movement times may be slowed and cognitive visuospatial skills impaired. The development of significant cognitive impairment and dementia in late stage PD will also preclude safe driving. The best way to assess a person's safety to drive is by a practical test. Several Driving Assessment Centres are located in the UK. Physical assessment and driving assessments are carried out and advice is also offered to passengers.

Handwriting skills

Handwriting is a vital communication skill. It is used to convey our thoughts, ideas and to record information. In PD handwriting can deteriorate to the extent of preventing adequate written communication and expression. In many cases the inability to sign a cheque can take away a vital part of the individual's autonomy. A specimen of a new signature can be given to financial institutions to authorize financial transactions. Writing, as group therapy or individual therapy, can be included as part of the programme of rehabilitation.

Counselling in PD

Most health professionals find themselves counselling at some point during the helping process. Each will have varying levels of skill. Counselling can be described as a way of being, rather than a set of skills (Egan 1990). A coming together of experience, awareness and communication is the most important part of the relationship between therapist and patient. The use of listening skills, allowing the patient to be heard, is an important aspect of this work. It is important to know your limitations and to know when to seek further advice from a psychologist. The onset of dependency in PD is a time when many patients may benefit from more formal counselling. Many patients will display fear, anger and shame at this time. Emotional adaptation appears to be an important part of a successful coping strategy in PD, yet is neglected by therapy interventions. Turnbull (1992) promotes a 'progressive paradigm' for referral in PD, with patients being referred before problems have developed, to promote emotional adaptation. More research is needed to explore which type of counselling approach is most effective in meeting the needs of patients and carers.

Stress, anxiety and depression

Anxiety is a common and disabling condition arising in PD. Social anxiety is particularly common in PD as patients are afraid of the reactions of others in social situations and withdraw from social life. Social isolation may also represent the onset of significant cognitive impairment. This, in turn, results in isolation and lack of opportunity to practice coping strategies and increases vulnerability to depression. Relaxation therapy can be effectively used in PD and needs to be explored more fully in group and individual treatments.

Depression is also common in PD and often coexists with anxiety. It is important for the therapist to recognize and detect depression as this can often be successfully treated by explanation, support, cognitive therapy and drug treatment. Patients described as having 'poor motivation' or 'needing a lot of prompting' usually are expressing cognitive problems, depression or a combination of the two.

Cognitive deficits

Cognitive problems are common in PD and result in reduction of activities and increased disadvantage. The assessment of cognitive function should increasingly become a role for the OT. Training in techniques of cognitive therapy, under the direction of neuropsychologists, will bring a much needed expertise to rehabilitation teams. Tiredness and fatigue exacerbate difficulties with concentration and memory and a rehabilitation programme must account for fatigue with a balance of rest and activity. Memory games and remedial reminiscence can be used to maintain cognitive function.

Evidence for the effectiveness of OT in PD

Unfortunately, there is very little published evidence of the efficacy of any of the approaches described above in the management of PD. There can be no doubt that OT 'works' given the known problems associated with PD. Patients with PD are still infrequently referred to OT (Meara and Hobson 1997) and patients have considerable unmet needs when first assessed (Beattie and Caird 1980). An early study of OT in PD was insufficiently detailed to interpret and suffered from serious methodological flaws (Gibberd et al. 1981). One study using a single blind and randomised design suggested practical benefit from group therapy intervention that persisted for over a year in the intervention group (Gauthier et al. 1987).

Summary

As a member of a multidisciplinary team the OT can make an important contribution to the successful management of the physical, functional, social, psychological, and emotional consequences of PD. Some of the difficulties surrounding assessment in PD have been discussed and some suggestions for treatment and rehabilitation programmes have been put forward. Whilst treatment should be knowledge and evidence based a stronger foundation for clinical practice is still required.

REFERENCES

Anthony M (1997) Challenging assumptions: Parkinson's disease and driving. *Occupational Therapy News*, April 1997, 12–13.

Beattie A, Caird FI (1980) The occupational therapist and the patient with Parkinson's disease. *British Medical Journal*, 280, 1354–5.

Collin C, Wade DT, Davis S, Horne V (1988) The Barthel ADL Index: a reliability study. *International Disability Studies*, 10, 61–3.

Egan G (1990) *The Skilled Helper*. California: Brooks Cole Publishing Company.

FIM (1993) *Guide to the Uniform Data Set for Medical Rehabilitation (Adult FIM)*. Buffalo New York: Research Foundation State University of New York at Buffalo.

Fisher AG (1995) *Assessment of Motor Processing and Skills*. Fort Collins Company: Three Star Press.

Gauthier L, Dalziel S, Gauthier S (1987) The benefits of group occupational therapy for patients with Parkinson's disease. *American Journal of Occupational Therapy*, 41, 360–5.

Gibberd FB, Page NGR, Spencer KM, Kinnear E, Hawksworth JB (1981) Controlled trial of physiotherapy and occupational therapy for Parkinson's disease. *British Medical Journal*, 282, 1196.

Hagedorn H (1992) *Occupational Therapy Foundations for Practice. Models, Frames of Reference and Core Skills*. London: Churchill Livingstone.

Law M, Polatajko H, Pollock N, McColl M, Carswell A, Baptiste S (1994) Pilot testing of the Canadian occupational performance measure: clinical and measurement issues. *Canadian Journal of Occupational Therapy*, 61, 191–7.

Meara RJ, Hobson JP (1997) Levels of service provision for people with Parkinson's disease: a survey of community registered patients' perceptions. *Journal of the British Association for Service to the Elderly*, 64, 3–10.

Turnbull G (1992) *Physical Management of Parkinson's Disease*. London: Churchill Livingstone.

Turner A (1992) *Occupational Therapy and Physical Dysfunction*. London: Williams and Wilkins.

Wade DT (1992) *Measurement in Neurological Rehabilitation*. Oxford: Oxford University Press.

14

Rehabilitation, speech and language therapy and elderly patients with Parkinson's disease

Sheena Round

Introduction

Speech and swallowing problems are common in elderly subjects with Parkinson's disease (PD). Patients and carers frequently cite communication difficulties as causing the greatest disability and handicap in PD (Oxtoby 1982). In one study around 70% of patients with PD complained of impairment of speech and voice and 41% reported difficulty with chewing and swallowing (Hartelius and Svensson 1994) and another study reported speech problems in over 60% of patients studied (Gibberd et al.1985). Dysphagia has been reported in 15–50% of patients with PD, with abnormalities on barium swallow being demonstrated in up to 95% of cases studied (Bramble et al. 1976, Robbins et al. 1986, Lieberman et al. 1980). A survey carried out by the Parkinson's Disease Society of the United Kingdom (UK) found that 40% of the PD patients contacted complained of drooling and 26% had difficulty swallowing (Oxtoby 1982). Aspiration pneumonia as a result of dysphagia is a common terminal event in late stage PD.

Despite the high prevalence of communication and swallowing problems very few patients with PD get referred to speech and language therapists (Oxtoby 1982, Mutch et al. 1986). Mutch et al. (1986) found that although 65% of patients in their study reported difficulties with speech less than 5% had been assessed by a speech and language therapist. A developing body of evidence exists supporting the efficacy of speech therapy in PD (Scott and Caird 1983, Robertson and Thomson 1984, Scott et al. 1985, Johnson and Pring 1990). This chapter aims to examine the symptoms most frequently seen by therapists working with elderly patients with PD, the methods of assessment used, and some of the therapy techniques used to treat PD.

What causes speech and language impairments and swallowing problems in PD?

The impairments that result in the characteristic speech of PD, which is often present early in the natural history of the disease and the involvement of swallowing, which is usually only seen in late stage disease, are poorly understood. Speech difficulties probably reflect rigidity and akinesia in the muscles involved in phonation and respiration. Speech requires rapid access to and execution of learnt motor plans. In PD the central motor deficit of akinesia disrupts speech and impairs communication. Loss of speech control due to akinesia must in turn reflect reduced striatal dopamine transmission. Clinically, certain elements of the speech disturbance of PD do improve after dopaminergic therapy though the temporal relationship between dose and effect is uncertain. Shea et al. (1993) found that selegiline could result in significant improvements in articulation and other speech problems. Swallowing problems occur in late stage disease and do not respond to dopaminergic drug treatment, though isolated case reports have claimed benefit from drug therapy. The association between swallowing problems, disease progression and late onset disease in older subjects suggest that these problems may result either from an interaction of dopamine loss and aging changes or to involvement of other non-dopaminergic pathways with disease progression.

Age and comorbidity

The elderly patient with PD has to contend with the recognized effects of aging, comorbidity and the effects of the disease itself on speech and swallowing mechanisms. These include physical, cognitive and perceptual changes linked to age and disease. It is important for the therapist treating the PD patient to be aware of these complex interactions (see Table 14.1). Communication and dysphagia often occur together in elderly patients and are the two main areas of intervention for the therapist.

Speech and language therapy impairments in elderly patients with PD

There are several aspects of speech and language that need to be assessed in patients with PD (see Table 14.2). Impairment of language includes loss of facial expression, loss of volume, reduced control over respiration and the rate of speech, reduction in the prosody and rhythm of speech and the presence of dribbling. The resulting motor symptoms are usually classified as a hypokinetic extrapyramidal dysarthria.

Communication disorders in PD

Communication itself is a two way process involving the imparting and exchange of information verbally and nonverbally. In PD communication can be disrupted in a number of ways from deficits that can include respiratory, phonatory, prosodic and articulatory features together with impaired body language.

Table 14.1 The impact of aging and disease on speech and swallowing in elderly patients with PD

- Age related changes include ossification of cartilages of the larynx, atrophy of the muscles of the vocal cords and stiffening of the crico arytenoid joints.
- Deteriorating vision may affect the interpretation of non verbal clues such as facial expression.
- Deafness is often a barrier to social interaction and personal adjustment despite the advances in hearing aids. Hearing aids, even when provided, are not always worn and even when in place are sometimes in a poor state of repair.
- Any respiratory disease that impairs vital capacity can affect speech. Respiratory disease is common in older people and will further impair speech in PD.
- Speech repetition and hesitation are recognized features of conversation in the elderly (Scott et al. 1985). These may augment the disruption in rhythm of speech often noted in elderly patients.
- Elderly patients are more likely to have cognitive impairments and dementia than the younger patients and communication skills are further impaired by dementia (Powell et al. 1995).
- Depression and anxiety, which are common features of aging, may increase the communication difficulties, social isolation and dependency resulting from language and swallowing difficulties caused by PD.
- Swallowing problems in PD may in elderly patients be further impaired by side effects of concurrent medication (dry mouth), poor dentition, ill fitting dentures and poor oesophageal motility

Table 14.2 Areas of speech and language and dysphagic assessment

- Facial expression
- Rate of speech
- Intonation
- Volume
- Intelligibility
- Respiration
- Swallowing
- Rhythm

Overall, the patients' communication difficulties may make them hard to understand and tiring to listen to. Reduced facial expression can be misinterpreted by carers, friends and professionals as indicating a lack of intelligence, hostility, coldness, depression, deafness or lack of interest on the patient's part. The intended message of the PD patient can, therefore, be misinterpreted due to the loss or reduction in the effectiveness of communication skills that were previously auto-matic.

Respiratory associated impairments in elderly patients with PD

Elderly patients frequently exhibit symptoms that suggest an underlying respira-tory deficit. Decreased expiratory air flow, short, shallow clavicular breathing, reduced lung capacity and air wastage before initiating an utterance are features of the impaired respiratory mechanism in elderly patients. As a result, respiratory associated functional symptoms may include shortness of breath when speaking and a reduction in volume. Difficulties coordinating respiration and phonation may result in reduction in control over the pace of speech, which can, in turn, result in abnormalities in rhythm. Breath may run out before a phrase or sentence has been completed.

Voice, volume and respiration

Respiration, in terms of breath support and breathing patterns, is inextricably linked to the volume, pacing of speech and phonation of the PD patient (Montgomery et al. 1972).

Clavicular breathing patterns can result in short, shallow episodes of inspiration and expiration. Breath support can then be inadequate to maintain phonation over a complete sentence and short phrasing results, or, typically, breath runs out before the end of the sentence and residual air is used whilst the patient continues to try to phonate.

The voice quality is breathy, indicating inefficient use of breath for phonation. Phonation cannot be maintained and there is a loss of vocal intensity. If tension of the laryngeal musculature is evident, the voice quality can become harsh and erratic as a result of a combination of 'breathiness' and tension. Voice production can be intermittent, with slowed onset of voice and pitch breaks.

Articulation

Although the PD patient is usually capable of producing speech sounds in isolation or within single words correctly with no phonological difficulties, inaccuracies often become apparent in conversation. Ill fitting dentures can also influence artic-ulatory accuracy and rate. The range and accuracy of the sophisticated, fine coor-dinated movements needed for speech are reduced due to muscular rigidity and tremor together with difficulties in initiation. This affects movements of the lip, tongue and jaw.

Multisyllabic words and consonant clusters are often articulated imprecisely with articulatory placements not always accurately achieved. Plosives (p,b,k,g,t,d) can be weak due to an impoverished air stream and some sounds and syllables may

Table 14.3 Prosodic features in PD

- The rate of speech in PD can be increased or decreased compared to age matched subjects and can exhibit festination as utterance length increases.
- There is often a lack of pausing or a reduced length of pausing.
- The incomplete production of sounds, together with lack of pausing and the elision of parts of consonant clusters or reduction of the number of syllables can give the impression that a faster rate of speech is being used.
- Voicing can be continuous.
- There can be a loss of word stress in polysyllabic words and a loss of syllable stress and contrastive stress.
- Use of stress can be inappropriate and there can be difficulty in both imitating and achieving different stress patterns.

be omitted. Articulatory contacts can be incomplete and repeated sounds can be produced with too short a duration and contrasts usually made between, for example, voiced and unvoiced phonemes (e.g. p/b) can be blurred, with continuous voicing evident. There is often a reduced duration of some phonemes compared to those produced by normal speakers. Some phonemes, syllables and words can be run together with complete elision of some phonemes or syllables. The resultant speech is often described as slurred or indistinct and assessed and treated as a hypokinetic dysarthria.

Prosody

Prosody is defined as the rhythm of speech. Prosodic features often affected in PD are rate, stress and intonation (see Table 14.3). The placing of correct stress patterns within words, phrases and sentences can affect intelligibility and semantics, including conveying emotion without altering the syntax. The overall result of the impairment of prosody can be a flat, monotonous voice, which further reduces the effectiveness of the patient's ability to communicate. Pitcairn et al. (1990) found that the tape recorded voice of patients with PD was interpreted by observers as cold, withdrawn and anxious and to relate poorly to the interviewer.

Rate of speech

Speech rate can be variable, often increased and festinant or slow with problems in initiation. Palilalia, the involuntary repetition of single words, may also be present. Hammen and Yorkston (1996) found that subjects with PD had a greater proportion of pauses occurring at syntactically inappropriate locations in comparison with age matched subjects. When speech rates were reduced, both groups showed a decrease in pauses located at appropriate syntactic boundaries.

Assessment of communication in PD

Assessments devised to tailor communication assessment to the individual profile of the patient are not yet widely used or available. The Parkinson's Disease Society of the UK has devised a Speech and Language Therapy checklist for PD patients. This assessment is service specific and in common with modality specific assessments (e.g. dysarthria assessments) does not take full account of the patients' or carers' perceptions of communication difficulties in functional terms. At present, standard multidisciplinary assessments that would allow us to form collaborative care pathways or establish mutual goals for patients, do not exist. As multidisciplinary teams emerge and develop, then so will the need for assessments that can be incorporated easily into this model of care. Ideally, assessment would be aimed at finding areas of difficulty from each discipline's perspective and then determining therapeutic goals. Goals should be based not only on the performance in a specific assessment test, but also on the perception and wishes of the patient and carer. What are the patient and carer's aims and aspirations? Are they the same as the therapist's? These aspirations may be at a different point of the denial curve for patient, carer and family at any one point in time. A patient may be at the point of denying the diagnosis, whilst the carer may have accepted it, causing a different emphasis in attitude to rehabilitation, which may affect functional outcome. Speech therapy assessments rarely include functional outcome measures such as quality of life, even though these are arguably the most important issues for the patient and carer.

Speech and language therapy treatment in PD

Present practice is for early intervention by therapists at the time of diagnosis to maintain function rather than intervening at a later stage to restore function. This has not been subject to any formal evaluation of effectiveness, but represents a growing clinical consensus of best practice. Intervention at this stage can also prevent unhelpful habits from forming. Early intervention is particularly important in elderly subjects who are at greatest risk of early decline in language function. Skills that were previously carried out automatically need to be relearned as taught behaviours. These include facial expression, diaphragmatic breathing, prosody, volume and the ability to self monitor. Video and audio recordings are often used to overcome problems patients may have in self-monitoring speech production and quality.

Speech therapy treatment as part of an exercise programme in PD

The PROPATH programme (Montgomery et al. 1994) was designed to improve functional outcome for PD patients through a programme of education and exercise. The study demonstrated that disease symptoms could be stabilized and self-efficacy and health confidence could be increased by this approach. This suggests that outcomes from therapy in PD may be improved by linking therapy exercise to more general physical exercise in a multidisciplinary rehabilitation programme

Intensive speech therapy in PD

A number of studies have suggested that therapy may be more effective when given intensively rather than in the traditional once weekly therapy model (Scott and Caird 1981, 1983, 1984, Robertson and Thomson, 1984, Le Dorze et al. 1992). These studies found that periods of intensive therapy can produce significant improvements in speech as assessed by scores for prosodic abnormality and intelligibility. Such improvements can last for several months after therapy stops. Carer perceptions in these studies also indicated that improvement in communication skills had occurred in the patients.

Treatment of respiratory related symptoms

Respiratory related symptoms can affect volume, pitch, segmentation of speech into phrases, rate of speech and the ability to control the rate and rhythm of speech. The treatment of respiratory related symptoms is aimed at increasing breath support, the control of respiration and the relaxation of respiratory musculature. Diaphragmatic breathing and total body relaxation are often used to achieve this.

Treatment of prosodic features

Patients with PD appear to experience difficulty in perceiving different prosodic features of intonation (Scott et al. 1984). Group therapy is often helpful since it allows the patient to experience multiple examples of the target and receive feedback from other group members, which aids self-monitoring. The Vocalite, a voice operated light source, has been used successfully to improve prosodic abnormality by increasing the patient's awareness of difficulties and allowing the practice of more normal patterns of intonation and conversational speech.

Treatment of abnormal speech rate

Pacing techniques are usually used to aid control over the delivery of speech. These include pacing boards (Helm 1979), with physical markers for the patient to use to pace their speech. Beukelman and Yorkston (1977) also targeted rate reduction by using an alphabet board where the first letter of each word spoken was pointed to on the alphabet board. They found that this slowed the rate and increased intelligibility. Rate of speech can often improve with the use of diaphragmatic breathing and the increased control over phonation that this provides due to the relaxation of the muscles used for respiration and phonation. Relaxation of the laryngeal musculature may increase their range and ease of movement and consequently the patient's level of control and pacing abilities in speech. Hanson and Metter (1980) used the technique of delayed auditory feedback for the same purpose.

Pacing boards and syllabic speech, where speech is paced in synchrony with a slow, tapped beat, both serve to help establish a learned, patterned response where there were previously automatic responses. Another method used is to introduce short pauses between words. Improvement in speech rate may not itself lead to meaningful gains in functional performance (Downie et al. 1981).

Every technique requires the motivation and cooperation of the patient. Without adequate self monitoring abilities, improvement may only be apparent to the patient when feedback is given by a member of the family or by the therapist.

Treatment to improve intonation

This is often reduced in the elderly patients due to a decreased ability to alter pitch, but may improve with therapy. The underlying deficit will remain unaltered, but where muscular rigidity is evident, therapy to reduce such rigidity can be effective. If the laryngeal muscles are rigid then the elongation and contraction of the vocal cords longitudinally is reduced and therefore the ability to alter pitch is impaired. Relaxation of these muscles through diaphragmatic breathing, laryngeal massage, use of 'hot packs', hydrotherapy and prosodic exercises can help to restore the range of movement of the muscles by relaxing them and reducing muscle spasm. This can result in an increased pitch range, which will have a positive effect upon pitch use for emphasis in sentences and stress within words. The ability to sing, tell jokes, recite poems and provide interest for the listener in the conversation of the patient can all be affected by loss of intonation and respond following prosodic therapy. If there are difficulties in recognizing and imitating a normal model then group therapy can again be helpful.

Visual feedback to improve self monitoring of speech

Caligiuri and Murray (1983) found that visual feedback allowed patients to monitor self-generated changes in intensity, duration or intraoral pressure of the stressed syllable or word. In the UK the Royal National Institute for the Deaf's Visispeech and the IBM Speechviewer computer programmes are used to provide visual feedback with regard to pitch, volume and intonation patterns.

How effective is prosodic therapy?

Research into prosodic therapy often describes the use of prosodic exercises without a description of any programme of therapy to reduce muscular rigidity. Scott and Caird (1983) examined the effects of therapy on specific prosodic

Table 14.4 Environmental adaptations to improve communication

- Use contextual clues to aid the listeners understanding of the communicated message
- Ensure a low level of background noise
- Maintain good lighting on the face of the speaker
- Keep the distance between speakers short
- Adopt a good posture
- Use external aids (e.g. amplifiers)

features. They found that abnormalities of intonation and rhythm, although universally present, only marginally improved after therapy. Abnormalities of vocal quality, rate and volume were present in 80% of patients and improved substantially and this improvement was largely maintained. Abnormalities of pitch and tone were present in around half of the patients studied and showed some improvement after therapy, though this was not maintained.

Treatment to improve volume

The elderly PD patient characteristically has a quiet voice. Fear of being inaudible can cause anxiety, which increases tension. The volume that can be produced with a sudden burst of energy such as a shout is often far removed from the patient's functional ability when conversing. This can be measured using a Sound Level Meter during assessment to determine habitual volume.

Diaphragmatic breathing as described above aids the patient not only in creating good breath support but also in facilitating maximum achievable volume for conversation, as respiration is synchronized with phonation.

Ramig et al. (1995) compared the effects of intensive speech therapy on respiration and on voice and respiration in PD. They concluded that intensive treatment of voice and respiration was more effective in improving volume than the treatment of respiration alone. Several environmental adaptations can facilitate communication when voice volume is reduced (see Table 14.4).

Where lack of volume is the main deficit, amplification systems for the patient have been found to be beneficial (Greene and Watson 1968). When this type of speech is amplified, a client will continue to match speech with the amplified output for some time after the latter has been switched off (Greene 1980). The benefits are reduction of anxiety, which reduces rigidity, tremor and akinesia, the psychological value and increased ability to monitor their own speech due to the auditory feedback. Sound Level Meters and visual displays of volume on computer programmes, such as the IBM Speechviewer, indicate at a glance the volume obtained by the patient, providing visual feedback and reinforcement to encourage self monitoring of volume as a therapeutic goal. However, if speech is not articulated well, increasing the volume may reduce the intelligibility.

There is now an impressive range of amplifiers on the market that include portable amplifiers and static more powerful amplifiers for use at home or for work. Amplifiers are particularly useful where the spouse has a hearing loss. Telephone amplifiers are also available.

Adams and Lang (1992) found that if white masking noise was presented at a sound pressure level of 90 decibels then there was a marked increase in voice intensity. Portable voice activated maskers such as the Edinburgh Masker may help to transfer this skill to daily conversation. The Lightwriter allows a simple message to be conveyed with the use of a voice synthesizer. Easy Keys is a laptop computer with a voice synthesizer, which can convey complex messages without the need for any vocal effort.

Nonverbal aspects of communication in PD

Facial expression in PD

Bradykinesia in conjunction with rigidity produces the typical mask-like facial expression. Pentland et al. (1988) found that reduced facial expression made patients with PD appear to have no strong feelings and seem less likeable to observers, appearing bored and unfriendly. Patients also appeared to be more anxious, hostile, suspicious, introverted and passive than the age matched subjects without PD. Overall patients were rated as 'less likeable'. Smiles were regarded as 'false smiles'. Consequently, the message that a PD patient is communicating is not necessarily that which was intended.

The improvement of facial expression is encouraged through facial exercises, relaxation and occasionally hydrotherapy to reduce the muscle rigidity. Scott and Caird (1981) found that proprioceptive neuromuscular facilitation (PNF) techniques were effective in improving impoverished facial expression. The kinaesthetic awareness of a patient's own facial expression is reduced, decreasing the effectiveness of self-monitoring skills. Mirrors may be used to aid self-monitoring. Group therapy encourages patients to monitor each other and so increase awareness of facial expression, relearning a previously automatic skill.

Additional nonverbal features

Altered posture may result in a stooped position with the upper body bent forward or deviating from the midline. Head control, eye contact and the ability to use normal gesture may all be affected in a way that reduces the ability to communicate. Communication can be variable, depending on factors such as fatigue, the time within their drug cycle, or stress. The patient can become a passive communicator, losing the desire and/or ability to initiate a conversation, argue or debate; responding to the communication of others rather than taking a shared responsibility for conversation. The temptation for the carer is then to speak 'for' the patient, further increasing the patient's role as a passive communicator.

The role of carers in speech therapy

Scott and Caird (1983) found that carers' frustrations arose from problems caused by the reduction in volume of the voice, difficulty maintaining a conversation because of monotonous responses, distress at the quality of the voice, difficulty following the disordered rate of speech, and embarrassment at their own inability to cope. When intervening therapeutically to increase functional performance, these aspects must be taken into account in the wider context of assessing the patient's communication needs. Carers need to feel that they are active participants in therapy programmes and only then will the maximal potential benefit from therapy be achieved. Carers also need to have a clear understanding of what therapy can and cannot achieve and feel confident in supporting the patient through the course of therapy.

Assessment and treatment of dysphagia in PD

Dysphagia results from tongue tremor with reduced initiation of lingual movement, repetitive tongue pumping action and lingual festination. Excessive tremor and dyskinesia may disguise the fact that a bolus is immobile. A dry mouth due to drug therapy can also affect the ability to form a bolus. Delayed initiation of the swallow and swallow rehearsals, when the swallow is repeated without progression of the bolus, are common findings. Poor postural control can increase the difficulty in successfully transporting the bolus posteriorly in the mouth in order to initiate the swallow reflex. As a consequence, there can be a delayed pharyngeal swallow, reduced pharyngeal peristalsis, multiple swallows to clear the pharynx of the bolus, inadequate laryngeal elevation and/or closure, laryngeal penetration, the presence of an ineffective cough and pharyngeal pooling. These impairments increase the risk of aspiration and aspiration pneumonia. Aspiration and choking are not infrequent in the late stage PD. The therapist can advise on safe consistency of diet and swallowing rehabilitation techniques.

Eating difficulties include the wider range of difficulties encountered rather than the swallowing process alone. Tremor and symptoms described below can increase the time it takes to eat and can cause embarrassment when eating in public. This results in reduced visits to restaurants or for social meals leading to social isolation and overprotection by the carer.

Dysphagia assessment

Dysphagia assessment would normally involve the therapist carrying out a standardized formal or informal assessment, including possible referral for videofluoroscopy. Videofluoroscopy can confirm the assessment findings and contribute to the dysphagia management of the patient. The effects of swallowing rehabilitation techniques can also be assessed while the patient is undergoing videofluoroscopy (e.g. the patient moving their head to a different position when swallowing).

The formal assessment may include oro-motor assessment, assessment of posture, and respiratory status. This would normally be followed by assessment of the oral and pharyngeal stages of the swallow to determine whether the patient is at risk of aspiration using different consistencies and amounts of liquids and/or solids. Recommendations on the safe consistency of food and liquid for the patient are then made. Laryngeal indicators of aspiration can include poor laryngeal elevation, absence of voice, 'wet' or 'gurgly' voice quality, the absence of a voluntary cough, a weak, unprotective cough and / or coughing as a result of swallowing.

Multidisciplinary management of dysphagia

Physiotherapists and speech therapists have developed techniques to improve the mobility of the tongue. Better mobility of the tongue will reduce difficulty retaining the bolus in the midline and will improve the retrieval of food from the bucchal sulcii and transportation of the bolus to trigger the swallow reflex. Dieticians and speech therapists must work closely together in managing dysphagia, with the dietician providing an individually tailored diet for the patient. Speech therapists must also liaise with occupational therapists to establish the most appropriate posture for feeding and the need for any feeding aids (see Chapter 13). Changes in the timing of antiparkinsonian medication may improve dysphagia (Bushmann et al. 1989, Fonda and Schwarz 1995).

Conclusions

The speech therapist has an important role in helping to improve the communication and swallowing problems of elderly patients with PD. This role is constantly evolving as more effective communication aids are developed, multidisciplinary working improves, new treatment becomes available and more research is undertaken into the clinical effectiveness of therapy interventions. Multidisciplinary assessments are needed to underpin these developments. The perceptions and goals of patients and carers are increasingly recognized as being important in directing effective therapy.

REFERENCES

Adams SG, Lang AE (1992) Can the Lombard effect be used to increase low voice intensity in Parkinson's disease? *European Journal of Disorders of Communication*, 27, 2, 121–7.

Beukelman DR, Yorkston KM (1977) A communicative system for the severely dysarthric speaker with an intact language system. *Journal of Speech and Hearing Disorders*, XL11, 257–64

Bramble MG, Cunliffe J, Dellipiani AW (1976) Evidence for a change in neurotransmitter affecting oesophageal motility in Parkinson's disease. *Journal of Neurology, Neurosurgery, and Psychiatry*, 41, 709–12.

Bushmann MM, Dobmeyer SM, Leeker L, Perlmutter JS (1989) Swallowing abnormalities and their response to treatment in Parkinson's disease. *Neurology*, 39, 1309–14.

Caligiuri MP, Murray T (1983) The use of visual feedback to enhance prosodic control in dysarthria. In: *Clinical Dysarthria*, ed. W Berry, pp. 267–282. San Diego: College Hill Press.

Downie AW, Low JM, Lindsay DD (1981) Speech disorders in parkinsonism – usefulness of DAF in selected cases. *British Journal of Disorders of Communication*, 16, 2, 135–9.

Fonda D, Schwarz J (1995) Parkinsonian medication one hour before meal improves symptomatic swallowing: A case study. *Dysphagia*, 10, 165–6

Gibberd FB, Oxtoby M, Jewell PF (1985) The treatment of Parkinson's disease: a consumer view. *Health Trends*, 17, 19–21.

Greene MC (1980) *The Voice and its Disorders*. London: Pitman Medical, 1980, 311–16.

Greene MC, Watson BW (1968) The value of speech amplification in Parkinson's disease. *Folia Phoniatrica*, 20, 250–7

Hammen VL, Yorkston KM (1996) Speech and pause characteristics following speech rate reduction in hypokinetic dysarthria. *Journal of Communication Disorders*, 29, 6, 429–44.

Hanson WR, Metter EJ (1980) DAF as instrumental treatment for dysarthria in a progressive supranuclear palsy: a case report. *Journal of Speech and Hearing Disorders*, 45, 268–76.

Hartelius L, Svensson P (1994) Speech and swallowing symptoms associated with Parkinson's disease and multiple sclerosis: a survey. *Folia Phoniatrica et Logopedica*, 46, 1, 9–17.

Helm NA (1979) Management of palilalia with a pacing board. *Journal of Speech and Hearing Disorders*, 44, 350–3.

Johnson JA, Pring TR (1990) Speech therapy and Parkinson's disease: A review and further data. *British Journal of Disorders of Communication*, 25, 183–94.

Le Dorze G, Dionne L, Ryalls J, Julien M, Ouellet L (1992) The effects of speech and language therapy for a case of dysarthria associated with Parkinson's disease. *European Journal of Disorders of Communication*, 27, 313–24.

Liberman AN, Honowitz L, Redmond P (1980) Dysphagia in Parkinson's disease. *Annals of Gasteroenterology*, 74,157–60.

Montgomery EB, Lieberman A, Singh G, Fries JF on behalf of the Propath Board (1994) Patient education and health promotion can be effective in Parkinson's disease: a randomised controlled trial. *American Journal of Medicine*, 97, 429–35.

Montgomery EB, Lieberman A, Singh G, O'Reilly F, Fallwright S, Davey Smith G, Ben-Obenour WH, Stevens PM, Cohen AA (1972) The causes of abnormal pulmonary function in Parkinson's disease. *American Review of Respiratory Disease*, 105, 3, 382–7.

Mutch WJ, Strudwick A, Roy SK, Downie AW (1986) Parkinson's disease: disability, review and management. *British Medical Journal*, 293, 675–7.

Oxtoby M (1982) *Parkinson's Disease Patients and their Social Needs*. London: Parkinson's Disease Society.

Pentland B, Pitcairn TK, Gray JM, Riddle WJR (1988) The effects of reduced expression in Parkinson's disease on impression formed by health professionals. *Clinical Rehabilitation*, 1, 307–13.

Pitcairn TK, Clemie S, Gray JM, Pentland B (1990) Impressions of parkinsonian patients from their recorded voices. *British Journal of Disorders of Communication*, 25, 1, 85–92.

Powell JA, Hale MA, Bayer AJ (1995) Symptoms of communication breakdown in dementia: carers' perceptions. *European Journal of Disorders of Communication*, 30, 65–75.

Ramig LO, Countryman S, Thompdon LL, Horii Y (1995) Comparison of two forms of intensive speech treatment for Parkinson's disease. *Journal of Speech and Hearing Research*, 38, 6, 1232–51.

Robbins JA, Logemann JA, Kirshner HS (1986) Swallowing and speech production in Parkinson's disease. *Annals of Neurology*, 19, 282–7.

Robertson SJ, Thomson F (1984) Speech therapy in Parkinson's disease: a study of the efficacy and long-term effects of intensive treatment. *British Journal of Disorders of Communication*, 19, 213–24

Scott S, Caird FI (1981) Speech for patients with Parkinson's disease. *British Medical Journal*, 283, 1088.

Scott S, Caird FI (1983) Speech therapy for Parkinson's disease. *Journal of Neurology, Neurosurgery, and Psychiatry*, 46, 140–4.

Scott S, Caird FI (1984) The response of the apparent receptive speech disorder of Parkinson's disease to speech therapy. *Journal of Neurology, Neurosurgery, and Psychiatry*, 47, 302–4.

Scott S, Caird FI, Williams BO (1984) Evidence for an apparent sensory speech disorder in Parkinson's disease. *Journal of Neurology, Neurosurgery, and Psychiatry*, 47, 840–3.

Scott S, Caird FI, Williams BO (1985) *Communication in Parkinson's Disease*. London: Croom Helm.

Shea BR, Drummond SS, Metzer WS, Krueger KM (1993) Effect of selegiline on speech performance in Parkinson's disease. *Folia Phoniatrica*, 45, 1, 40–6.

Index

Note: page numbers in *italics* refer to figures and tables

acetazolamide 89
acetylcholinesterase inhibitors 42
Achilles tendon stretch 206
activities of daily living (ADL)
   assessment 218, 220
   scales 186
affect–arousal 173
age/aging 27
   at diagnosis of PD 28–9
   clinical heterogeneity of PD 27–30
   essential tremor 82
   neurodegenerative disease 111
   prevalence of PD 112
   risk of PD 114–15, 118
   speech and language problems 227, *228*
agranulocytosis, fatal 65–6
akinesia 1, 4, *5*, 24, 25, 227
   diagnosis 6
   diagnostic criteria 7
   dopamine agonists 149
   progressive supranuclear palsy 9
   swallowing mechanism 46
alcohol, essential tremor 15, 85–6
alprazolam 89
Alzheimer's disease (AD) 7, 8, 9
   age associated risk 111
   concurrent 8
   dementia with Lewy bodies 41
   diagnostic errors 8
   extrapyramidal signs 117–18
   Lewy bodies 23
   senile plaques 23
amantadine 145–6, 157
   essential tremor treatment 89–90
amiodarone 72
amisulpride 66
amitriptyline 65, 154
amphoterocin B, DIP 73
amplifiers 235

anaesthesia 193
anismus 158, 192
ankle dorsiflexor stretch 207
   reflex 208
anti-emetics 71
anticholinergic drugs 146
   bladder dysfunction 10
   constipation 10
   gastric motility inhibition 158
   hallucinations 157
   neuroleptic-induced parkinsonism treatment 71
   psychosis 42
   urge incontinence 154, 155
antidepressants 38, 224
   impotence 156
anxiety 223–4
   assessment 200
   dependency 168
   disability determinant 173
apomorphine 34, 45, 50–3, 135
   administration 51, 52
   challenge test 52, 187
   injection site nodules 53
   patient assessment 187
   patient selection criteria 51–2
   surgical patients 194
apoptosis, selegiline inhibition 145
articulation 229–30
   impairment 227
articulatory contacts 230
aspiration 226, 236
   laryngeal indicators 237
   perioperative 193
Assessment of Motor Processing and Skills 220
assessment of patients 30, 32
assessment tools, standardized 186
assets 168
Association of Chartered Physiotherapists
      Interested in Neurology (ACPIN) 199

Association of Chartered Physiotherapists with a
　　Special Interest in Elderly People (ACSIEP)
　　199
atenolol 87
Attendance Allowance 190
attention deficit, selective 173
autonomic dysfunction, severe 10
autonomic failure 35
autonomic function 43

Babinski sign, vascular parkinsonism 13
balance 47
　　evaluation 208–9
　　impaired 190
　　patient status assessment 200
　　physiotherapy 208–9
　　problems in elderly 33
Balance Performance Monitor 209
balance problems 34, 49
Barthel Scale/Index 31, 186, 220
basal ganglia 102, 103, 104
　　dopamine mediated gene regulation 34
bathing 221
benign essential tremor 83
benserazide 135
benzodiazepines 88–9
benzquinamide 71
benztropine 146
Berg Scale 208
beta adrenergic blockers 87–8
betahistine, neuroleptic substitute 70–1
bethanechol 72
Binswanger's disease 13, 101
blood pressure 43
Bobath approach 201
body language, impaired 227
body weight maintenance 191
botulinum toxin injection 90
bowel symptoms 45–6
bradykinesia 235
　　medication strategy 149
breathing
　　clavicular patterns 229
　　control 187
　　diaphragmatic 232
　　see also respiration
bromocriptine 137, 138–9
bupropion 38

cabergoline 137, 140, 154
calcium channel blockers 72
CAMCOG cognitive function assessment 31,
　　32
Canadian Occupational Performance Measures
　　(COPM) 218

carbidopa 135, 136
　　controlled release 137
carbonic anhydrase inhibitors 89
care
　　quality 30
　　rehabilitation activity 166
carers
　　asset value 168
　　communication for patient 236
　　dependency 168
　　distress 39
　　ill health 179
　　needs 128–9
　　　palliative care 131
　　physiotherapy implications 204
　　psychological support 186
　　role in speech and language therapy 236
catechol-*O*-methyltransferase (COMT)
　　central inhibition 142–3
　　inhibitors 142–4, 153
　　medication strategy 149
　　peripheral inhibition 142
cephaloridine, DIP 73
cerebral cortex, Lewy bodies 23
cerebral multi-infarct states (CMIS) 98, 100–1,
　　104–5
cerebrospinal fluid (CSF) shunt 14
chin, tremor 85
chlorpromazine 65
chromosome 4q21–22 116–17
cinnarizine 72
cisapride 46
　　gastric motility 158
clasp knife rigidity 5, 13
clinical criteria, diagnostic 7
clinical effectiveness evidence 129
clinical guidelines 199
clinical manifestations, essential tremor 82
clinical trials 134–5
clinics, specialist 126, *127*, 130
clonazepam 89
clozapine 42, 65–6
　　hallucination control 157
　　tremor control 148
co-beneldopa 135, 137
co-careldopa 135
　　controlled release (CR) 136–7, 149
co-danthramer 46
cogentin 146
cognitive function assessment 200
　　occupational therapists 224
cognitive impairment 34, 39, 134, 199, 224
　　cortical 41
　　dementia risk 40
　　depression 36–7

cognitive impairment (*cont.*)
  motor disability link 173
  palliative care 49
  subcortical 41
cognitive therapy 224
cogwheel rigidity 3, 15
  lithium 72
colon, myenteric plexus 158
communication
  assessment 200, 231
  disorders 226, 227–30
  environmental adaptations 234
  nonverbal aspects 235–6
  nursing care 187, 189
  passive 236
  sexuality 192–3
  variability 235–6
communicative impairment 173
comorbidity, speech and language problems 227
compensatory strategies, physiotherapy 204
complementary therapies 179
computed tomography (CT) 16, 17
conductive education programmes 201, 222
confusion, benzodiazepines 89
constipation 10, 45–6, 158
  nursing care 192
  occupational therapy interventions 221
continence advisor 45
corollary discharges 198
cortical loops 24–5
corticobasal ganglionic degeneration (CBDG) 8
  dopaminergic drugs 10
  motor sign asymmetry 11
  neuroimaging 17
counselling 223
Creutzfeldt–Jakob disease 8
cytoplasmic inclusion bodies *see* Lewy bodies

delayed auditory feedback 233
delirium 134
  drug-induced 42
delusional ideas/delusions 36, 39, 42
dementia 39–42, 173
  causes 40
  clinical characteristics 8–9
  early 8–9
  epidemiology 39–40
  levodopa/PDI 149
  with Lewy bodies 3, 8, 9, 40–1
  management 42
  neuropsychological features 41–2
  normal pressure hydrocephalus 13, 14
  nursing home admission 114
  risk factors 40
demographic change 122–3

dentures 191
  speech 229
dependency 167–8
  recognition 176
deprenyl 144
depression 35–9, 157–8, 223–4
  assessment 200
  associated features with PD 36–7
  cognitive impairment 36–7
  dementia risk 40
  dependency 168
  detecting 38
  diagnostic criteria 35
  disability determinant 173
  dopamine 37
  DSM-III criteria 36
  epidemiology 35–6
  medial prefrontal cortex 38
  psychotic features 36
  sleep disorders 154
  treatment 38–9
desmopressin 45, 155
diagnosis
  accuracy 6–7
  atypical features 7–12
  communication 177–8
  milestones in PD 176, 177–9
  progression to disability 177–9
diagnostic accuracy 23, 111
diagnostic criteria 30
  predictive value 7
diaphragmatic breathing 232
diary keeping 151, *152*
diazepam
  DIP 73
  essential tremor treatment 89
dietician 221
diphasic dystonia/dyskinesia (D-I-D) dystonia 153
disability
  early 179, *180*
  impact of daily life 176
  late stage 179, *181*
  variability 173–4
disability organizations 176
  see also Parkinson's Disease Society
disadvantage 166, 167
disease aetiology theories 116
disease progression, treatment strategy 149–50
dizziness, treatment 70–1
domperidone 33, 135
  blood pressure 44
  levodopa absorption 136
  nausea control 136
  neuroleptic substitute 70–1
  surgical patients 194

donazepil 42
dopamine
  deficiency 1, 23, 198
  depression 37
  loss 25
  storage inhibitors 71–2
  striatal depletion 69
  striatal levels with COMT inhibitors 142–3
  transport inhibitors 71–2
dopamine agonists 137–8, 153
  akinesia 149
  orthostatic hypotension 44
  psychosis 42
  side effects 138
  see also apomorphine
dopamine-mediated gene regulation, basal ganglia
    34
dopaminergic drugs 10–11
  adverse reactions in PD 65
dorsiflexion, active 207
dorsiflexor stretch, reflex 208
dosette 187
dreams, vivid 47, 154
dressing 220–1
drinking 221
driving ability 190, 222–3
Driving Assessment Centres 223
drooling *see* sialorrhoea
drug therapy 134–5
  cost/cost benefits 129
  medication strategies 148–51, *152*, 153–8
  surgical patients 194
  see also individual drugs
drug-induced parkinsonism (DIP) 2, 49, 64, 72–3,
    117
  calcium channel blockers 72
  dopamine storage/transport inhibitors 71–2
  gender 69
  genetic influence 69
  metabolic defect 69
  neuroleptic-induced 65–71
  PD distinction *68*
  subclinical PD 69–70
dry mouth 191
dyskinesia 47, *153*
  peak dose 150–1
  sleep disturbance 154
dysphagia 226, 236–7
  see also swallowing difficulties
dysthymic disorder 35
dystonia
  anismus 158
  off period 34
  physiotherapy 209–10
  wearing off 151, 153

Easy Keys 235
eating 221
  aids 237
  difficulties 191, 236–7
  posture 237
  see also nutrition
Edinburgh Masker 235
educational programmes 126
Eldepryl™ 144
elderly patients, assessment of PD 30–2
electroconvulsive therapy (ECT) 33, 38
  neuroleptic-induced parkinsonism treatment
      71
emotionalism 35
end of dose
  deterioration 32–3
  motor fluctuations 34, 150–1
entacapone 142, 144
environment 166
  modification 167
  safe 221
environmental adaptations, communication 234
environmental risk factors for PD 115
epidemiology of parkinsonism 117–18
  evaluation of studies *112*
epidemiology of PD 111–12
  risk factors 114–17
equilibrium apraxia 106
equipment
  feeding aids 237
  provision 222
erectile dysfunction 155, 192
essential tremor (ET) 3, 14–15
  age 82
  alcohol 15, 85–6
  beta adrenergic blockers 87–8
  clinical manifestations 82–5
  clinical variants 84–5
  differential diagnosis 84
  disability 83–4
  epidemiology 80
  factors influencing 82–3
  genetics 80–1
  prevalence 80, *81*
  treatment 85–91
  tremor progression 82
etat crible 13
ethics, life sustaining measures 182
exercise 189
  early PD 202–3
  mortality 212
  physiotherapy 201
  stretching 206
exercise programme 178
  speech and language therapy 231–2

exercise tolerance 210
  assessment 200
external cues 108
externally cued movements 106
extrapyramidal reactions, piperazine derivatives 72
extrapyramidal signs 117–18
extrapyramidal syndromes, neuroleptic-induced
  70
eye of the tiger sign 17

facial expression 235
  loss 227
faecal impaction 46
falls 9–10, 34, 47, 190
  benzodiazepines 89
  late stage PD 179
  management 209
  multisystem degeneration parkinsonism 49
  orthostatic hypotension 43
  physiotherapy 208
  prevention 172
familial parkinsonism, autosomal dominant 111
family history, risk factor 116
features, atypical 7–12
feeding see eating; meals; nutrition
financing of health care 123
Flewitt–Handford approach 201
fludrocortisone 44, 156
fluid intake 155, 156
flunarizine 72
5-fluorouracil, DIP 73
fluoxetine 38
  DIP 73
flurbiprofen 44
focal infarction, single 13
foot care 189, 208
fractures, late stage PD 179
free radical theory of cell death in PD 116
freezing 9, 153–4
  episodes 6, 47
frontal fields 102
functional disability, symptomatic therapy 148–9
Functional Independence Measure 220
Functional Limitations Profile 200
funding systems 129

gait 6, 9–10
  deterioration 47
  disturbance 206–7
  freezing 9
  problems 33, 34
  re-education 207–8
  senile 15–16
gait apraxia 3, 14, 98
  syndrome 98–100

gait disorders
  classification 101–2
  normal pressure hydrocephalus 13–14
  severe isolated 9
  treatment 107
  vascular disease 50
  vascular parkinsonism 100–1
  see also vascular higher-level gait disorders
gait ignition 102–4
  impairment 105
gastric motility 158
gastrocolic reflex loss 46
gegenhalten 5, 13
general practitioner (GP) 123
genetic anticipation, essential tremor 81
genetic risk of PD 116–17, 118
Geriatric Depression Scale (GDS-15) 32, 35
'Get up and Go' test 208
globus pallidus 24, 25, 26
  eye of the tiger sign 17
glottal area tremor 210
glycopyrrolate 155
goal setting, joint 201
grooming 220–1
group programmes 204
group therapy 222, 223
  facial expression awareness 235
  prosody 232, 233–4

Hallervorden–Spatz disease 12, 17
hallucinations 9, 36, 39, 47
  drug-induced 157
  levodopa/carbidopa CR 137
  nursing home admission 114, 134
hallucinosis 42
  impaired vision/hearing 190
  levodopa-induced 34
haloperidol 65
hand, essential tremor 82, 83
handwriting 189
  skills 223
  see also writing tremor
head
  control 235
  essential tremor 82, 84, 87
  injury risk factor 116
  tremor 11
health promotion 172
Health Status Questionnaire 12 (HSQ-12) 32
healthcare delivery 123
healthcare needs 122, 171
healthcare professionals
  patient relationships 177
  roles 174–5
hearing 190

heel strike 207
hemiballism 26
hemiparkinsonism 37
hemiparkinsonism hemiatrophy 11
higher-level gait disorders 101–2, 108
  see also vascular higher-level gait disorders
HLA B44 69
hospital admission, nursing care 193–4
Huntington's disease 12
  patient needs 171
hydrocephalus, normal pressure 8, 13–14
  levodopa 10–11
  neuroimaging 17
hydrotherapy 205
hyperkinesia, tetrabenazine therapy 71
hyperreflexia, vascular parkinsonism 13
hypnotic drugs 47–8, 154
hypotension, orthostatic 43–4
hyrocephalus, normal pressure 9

ignition apraxia 105–6, 108
immobility 47
impotence 155, 192
incidence of PD 111, 113
inclusion bodies *see* Lewy bodies
incontinence *see* urinary incontinence
independence
  medical management quality 172
  PILS scheme 167–8, 170
information
  access to 176
  availability 176–7
  inaccurate 177
  leaflets 176–7, 179, 189, 203
  misconstrued 177
  nurse provision 189
  provision to patients 172
institutional care 113–14, 134
interventions
  effectiveness 169–70
  multidisciplinary 169
  palliative 166
  participation 169
  physiotherapy 198
  relevance 165
intubation 193

kinaesthetic information 198–9

lactulose 46
language
  impairments 226–7
  see also speech and language problems; speech
    and language therapy
laryngeal muscle relaxation 233

laxatives 46, 192
lead-pipe rigidity 5, 13
leaflets, information 176–7, 179, 189, 203
leg cramps 154
levodopa 10–11, 135–7
  bioavailability 135–6
  controlled release 135, 136–7, 149, 153
  dementia management 42
  dosage level 33, 136
  formulations 33, 34
  long-term therapy 134
  metabolism 135
  multisystem degeneration parkinsonism 49
  orthostatic hypotension 44
  peripheral decarboxylase inhibitor combination
    135–6, 149, 153
  side effects 33, 136
  sustained release 154
  terminal care 49
  L-tryptophan addition 37
  vascular parkinsonism 13
Lewy bodies 1, 3, 23
  Alzheimer's disease 23
  brainstem 41
  cortical 41
  dementia 40–1
  motor neurone disease 23
  myenteric plexus of colon 158
  see also dementia, with Lewy bodies
life event risk factors for PD 115, 116
life sustaining measures, ethics 182
lifestyle
  PILS scheme 167, 168, 169, 170
  risk factors for PD 115, 116
Lightwriter 235
limb oedema 211
lithium 72–3
long-term care 113–14

Machado–Joseph disease 12
Madopar™ 135
magnetic resonance imaging (MRI) 16, 17
masker, voice activated 235
meals 221
medial prefrontal cortex, depression 38
medication
  nursing care 187
  strategies 148–51, *152*, 153–8
meperidine, DIP 73
metclopramide 136
methazolamide 89
1-methyl-4-phenyl-1,2,3,6-tetrahydropyridine *see*
    MPTP
alpha-methyldopa 71–2
metoclopramide 67

metoprolol 87
micturition
    urgency 221
    see also nocturia; urinary incontinence
midodrine 156–7
mineralocorticoids 156
Mini-Mental State Examination (MMSE) 31, 32,
    200
misdiagnosis of PD 117, 118
mixed gait apraxia 106–7
mobility 189–90, 222
    deterioration 190
    fluctuation 190
    medical management quality 172
    nursing care 189–90
    visual cues 207–8
monoamine oxidase-B inhibitors 144–5, 146–7
mood
    disorders 200
    disturbances 37, 173
mortality
    exercise 212
    from PD 111, 113
motor blocks 6
motor disability 37
    cognitive impairment link 173
    rehabilitation 33
motor disorder, pathophysiology 198–9
motor fluctuations 33–4
    medication strategy 149–51, *152*, 153–4
motor neurone disease
    age associated risk 111
    Lewy bodies 23
    patient needs 171
motor programming failure 104
motor signs
    asymmetry 11
    drug resistant 33
motor syndromes 32–5
motor tricks 153–4
movement
    internal sense 198
    patient status assessment 200
    practice 207
    rotational components 205–6
movement disorders
    clinics 126, *127*
    social isolation 203
MPTP 146–7
multi-infarct disease 13
multidisciplinary team 123, 126
    goals 179
    physiotherapist liaison 204
multiple pathologies 171
multiple sclerosis, patient needs 171–2

multiple system atrophy (MSA) 7, 9, 10
    autonomic function 43
    epidemiology 117
    levodopa response 10
    parkinsonism 49, 50
    rehabilitiation 180, 182
    striato nigral variant 50
multisystem degenerative diseases, epidemiology
    117
multisystem neurodegenerative disease,
    parkinsonism 2–3
muscle
    changes in immobilized 206
    flexor 206
    strengthening 207
    stretch 206
    tone 200

nadolol 87
natural history of PD 111
nausea treatment 70–1
needs, perceived 176
neurofibrillary tangles 41
neuroimaging 16–18
neuroleptic agents
    atypical 66
    DIP 65–7
neuroleptic-induced parkinsonism 64–5, 65–71
    agents 65–7
    clinical features 67–8
    duration 68
    incidence 69
    pathogenesis 69–70
    susceptibility 69
    treatment 70–1
neuropathology
    coexisting with PD 23
    PD 22–3
neurophysiological tests 16–18
neurophysiology of PD 24–6
neurosurgery 34–5
    cost of procedures 129
    see also surgery
neutropenia, neuroleptic-induced 66
nightmares 154
nigrostriatal tract 23, 25, *26*
nimodipine 72
nocturia 154, 155
nurse, specialist PD 126, *127*, 174–5, 195
    inpatient management guidelines 194
nurses
    community 175
    psychological support 186
nursing
    assessment 186–7

plan *188*
service purchasing 195
team 185
nursing care 185–6
communication 187, 189
components 187, *188*, 189–95
continuity 185
elimination 191–2
hospital admission 193–4
information provision 189
medication 187
mobility 189–90
nutrition 191
palliative care 195
planning 185–6
sexuality 192–3
nursing home residents 114, 134
nutrition
nursing care 191
problems in late stage PD 179
see also eating; meals

occupational therapy 126, *127*, 217
aims 217, *218*
assessment 218, 220
dysphagia 237
evidence for effectiveness 224
frame of reference 218, *219*
interventions 220–4
model of practice 218, *219*
off period
disability 35
dystonia 34
olanzapine 42, 66
on–off mood swings 37
ondansetron 71
oral hygiene 191
Orem's Model of nursing care 187
oro-motor assessment 237
orthostatic hypotension 211
oxybutynin 45

palilalia 230
palliative care 48–9, 130–1, 166
nursing care 195
physiotherapy 204
parkinsonism 1
autosomal dominant 12
diagnosis 4, 5
drug-induced 12, 38
lower body 9, 13
multisystem neurodegenerative disease 2–3
post-encephalitic 12
pyramidal tract signs 11
rest tremor 6

unilateral acute onset 11
vascular 2, 13
levodopa 10–11
see also drug-induced parkinsonism (DIP)
Parkinson's disease (PD) 1–2
age at diagnosis 28–9
basal ganglia disordered cueing 104
clinical expression *28*
clinical signs 4–7
coexisting neuropathology 23
concurrent Alzheimer's disease 8
conditions mimicking 12–16
with dementia 40
DIP distinction *68*
heterogeneity *29*
late onset 2, 29–30, 33
late stage 2, 28
neuropathology 22–3
neurophysiology 24–6
rapidly progressing 29
subclinical 69–70
subtypes 28–9
tremor dominant 7
Parkinson's Disease Society 176, 193, 212
physiotherapy assessment 200
scale 200
Speech and Language Therapy checklist 231
paroxetine 38
DIP 73
participation 169
pathology of PD 111
patients
health care professionals relationships 177
psychological support 186
PDQ-39 32, 200
PDQL 32, 200
percutaneous endoscopic gastrostomy (PEG)
feeding 182
pergolide 45, 137, 139–40
peripheral decarboxylase inhibitor (PDI) 135–6
permissive exposure, latent period 116
perphenazine 65
pesticide use, risk factor 116
pharynx, dysphagia 236
phenelzine 73
phenobarbital 89
phenothiazines 66
fluorinated 65
phonation 229
phonemes, elision 230
physical deficit combination with psychological
deficit 173
physical therapy 126
physiotherapy 34, 126, *127*, 166, 178
assessment 199–201

physiotherapy (*cont.*)
  balance 208–9
  breathing control 187
  clinical guidelines 199
  compensatory strategies 204, 207–8
  disease progression 203–4
  domiciliary 204–5
  dystonia 209–10
  early PD 202–3
  environment 204–5
  evidence base 211–12
  exercise tolerance 210
  falls 208
  gait disturbance 206–7
  hospital 205
  intervention 198
  late stage PD 204
  management cycle *202*
  movement component treatment 205–11
    range 206
    rotational 205–6
  muscle shortening 206
  muscle strengthening 207
  occupational therapy interventions 222
  palliative care 204
  respiratory function 210–11
  review 202
  tongue mobility 237
  treatment approaches 200–4
  walking aids 209
PILS scheme 167–8
  evidence for intervention effectiveness 169–70
pindolol 87
piperazine
  derivatives 72
  neuroleptic-induced parkinsonism 65
pneumonia, aspiration 226, 236
podiatry 189, 208
positron emission tomography (PET) 17–18
postural hypotension 156–7
  multiple system atrophy 182
postural instability 6, 9–10
postural reflexes
  absent 6
  impaired 47
posture
  advice 206
  altered 235
  assessment 237
  feeding 237
  patient status assessment 200
pramipexole 137, 140–1
pre-dementia 41
premotor area (PMA) 102, 103–4
pressure sores 190
  late stage PD 179

prevalence of PD 111, 112–13
prevention, PILS scheme 167, 170
primary health care teams 195
primary motor cortex (M1) 102, 103, 104
primidone, essential tremor treatment 88
private sector 176
procaine 73
prochlorperazine 136
progression of disease 171–2
progressive neurological disorders, needs 171–2
progressive supranuclear palsy (PSP) 7, 8, 9
  epidemiology 117
  levodopa response 10
  neuroimaging 17
  parkinsonism 49–50
  rehabilitiation 180
PROPATH programme 231–2
propiverin 155
propranolol 71
  essential tremor treatment 87, 88
proprioceptive neuromuscular facilitation 235
prosodic cue perception 173
prosodic therapy 232, 233–4
prosody 230
psychiatric disorders 173
psychiatric disturbance, bromocriptine 139
psychological deficit combination with physical
      deficit 173
psychosis 42–3
  drug-induced 42
putamen, cortical input 25
pyridostigmine 72
pyridoxine 71

quality of care 30
quality of life
  essential tremor 83
  health related measures 32, 130
quetiapine 66

Reed and Sanderson model 218, *219*
referral, progressive paradigm 223
rehabilitation 165
  apomorphine 52
  assets 168
  complexity 168–9
  concepts 165–6
  degenerative parkinsonian syndromes 180, 182
  disadvantage 166, 167
  effectiveness 169–70
  goals 166
  implementation 166–9
  intensive inpatient 176
  motor disability 33
  multisystem degeneration parkinsonism 50
  needs specific to PD/parkinsonism 172–4

nursing assessment 186–7
resources 174–6
service matching to needs 170–6
speech and language therapy exercise
programme 231–2
strategies 176–9, *180–1*
structured process 169
swallowing 236
virtual reality images 104–5
writing 223
relaxation
therapy 223
total body 232
REM behaviour disorder 48
reserpine 71
resources, rehabilitation 174–6
respiration
associated impairments 229
reduced control 227
related symptoms and speech and language
therapy 232
respiratory function
assessment 200
physiotherapy 210–11
respiratory muscle training 211–12
respiratory status assessment 237
respiratory support, speech 211
rest tremor 7
absence 11–12
vascular parkinsonism 13
rigidity 1, 4–5, 24
diagnostic criteria 7
essential tremor 15
facial expression 235
lithium 72
medication strategy 149
swallowing mechanism 46
vascular parkinsonism 13
see also gegenhalten
risk factors for PD 114–17
risperidone 66
ropinirole 137, 141

seborrhoea 155
secondary care 126
selective attention 173
selective serotonin reuptake inhibitors (SSRIs) 38,
39, 157, 158
DIP 73
impotence 156
serotonin syndrome 145
selegiline 38, 144–5, 148, 154, 157
neuroprotection 146–7
orthostatic hypotension 44
psychosis 42
speech and language problems 227

self-efficacy, subjective sense 172, 178–9
self-funding treatment 129
senile plaques 41
Alzheimer's disease 23
serotonin 37, 38
precursors 37
syndrome 145
sertindole 66
sertraline 38, 158
service organization/provision 123, *124–5*, 126
economic appraisal 129
quality assessment 129–30
utilization *128*
services
access to 176
diagnosis specific 170–4
matching to needs 170–6
requirements in progressive neurological
disorders 172
sexual desire 192
sexual dysfunction 48, 155–6
sexuality, nursing care 192–3
Short-Form 36 (SF-36) 32, 130
sialorrhoea 42, 46, 146, 155, 191, 226
Sinemet™ 135
sitting exercises 189
skin care 191
sleep
abnormalities 154
disturbance/fragmentation 47–8
smoking 116
social isolation 203, 223
social needs 122, 171
social networks 126, 128
social resources, PILS scheme 167, 168, 170
social support 36, 126, 128
soft tissue length/extensibility 200
sotalol 87
Sound Level Meter 234
spasticity 5
speech
abnormal rate treatment 232–3
articulation 229–30
coordination 229
difficulties 46
disorders in progressive supranuclear palsy 50
impairments 226–7
intonation improvement 233
rate 230
respiratory support 211
self monitoring 233
visual feedback 233
volume 234–5
loss 227, 229
speech and language problems
age 227, *228*

speech and language problems (*cont.*)
  comorbidity 227
speech and language therapist 187
speech and language therapy 126, *127*, 210, 226
  carer role 236
  exercise programme 231–2
  intensive 232
  respiratory related symptom treatment 232
  treatment 231–4
Speechviewer (IBM) 234–5
spino bulbar muscular atrophy, X-linked 81
standing exercises 189
state disability allowances 190
state funding 129
stress 36, 223
stress incontinence 192
substantia nigra
  cell loss 22
  gliosis 22
  nigrostriatal tract 23
  pars compacta 22, 23, 25
    cell degeneration 1
  pars reticulata 22, 24, *25*
subthalamic nucleus 25–6, *26*
supplementary motor area (SMA) 102, 103
  infarction 104
supraglottal area tremor 210
surgery 193
  drug treatment 194
  see also neurosurgery
swallowing difficulties 226–7, *228*, 236–7
  disease progression 46
  dopaminergic therapy 155
  drooling 155
  impairment in progressive supranuclear palsy 50
  late stage PD 179
  multiple system atrophy 182
  rehabilitation techniques 236
syllables, elision 230
symptom diary 151, *152*
syncope 43, 44
alpha-synuclein 117

tablet containers 187
tacrine 42
tardive dyskinesia 70, 71
teamwork 174–6
telephone amplifiers 235
terminal illness 130–1
  see also palliative care
tetrabenazine 71
thalamic inhibition 24–5
thalamic stimulation
  essential tremor treatment 91
  refractory tremor 148

thalamotomy
  essential tremor treatment 90
  refractory tremor 148
thioridazine 65
thioxanthenes 66
timolol 87
tocopherol 147
toileting 221
tolcapone 34, 142, 143
tolterodine 155
tongue
  essential tremor 87
  mobility 237
  tremor 85, 236
torsion dystonia, autosomal dominant idiopathic 81
training provision to patients 172
transcutaneous nerve stimulation (TENS) 211
treatment
  individualized plan 201
  nursing care regimes 187
  problem solving approach 200–1
tremor 1, 24
  diagnostic criteria 7
  drug treatment 148
  essential 7, 11–12
  glottal area 210
  head 11
  lithium 72
  medically undiagnosed 117
  medication strategy 148, 149
  pill-rolling 6
  postural 72
  rest 5–6
  supraglottal area 210
  task-specific 84, *85*
  tongue 236
  writing 84
  see also essential tremor (ET); rest tremor
tricyclic antidepressants 38, 154, 157
trihexylphenidyl 146
trunk mobility exercises 210
trunk mobilization techniques 207
L-tryptophan 37

Unified Parkinson's Disease Rating Scale (UPDRS) 30–1, 186
  score 211
urethral sphincter electromyography 10
urge incontinence 154–5, 191–2
urinary bladder symptoms 45
urinary incontinence 10, 154–5
  multiple system atrophy 180
  normal pressure hydrocephalus 13, 14
  nursing care 191–2
urodynamic studies 10

vaginismus 192
vascular higher-level gait disorders 98, 102, 104–5
   classification 105–7, 108
   disequilibrium 105
   equilibrium apraxia 106
   ignition apraxia 105–6
   mixed gait apraxia 106–7
   physiotherapy 107
   treatment 107–8
vascular parkinsonism 100–1
ventilation during surgery 193
videofluoroscopy 237
videotapes 189, 203
vincristine/adriamycin combination, DIP 73
virtual reality images, rehabilitation 104–5
vision 190
visual cues, mobility 207–8
visual feedback, speech 233
visual impairment, progressive supranuclear palsy
   50, 180
vitamin C, protective effect for PD 116
vitamin E *see* tocopherol
vocal cords, abduction/adduction 210
Vocalite 232
voice
  essential tremor 87
  tremor 82, 83, 85
  volume 227, 229, 234–5

voluntary motor control loss 24
voluntary organizations 176

walking 189
  aids 204, 209
  confidence 206
  elderly 15–16
walking frames 209
walking sticks 209
washing 221
wearing off
  dystonia 151, 153
  motor fluctuations 150–1
Webster Scale 200
welfare workers 176
wheelchair 222
Wilson's disease 12
World Health Organization Classification of
      Impairments, Disabilities and Handicaps
      166
writing tremor
  primary 84
  see also handwriting

ziprasidone 66
zolpidem 154
zotepine 66